Antimicrobial Resistance and Implications

Antimicrobial Resistance and Implications

Editor: Steven Blair

AMERICAN
MEDICAL PUBLISHERS
www.americanmedicalpublishers.com

AMERICAN
MEDICAL PUBLISHERS
www.americanmedicalpublishers.com

Cataloging-in-Publication Data

Antimicrobial resistance and implications / edited by Steven Blair.
p. cm.
Includes bibliographical references and index.
ISBN 978-1-63927-208-2
1. Drug resistance in microorganisms. 2. Anti-infective agents. 3. Antibiotics--Effectiveness.
4. Emerging infectious diseases. 5. Immunology. I. Blair, Steven.
QR177 .A58 2022
616.904 1--dc23

American Medical Publishers,
41 Flatbush Avenue,
1st Floor, New York,
NY 11217, USA

ISBN 978-1-63927-208-2 (Hardback)

Contents

Preface

The resistance of a microorganism to an antimicrobial drug that was once able to treat it is known as antimicrobial resistance. Antimicrobial resistance also develops through the natural resistance in certain bacteria, genetic mutation or one species can acquire resistance from another species. Antibiotic resistance is a subset of antimicrobial resistance which is related to pathogenic bacteria. It is sub-divided into microbiological and clinical resistance. The microbiologically linked resistance occurs from genes that enable the bacteria to resist the mechanism associated with certain antibiotics. Resistant microbes are difficult to treat and require alternative medication or a high dose of antimicrobials. Clinical resistance occurs through the failure of many therapeutic techniques where the bacteria that were likely to be treated, become resistant after surviving the treatment. This book contains some path-breaking studies in the field of antimicrobial resistance. It consists of contributions made by international experts. Those in search of information to further their knowledge will be greatly assisted by this book.

All of the data presented henceforth, was collaborated in the wake of recent advancements in the field. The aim of this book is to present the diversified developments from across the globe in a comprehensible manner. The opinions expressed in each chapter belong solely to the contributing authors. Their interpretations of the topics are the integral part of this book, which I have carefully compiled for a better understanding of the readers.

At the end, I would like to thank all those who dedicated their time and efforts for the successful completion of this book. I also wish to convey my gratitude towards my friends and family who supported me at every step.

Editor

Carriage of antibiotic-resistant *Enterobacteriaceae* in hospitalised children in tertiary hospitals in Harare, Zimbabwe

Marcelyn T. Magwenzi[1*], Muchaneta Gudza-Mugabe[2], Hilda A. Mujuru[3,4], Mutsa Dangarembizi-Bwakura[3,5], Valerie Robertson[1,6] and Alexander M. Aiken[6,7]

Abstract

Background: Extended-spectrum β-lactamase-producing and gentamicin resistant *Enterobacteriaceae* are increasingly recognised as a major cause of infection in low-income countries. We assessed the prevalence of gastrointestinal carriage of these bacteria in hospitalised children in Harare, Zimbabwe.

Methods: We conducted a cohort study in paediatric inpatients at two tertiary-referral hospitals between May and July 2015. Rectal swabs and faecal samples were collected within 24 h of admission and further follow-up samples were collected on alternate days during hospitalization. Disc-based, selective and enrichment methods were used to detect carriage of these two forms of resistance. Standard methods were used to confirm resistance status and determine the susceptibility of resistant isolates to other commonly-used antibiotics.

Results: One hundred and sixty four paediatric inpatient admissions (median age = 1.0 year, IQR = 0.2–2.2years) were enrolled, and an average of 1.9 faecal samples per patient were collected. On admission, 68/164 (41%) patients had both ESBL and gentamicin-resistant *Enterobacteriaceae* detected, 18 (11%) had ESBL only, 17 (10%) had gentamicin resistance only and 61 (37%) had negative screening for both forms of resistance. During hospitalisation, 32/164 (20%) patients were found to have a type of resistant organism which was not present in their admission sample. We found that faecal samples and use of a selective enrichment broth enhanced the detection of resistant organisms. Amongst resistant bacteria isolated, there were high levels of resistance to ciprofloxacin and chloramphenicol, but not ertapenem.

Conclusions: More than half of children had enteric carriage of a clinically-relevant form of antibiotic resistance on admission to public-sector hospitals in urban Zimbabwe. Additionally, a fifth of children acquired a further form of resistance during hospitalisation. Urgent action is needed to tackle the spread of antibiotic resistant enteric bacteria in African hospitals.

Keywords: *Enterobacteriaceae*, ESBL, Antibiotic resistance, Colonization, Children

Background

Clinically significant levels of resistance to various antibiotic classes have developed in most Gram-negative bacteria, though there is marked geographic variation in the prevalence of resistance [1]. Historically, many forms of antibiotic resistant organisms emerged in and were disseminated from healthcare facilities in high-income settings, but in more recent times, hospitals in low and middle-income settings appear to have been the origin and amplifiers of several forms of resistance [2–4]. Weak antibiotic stewardship and limited infection control resources promote the spread of antibiotic resistant organisms in hospitals, especially where there are no microbiological diagnostic services for the identification of resistance [5].

In the family of *Enterobacteriaceae*, organisms such as *Escherichia coli* and *Klebsiella pneumoniae* can produce extended-spectrum β-lactamase (ESBL) enzymes, which

* Correspondence: mmagwenzi@yahoo.com
[1]College of Health Sciences, Department of Medical Microbiology, University of Zimbabwe, PO Box A178, Harare, Zimbabwe
Full list of author information is available at the end of the article

confer resistance to third generation cephalosporins and most penicillins but are inhibited by agents such as clavulanate. These types of resistant bacteria are increasingly implicated as causes of both community- and hospital-acquired infections [6, 7] and are associated with higher levels of mortality than non-ESBL producers [8]. Across sub-Saharan Africa, a limited number of studies have described high levels of ESBL faecal carriage in children in association with hospital facilities [9–13]. Gentamicin is an aminoglycoside antibiotic that has been used for the treatment of Gram-negative infections for more than 40 years [14]. Its low-cost and broad spectrum of activity means that it is widely used for treatment of severe infections in many low-income countries.

The gastrointestinal tract is the principal ecological niche for *Enterobacteriaceae*. In this environment, inter- and intra-species exchange of resistance genes can occur and under appropriate selective pressure, resistant species can rapidly emerge and dominate [15]. While faecal carriage of antibiotic resistant bacteria is not an immediate threat to a healthy individual, it poses two risks—firstly, when auto-infection of a sterile body-site subsequently occurs (for example, hospital-acquired bacteraemia [16]) treatment is substantially more difficult and secondly, there may be transmission of the resistant organism to other individuals [17].

In order to describe levels of carriage of Gram-negative antibiotic resistance amongst hospitalised children in Zimbabwe, we aimed to measure 1) the prevalence of carriage of ESBL producing and gentamicin-resistant enteric bacteria in paediatric patients at the time of admission to hospital and 2) the risk of acquisition for the same types of bacteria during the corresponding time of hospitalization. We also sought to evaluate different methods for screening for the presence of these resistant organisms.

Methods

Study design

This was a prospective observational cohort study conducted in paediatric wards at two tertiary government hospitals in Harare, Zimbabwe between May and July 2015. Paediatric patients were recruited within 24 h of admission to hospital and remained in the study until discharge from hospital or death. All paediatric patients were eligible for inclusion in the study regardless of their presenting illness, provided that they remained in hospital for at least one night. These hospitals had paediatric wards divided into cubicles of 6 to 8 beds and limited isolation rooms. Each cubicle or room had a single hand-wash basin; alcohol-based hand sanitizers were not consistently available. There was no established practice of screening for carriage of resistant organisms in these wards at the time of this study.

Screening for ESBL and gentamicin resistance

Two rectal swabs and/or a stool sample were collected within 24 h of admission. Further similar samples were collected three times per week for all participants. The swabs and stool samples were directly inoculated onto a range of screening plates in the Department of Medical Microbiology laboratory, University of Zimbabwe, as follows:

1) MacConkey agar without salt (Oxoid, UK) plates with either a Cefpodoxime (10 μg) or a Gentamicin (10 μg) disc placed on the plate. The plates were incubated at 37 °C for 24 h. Growth within 5mm of the margin of the disc was considered potentially significant.
2) Selective ChromID ESBL-agar (Biomerieux, France) and Gentamicin-MacConkey plates. The latter was prepared in-house by adding 800 μl Gentamicin 10 mg/ml (Gibco, UK) in 1 L of MacConkey agar without salt. Any growth on these plates was considered potentially significant.
3) Samples were selectively enriched overnight in 5 ml nutrient broth with either a Cefpodoxime (10 μg) or a Gentamicin (10 μg) disc added to the bijou bottle. These enriched samples were sub-cultured the following day and then handled in the same way as the direct methods above.

Where results were discordant between different sample types from the same patient using the screening methods, any detection of a resistant organism was considered to be the correct identification. A single colony of each distinguishable type (up to three per sample) was picked from a resistance screening plate, grown on a purity plate and subsequently tested as described below.

Identification of isolates

Bacterial isolates expressing either ESBL or Gentamicin resistance or both were obtained. An oxidase test was performed (Remel Bactidrop, UK) for all isolates. Oxidase-negative isolates were identified to the family/genus level using API10S kits (Biomerieux, France) according to the manufacturer's instructions; this system does not consistently provide identification to the species level. The ESBL phenotype was confirmed by paired disc tests [18] according to the manufacturer's instructions (Mast Diagnostics, UK). Where a sample had no isolates confirmed as ESBL producers by paired disc testing, we considered the sample to be negative for that type of resistance throughout the analysis.

Antimicrobial susceptibility testing

Overnight pure cultures confirmed to be ESBL positive or gentamicin resistant had further susceptibility testing performed using the standard disc diffusion method based on Clinical Laboratory Standards Institute (CLSI) breakpoints for susceptibility testing. The antibiotics tested were gentamicin (10 μg), chloramphenicol (30 μg), ciprofloxacin (1 μg), ertapenem (10 μg), cefpodoxime (10 μg) and ampicillin (10 μg) (Oxoid, England). Reference strains *E. coli* ATCC25922 (fully susceptible) and *E. coli* NCTC13353 (ESBL CTX-M type and gentamicin resistant) were used as control organisms. Data were recorded in a Microsoft Access database and STATA v13 was used to calculate prevalence and acquisition rates of resistance carriage and perform tests of association.

Results

Admissions

A total of 164 paediatric inpatients were recruited to the study out of a total of 1757 paediatric admissions to these two hospitals in the study period. Most patients (142/164, 87%) were recruited on the day following their admission to hospital (hence after spending one night in hospital), but all within 24 h of their admission. A summary of these patients is shown in Table 1. The median age was 1.0 years (IQR 0.2 to 2.2 years). The most commonly recorded admission diagnoses were "severe pneumonia", "sepsis" and "severe malnutrition". The average duration of hospitalization was 5.6 days (IQR 2–7.5 days; range 1–32 days) and the inpatient mortality was 8% (13 deaths/164 admissions).

Table 1 Summary of study admissions

	Number (n =164)	%
Age of child		
0–28 days	19	12%
29 days–1 year	63	38%
1–5 years	64	39%
Over 5 years	18	11%
Ward of recruitment		
Harare Childrens Hospital, ward B1	41	25%
Harare Childrens Hospital, ward B2	63	38%
Parirenyatwa Hospital, admission unit	3	3%
Parirenyatwa Hospital, ward A4 General	22	22%
Parirenyatwa Hospital, ward A4 Special	24	24%
Parirenyatwa Hospital, ward A5	11	11%
Enteric carriage of resistance on admission		
Both ESBL and gentamicin resistance	68	41%
ESBL resistance only	18	11%
Gentamicin resistance only	17	10%
Neither form of resistance	61	37%
Outcome of admission		
Discharged	151	92%
Died	13	8%

Carriage of antibiotic resistance on admission

The prevalence of ESBL carriage was 52% (86/164) and gentamicin resistance carriage was 52% (85/164), on the initial sample taken from patients, with 41% of all patients having both forms of resistance. On admission, ESBL carriage was higher amongst children in the age groups 29 days-1 year (39/63; 62%) and 1–5 years (37/64; 58%) and lower in the younger (0–28days (7/19; 37%)) and older (5+ years (3/18; 18%) age groups; (Fishers exact test across these categories $p = 0.001$). We found no difference in carriage rates by age group for gentamicin resistance on admission to hospital. Only 37% of children had neither form of resistance detectable—see Table 1. There was no association between hospital of admission and prevalence of carriage of ESBL (χ^2-test $p = 0.23$) or gentamicin resistance ($p = 0.32$). Death as an inpatient was associated with ESBL carriage on admission (Fisher's exact test $p = 0.02$) but not with gentamicin resistance ($p = 0.25$).

Acquisition of carriage during admission

An average of 1.9 samples were obtained per patient (range = 1 to 8) with 91 patients having two or more samples collected. A total of 32 admissions were detected to have a new form of resistance during their hospital admission: 17 gained both ESBL and gentamicin-resistance, 12 gained ESBL only and 3 gained gentamicin resistance only (see Table 2). There was no association between hospital and acquisition of resistance during admission for either ESBL (χ^2-test $p = 0.40$) or gentamicin resistance (χ^2-test $p = 0.40$). The probability of any sample containing a resistant organism was closely related to the time since admission to hospital—see Fig. 1. After a patient had been hospitalised for five or more days, there was over 90% probability (86/93 samples) that carriage of both ESBL and gentamicin-resistant organisms would be detected in a faecal specimen.

Screening methods for detection of resistant organisms

A total of 312 samples were collected, of these 143 were rectal swabs only, 23 were faecal samples only and 146 had both types of specimen. In the samples with both rectal swabs and faecal samples, the sensitivity of the

Table 2 Summary of ESBL or Gentamicin resistance acquisition status during admissions

>1 faecal sample taken during hospital admission	91/164 (55%)
New detection of ESBL during admission	29/164 (18%)
New detection of gentamicin resistance during admission	20/164 (12%)
New detection of either form of resistance	32/164 (20%)
New detection of both forms of resistance	17/164 (10%)

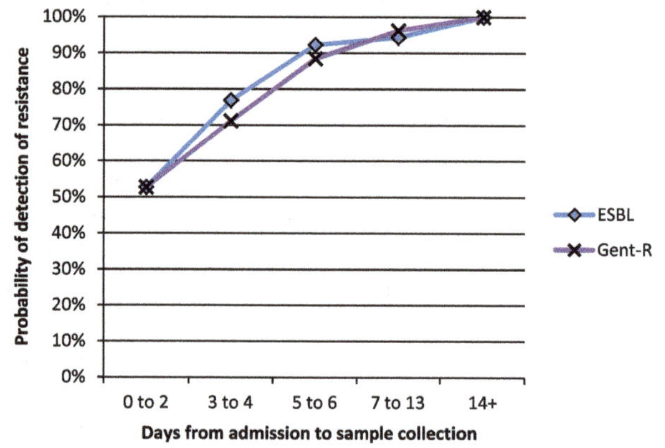

Fig. 1 Probability of detection v time-to-sample

different detection techniques is shown in Table 3. Broadly speaking, we found that higher sensitivity was achieved with faecal samples and inclusion of the enrichment broth step. Use of selective media did not achieve substantially higher sensitivity, but was noted to be practically easier to use in the laboratory. Out of the oxidase-negative Gram-negative isolates detected by the ESBL screening methods and confirmed as *Enterobacteriaceae*, the large majority (190/214; 89%) were confirmed as ESBL by both disc pairs (cefotaxime/clavulanate pair and ceftazidime/clavulanate pair) and some were confirmed by only a single pair of ceftazidime/clavulanate (16/214; 7.5%). A small number of isolates were not confirmed as ESBL-producers by either disc pair (8/214; 4%).

Antibiotic resistance profiles

Amongst the isolated *Enterobacteriaceae* that were confirmed ESBL ($n = 206$) or gentamicin resistant ($n = 146$), we examined the co-resistance to other commonly used antibiotics—see Tables 4 and 5. We found high levels of co-resistance to ampicillin, ciprofloxacin and chloramphenicol, but virtually no co-resistance to ertapenem.

Discussion

Our study investigated enteric carriage of ESBL-producing and gentamicin resistant enteric bacteria in a sample of 164 hospitalised children drawn from two tertiary public-sector hospitals in Harare, Zimbabwe over a 3 month period. The main findings were high rates of carriage of ESBL and gentamicin resistant bacteria on admission to hospital and high rates of acquisition for the same resistance types during the inpatient period.

An initial sample was collected within 24 h of hospital admission for each patient, so these samples are likely to represent the carriage status prior to the current hospital admission. Other studies of ESBL prevalence around the time of admission to hospital have found carriage rates of 33% (133/408) in Guinea Bissau [9], 34% (37/110) in Gabon [12] and 22% (54/244) in Madagascar [11]. Amongst neonates in Tanzania, 25% (32/126) were found to have ESBL carriage, predominantly *Klebsiella pneumoniae* [13]. In a study conducted in a renutrition centre in Niger [10], ESBL carriage was 31% (17/55 patients) on admission and by time of discharge a further 15/16 children had acquired carriage. Our study, showed a higher prevalence of carriage than those previously described levels, though our methods of screening were probably more sensitive than the direct plating of rectal swabs used elsewhere. We are not aware of any previous African studies specifically investigating carriage of gentamicin resistance in hospitalised children. Carriage of resistance amongst hospital admissions is liable to be higher than carriage in the general community, as sick individuals probably have exposure to various healthcare-related risk factors prior to admission, so we cannot compare these results to truly community-based studies. However, the extremely high levels of carriage rates found suggest that circulation of ESBL and gentamicin resistance probably occurs in the community in Harare. Although we found an association between ESBL carriage and inpatient death, we were not able to assess for the confounding effects and hence it remains uncertain whether this is a causal association.

Collection of multiple follow-up samples during the inpatient period allowed us to observe acquisition of carriage of resistance over time. An important question is whether these in-hospital acquisitions are occurring via endogenous (arising from undetectably low levels already present in the gastrointestinal tract) or exogenous (arising

Table 3 Sensitivity of screening methods for resistant organisms ($n = 146$ samples)

	ESBL		Gentamicin-resistant	
Sample type	Rectal swab	Faecal sample	Rectal swab	Faecal sample
Plate with disc	73%	84%	66%	83%
Selective plate	75%	87%	70%	82%
Enrichment broth THEN plate with disc	90%	96%	87%	95%
Enrichment broth THEN selective plate	90%	96%	84%	96%

Table 4 Susceptibility profiles of confirmed ESBL-producing isolates ($n = 206$)

Antibiotic	Number resistant	% Resistant	Total tested
Gentamicin	130	65	199
Ampicillin	199	100	199
Ciprofloxacin	162	82	198
Chloramphenicol	105	53	198
Ertapenem	2	1	199

from cross-infection from an external source) routes. This distinction has important implications for antibiotic stewardship and infection control measures. For endogenous routes of acquisition, antibiotic stewardship activities focussing on reducing the selective pressure from antibiotic prescribing are important. For exogenous acquisition, measures to minimise cross-infection, such as improved hand hygiene, are priorities. Whilst we cannot be certain, we feel that both routes are likely to be contributing to the high levels of nosocomial acquisition seen here. Our screening methods included an enrichment step so that we should have been able to detect small quantities of resistant bacteria, making endogenous acquisition less likely, though a single faecal specimen is not a representative sample of the estimated 10^{14} cells in the intestinal microbiome. Enrichment broths with supplementary antibiotics have been used elsewhere to aid detection of resistant organisms in faecal samples [18]. Our clinical experience in these hospitals suggests there are substantial challenges with over-crowding, limited access to hand-hygiene facilities and high patient:staff ratios. With regard to hand-hygiene, at the time the study was conducted, water supplies in these wards were sporadic and alcohol-based hand rub (ABHR) was not widely available. Concurrent work conducted in the same wards as a separate part of this pilot study showed that hands of adult carers were frequently contaminated with Gram-negative antibiotic resistant bacteria [19]. These are all factors that might be expected to contribute to exogenous routes of transmission.

In line with findings from other studies, we found that most ESBL-producing bacteria from these children were also resistant to several other clinically-relevant antibiotic classes [9–13]. This represents a substantial clinical challenge for empirical treatment of suspected hospital-acquired infections—ciprofloxacin (for severe urinary sepsis) and chloramphenicol (for bacteraemia and meningitis) represent important and widely used second-line treatment options in many African hospitals. The level of carbapenem resistance amongst resistant isolates was very low, but as these agents are not currently routinely available through public-sector pharmacies in Zimbabwe, this information is of limited practical value for local clinicians.

Table 5 Susceptibility profiles of Gentamicin resistant isolates ($n = 146$)

Antibiotic	Number resistant	% Resistant	Total tested
Cefpodoxime[a]	126	86	146
Ampicillin	144	99	146
Ciprofloxacin	112	77	146
Chloramphenicol	77	53	146
Ertapenem	0	0	145

[a]These isolates were not formally confirmed as ESBL-producers by double disc testing

Due to rapid turnover of patients, we were only able to collect follow-up samples in a moderate number of patients; 73 patients had only a single sample collected. Whilst this does not affect estimates for the time of admission, it limits the ability of the study to detect new acquisition of carriage—in reality, probably even more children became carriers of resistance during admission than we detected. Ideally, an additional sample on the day of discharge would have been collected for all patients. Our simple screening and identification methods meant that we could not distinguish the simultaneous carriage of multiple different resistant organisms. Again, this means that the acquisition risk described here may underestimate the true in-hospital acquisition risk. We did not make use of molecular techniques for identification of resistance mechanisms or for investigating transmission of resistance. In this preliminary study, we were not able to evaluate clinical impacts of antibiotic resistance, either during hospital inpatient stay or after discharge. Whilst we did find some evidence that carriage of ESBL resistance was associated with inpatient mortality, investigating whether carriage of resistance was followed by clinical infection with the same organisms was beyond the scope of the study.

Future research is needed to better understand and tackle these high levels of antibiotic resistance. This will take many forms. We did not collect information on risk factors associated with carriage of resistance—this would be a valuable first step in understanding why this is occurring. In other settings, prior use of antibiotics and recent hospital admission have been associated with carriage of resistance [20]—we do not know if this is the case in Zimbabwe. More work is needed to identify the enzyme types and genes responsible for the forms of resistance that we detected—this will enable us to start to understand the dynamics of resistance transmission. Screening for drug-resistance on admission and cohorting or isolating patients can result in improved patient outcomes [21]—but no modelling work has ever been conducted to explore the value of this in the setting of African hospitals. We do not know how the acquisition of antibiotic resistance in hospitals relates to resistance in the community in Zimbabwe [22], nor do we know the wider impact of antibiotic resistance in terms of mortality, morbidity and costs in sub-Saharan African countries, though we suspect these to be substantial [23]. Given that many African hospitals have limited access to carbapenems, infections caused by ESBL-producers might have a substantially greater impact than has been seen in high-income settings [8].

At a more practical level, immediate action can be taken in a number of areas such as improving infection control practices, especially hand hygiene, which has been shown to reduce infections caused by antibiotic-resistant Gram-negative bacteria in high-income settings [24]. The use of alcohol-based hand rub as part of the WHO 5 moments for hand hygiene approach is a low-cost technology that could be much more widely adopted in African hospitals. Ideally, a rigorous evaluation of the implementation of such new practices would contribute to the evidence-base for these measures in low-income settings, which is currently extremely limited [25].

Conclusion

The rising level of antimicrobial resistance is of great concern worldwide. These high rates of ESBL and gentamicin resistance carriage found amongst paediatric inpatients in Zimbabwe are particularly worrisome. These bacteria pose risks of multi-drug resistant infections and transmission to other hospital inpatients. The high levels of carriage at the time of hospital admissions suggest that they are already in widespread circulation in the general community. Relevant infection control measures such as access to alcohol-based hand rub should be urgently scaled up in these hospitals and beyond, so that children who arrive at hospital without carriage of antibiotic resistant bacteria can remain free of these for the duration of their admissions.

Abbreviations

ABHR: Alcohol-based hand rub; CLSI: Clinical Laboratory Standards Institute; ESBL: Extended- spectrum β-lactamase; IQR: Inter-quartile range

Acknowledgements

We are grateful to the study nurses Dorah Kaisi and Phillipa Dingiswayo from the Department of Paediatrics and Child Health UZ for their diligent work on recruitment of patients and collection of samples. We would like to thank patients, parents and staff in the participating wards for their assistance with this work. We thank staff in the Department of Medical Microbiology, University of Zimbabwe and the Biomedical Research and Training Institute for their support.

Funding

This work was funded by an Academy of Medical Sciences Starter Grant for Clinical Lecturers (AA, grant reference AMS-SGCL11-AikenA). This work formed part of a pilot study ahead of a cluster-randomised trial of a hand-hygiene intervention in hospitals in sub-Saharan Africa.

Authors' contributions

Conceived and designed the experiments: MM, MGM, HAM, MBD, VR, AA. Performed the experiments: MM MGM. Analysed the data: MM AA. Contributed reagents/materials/analysis tools: VR AA. Wrote the manuscript: MM AA. All authors read and approved the manuscript.

Competing interests

The authors declare that they have no competing interests.

Consent for publication

Not applicable—the manuscript does not include details, images, or videos relating to individual participants but rather presents analysis of aggregated data on the study population.

Author details

[1]College of Health Sciences, Department of Medical Microbiology, University of Zimbabwe, PO Box A178, Harare, Zimbabwe. [2]National Microbiology Reference Laboratory, Harare Central Hospital, Harare, Zimbabwe. [3]College of Health Sciences, Department of Paediatrics and Child Health, University of Zimbabwe, Harare, Zimbabwe. [4]Harare Central Hospital, Harare, Zimbabwe. [5]Parirenyatwa Group of Hospitals, Harare, Zimbabwe. [6]Biomedical Research and Training Institute, Harare, Zimbabwe. [7]London School of Hygiene and Tropical Medicine, London, UK.

References

1. WHO. Worldwide country stiuation analysis: response to antimicrobial resistance. 2015.
2. Ma X, Wu Y, Li L, Xu Q, Hu B, Ni Y, et al. First multicenter study on multidrug resistant bacteria carriage in Chinese ICUs. BMC Infect Dis. 2015;15:358.
3. Yong D, Toleman MA, Giske CG, Cho HS, Sundman K, Lee K, et al. Characterization of a new metallo-beta-lactamase gene, bla(NDM-1), and a novel erythromycin esterase gene carried on a unique genetic structure in Klebsiella pneumoniae sequence type 14 from India. Antimicrob Agents Chemother. 2009;53(12):5046–54.
4. Carrer A, Poirel L, Yilmaz M, Akan OA, Feriha C, Cuzon G, et al. Spread of OXA-48-encoding plasmid in Turkey and beyond. Antimicrob Agents Chemother. 2010;54(3):1369–73.
5. Allegranzi B, Bagheri Nejad S, Combescure C, Graafmans W, Attar H, Donaldson L, et al. Burden of endemic health-care-associated infection in developing countries: systematic review and meta-analysis. Lancet. 2011;377(9761):228–41.
6. Thaden JT, Fowler VG, Sexton DJ, Anderson DJ. Increasing incidence of extended-spectrum beta-lactamase-producing Escherichia coli in community hospitals throughout the Southeastern United States. Infect Control Hosp Epidemiol. 2016;37(1):49–54.
7. Lukac PJ, Bonomo RA, Logan LK. Extended-spectrum beta-lactamase-producing enterobacteriaceae in children: old foe, emerging threat. Clin Infect Dis. 2015;60(9):1389–97.
8. de Kraker ME, Wolkewitz M, Davey PG, Koller W, Berger J, Nagler J, et al. Burden of antimicrobial resistance in European hospitals: excess mortality and length of hospital stay associated with bloodstream infections due to Escherichia coli resistant to third-generation cephalosporins. J Antimicrob Chemother. 2011;66(2):398–407.
9. Isendahl J, Turlej-Rogacka A, Manjuba C, Rodrigues A, Giske CG, Naucler P. Fecal carriage of ESBL-producing E. coli and K. pneumoniae in children in Guinea-Bissau: a hospital-based cross-sectional study. PLoS One. 2012;7(12):e51981.
10. Woerther PL, Angebault C, Jacquier H, Hugede HC, Janssens AC, Sayadi S, et al. Massive increase, spread, and exchange of extended spectrum beta-lactamase-encoding genes among intestinal Enterobacteriaceae in hospitalized children with severe acute malnutrition in Niger. Clin Infect Dis. 2011;53(7):677–85.
11. Andriatahina T, Randrianirina F, Hariniana ER, Talarmin A, Raobijaona H, Buisson Y, et al. High prevalence of fecal carriage of extended-spectrum beta-lactamase-producing Escherichia coli and Klebsiella pneumoniae in a pediatric unit in Madagascar. BMC Infect Dis. 2010;10:204.
12. Schaumburg F, Alabi A, Kokou C, Grobusch MP, Kock R, Kaba H, et al. High burden of extended-spectrum beta-lactamase-producing Enterobacteriaceae in Gabon. J Antimicrob Chemother. 2013;68(9):2140–3.

13. Nelson E, Kayega J, Seni J, Mushi MF, Kidenya BR, Hokororo A, et al. Evaluation of existence and transmission of extended spectrum beta lactamase producing bacteria from post-delivery women to neonates at Bugando Medical Center. Mwanza-Tanzania BMC Res Notes. 2014;7:279.
14. Chen C, Chen Y, Wu P, Chen B. Update on new medicinal applications of gentamicin: evidence-based review. J Formos Med Assoc. 2014;113(2):72–82.
15. Carlet J. The gut is the epicentre of antibiotic resistance. Antimicrob Resist Infect Control. 2012;1(1):39.
16. Aiken AM, Mturi N, Njuguna P, Mohammed S, Berkley JA, Mwangi I, et al. Risk and causes of paediatric hospital-acquired bacteraemia in Kilifi District Hospital, Kenya: a prospective cohort study. Lancet. 2011;378(9808):2021–7.
17. Donskey CJ. The role of the intestinal tract as a reservoir and source for transmission of nosocomial pathogens. Clin Infect Dis. 2004;39(2):219–26.
18. Thomson KS. Extended-spectrum-beta-lactamase, AmpC, and Carbapenemase issues. J Clin Microbiol. 2010;48(4):1019–25.
19. Gudza-Mugabe M, Magwenzi MT, Mujuru HA, Bwakura-Dangarembizi M, Robertson V, Aiken AM. Decontamination of hands using locallymanufactured alcohol-based hand rub in paediatric wards in Harare, Zimbabwe. Antimicrob Resist Infect Control, in press.
20. Pop-Vicas AE, D'Agata EM. The rising influx of multidrug-resistant gram-negative bacilli into a tertiary care hospital. Clin Infect Dis. 2005;40(12):1792–8.
21. Tacconelli E, Cataldo MA, Dancer SJ, De Angelis G, Falcone M, Frank U, et al. ESCMID guidelines for the management of the infection control measures to reduce transmission of multidrug-resistant Gram-negative bacteria in hospitalized patients. Clin Microbiol Infect. 2014;20 Suppl 1:1–55.
22. Hilty M, Betsch BY, Bogli-Stuber K, Heiniger N, Stadler M, Kuffer M, et al. Transmission dynamics of extended-spectrum beta-lactamase-producing Enterobacteriaceae in the tertiary care hospital and the household setting. Clin Infect Dis. 2012;55(7):967–75.
23. Aiken AM, Allegranzi B, Scott JAG, Mehtar S, Pittet D, Grundmann H. Letter responding to "Antibiotic resistance - the need for Global Solutions" by Laxminarayan et al. Lancet Infect Dis. 2014;14(July):550-1.
24. Johnson PD, Martin R, Burrell LJ, Grabsch EA, Kirsa SW, O'Keeffe J, et al. Efficacy of an alcohol/chlorhexidine hand hygiene program in a hospital with high rates of nosocomial methicillin-resistant Staphylococcus aureus (MRSA) infection. Med J Aust. 2005;183(10):509–14.
25. Luangasanatip N, Hongsuwan M, Limmathurotsakul D, Lubell Y, Lee AS, Harbarth S, et al. Comparative efficacy of interventions to promote hand hygiene in hospital: systematic review and network meta-analysis. BMJ. 2015;351:h3728.

Higher third-generation cephalosporin prescription proportion is associated with lower probability of reducing carbapenem use

Allison Muller[1,2], Xavier Bertrand[1,2], Anne-Marie Rogues[3,4], Muriel Péfau[4], Serge Alfandari[5], Rémy Gauzit[6], Catherine Dumartin[3,4], Houssein Gbaguidi-Haore[1,2,7*] and on behalf of the ATB-RAISIN network steering committee

Abstract

Background: The ongoing extended spectrum β-lactamase-producing *Enterobacteriaceae* (ESBL-PE) pandemic has led to an increasing carbapenem use, requiring release of guidelines for carbapenem usage in France in late 2010. We sought to determine factors associated with changes in carbapenem use in intensive care units (ICUs), medical and surgical wards between 2009 and 2013.

Methods: This ward-level multicentre retrospective study was based on data from French antibiotic and multidrug-resistant bacteria surveillance networks in healthcare facilities. Antibiotic use was expressed in defined daily doses per 1000 patient-days. Factors associated with the reduction in carbapenem use (yes/no) over the study period were determined from random-effects logistic regression model (493 wards nested within 259 healthcare facilities): ward characteristics (type, size…), ward antibiotic use (initial antibiotic use [i.e., consumption of a given antibiotic in 2009], initial antibiotic prescribing profile [i.e., proportion of a given antibiotic in the overall antibiotic consumption in 2009] and reduction in the use of a given antibiotic between 2009 and 2013) and regional ESBL-PE incidence rate in acute care settings in 2011.

Results: Over the study period, carbapenem consumption in ICUs ($n = 85$), medical ($n = 227$) and surgical wards ($n = 181$) was equal to 73.4, 6.2 and 5.4 defined daily doses per 1000 patient-days, respectively. Release of guidelines was followed by a significant decrease in carbapenem use within ICUs and medical wards, and a slowdown in use within surgical wards. The following factors were independently associated with a higher probability of reducing carbapenem use: location in Eastern France, higher initial carbapenem prescribing profile and reductions in consumption of fluoroquinolones, glycopeptides and piperacillin/tazobactam. In parallel, factors independently associated with a lower probability of reducing carbapenem use were ICUs, ward size increase, wards of cancer centres, higher initial third-generation cephalosporin (3GC) prescribing profile and location in high-risk regions for ESBL-PE.
(Continued on next page)

* Correspondence: hhgbaguidihaore@chu-besancon.fr
[1]University Hospital of Besançon, Infection Control Department, F-25030 Besançon, France
[2]University Bourgogne-Franche-Comte, UMR 6249 Chrono-Environnement, F-25030 Besançon, France
Full list of author information is available at the end of the article

(Continued from previous page)

Conclusions: Our study suggests that a decrease in 3GCs in the overall antibiotic use and the continuation of reduction in fluoroquinolone use, could allow reducing carbapenem use, given the well-demonstrated role of 3GCs and fluoroquinolones in the occurrence of ESBL-PE. Thus, antibiotic stewardship programs should target wards with higher 3GC prescription proportions to reduce them.

Keywords: Carbapenem, Antibiotic use, Antibiotic stewardship, ESBL, Multidrug-resistant bacteria

Background

The ongoing extended spectrum β-lactamase (ESBL)-producing *Enterobacteriaceae* (ESBL-PE) pandemic, mainly *Escherichia coli,* has led to an increasing use of carbapenems, which are considered as 'last-line' treatment against these multidrug-resistant (MDR) bacteria. This increasing carbapenem consumption worldwide [1–3], has accelerated the occurrence and spread of carbapenemase-producing *Enterobacteriaceae* (CPE) [4], which can lead to situations of therapeutic dead end. In France, the number of CPE cases has been increasing since 2010, and in an epidemic pattern in some regions [5]. In addition, more and more cases are no longer related to a foreign country [6]: from 29% of cases in 2010 to 58% in 2015. Lastly, according to the classification of the European survey of CPE (EuSCAPE), France is currently at epidemiological stage 4 of CPE spread [7], which corresponds to 'multiple epidemiologically-related outbreaks occurring in different health districts, suggesting an interregional autochthonous inter-institutional transmission'. Saving antibiotic resources, particularly carbapenems, has become a global public health priority [8, 9], especially since the pipeline of new antibiotics is drying up [10]. Therefore, French guidelines for carbapenems have been released in late 2010 to limit their use and improve the prescribing practices of this antibiotic class [11]. In French healthcare facilities (HCFs), carbapenem consumption has undergone a significant rise of 145% between 2000 and 2013 [12]: from 0.014 to 0.033 defined daily doses (DDDs) per 1000 inhabitants and per day. This high consumption level is mainly observed in intensive care units (ICUs) [13], although carbapenem use according to hospital wards has been scarcely studied. In this study, we sought to evaluate changes in carbapenem use in ICUs, medical and surgical wards of French HCFs between 2009 and 2013, and to determine factors associated with the reduction in use of this antibiotic class.

Methods

Design, setting and study period

This multicentre retrospective study at the ward level was mainly based on data from the ATB-RAISIN network (RAISIN stands for network for warning, investigation and surveillance of nosocomial infections), which is responsible for the surveillance of antibiotic consumption in French HCFs. We included a stable cohort of ICUs, medical and surgical wards of HCFs that participated in the surveillance every year from 2009 to 2013 on a voluntary basis. The geographical location of these HCFs refers to Coordinating Centres for Nosocomial Infection Control, distributed in five areas (North, West, South-west, East and South-east), each including several administrative regions.

Data collection

The ATB-RAISIN surveillance network retrospectively collected each year various types of data: (i) ward characteristics (type, size in number of beds, type of HCF from which it was derived, geographical location, and activity, expressed in number of patient-days), and (ii) inpatient antibiotic use, expressed in DDDs per 1000 patient-days (PD), in accordance to the Anatomical Therapeutic Chemical-DDD classification from the WHO [14]. Data on antibiotic use (dispensing data) were retrieved from pharmacy records, as described elsewhere [15]. Such data related to all antibiotic prescriptions whatever the context of treatment initiation (empirical or based on bacteriological results). Besides carbapenems (J01DH) and the overall antibiotic consumption (J01 + P01AB + J04AB02), the following antibiotics were studied: third-generation cephalosporins (3GCs, J01DD + J01DE + J01 DC07), fluoroquinolones (J01MA), aminoglycosides (J01G), aminopenicillins ± β-lactamase inhibitors (J01CA01 + 02 + 04 + J01CR01 + 02), imidazoles (J01XD + P01AB), glycopeptides (J01XA), piperacillin/tazobactam (J01CR05) and other potential alternatives to carbapenems for treating ESBL-PE infections (fosfomycin J01XX01, nitrofurantoin J01XE01, pivmecillinam J01CA08, temocillin J01CA17, tigecycline J01AA12 and cefoxitin J01 DC01) [16]. Moreover, the BMR-RAISIN network, which is responsible for the national surveillance of MDR bacteria in HCFs, provided data on ESBL-PE in acute care settings aggregated at the level of French regions. These data allowed taking into account the regional context in which a given ward operated in terms of ESBL-PE risk. Data generated from the laboratory, including antimicrobial susceptibility test results were only available for a few HCFs. Therefore, these data could not be considered in this work.

Data analysis

Temporal trends in carbapenem use within wards were explored by calculating two indicators: the relative change (and its 95% confidence interval [CI]) and the annual growth rate of this consumption (obtained by dividing the relative change by the number of years of the relevant time period). These indicators were computed for various time periods: before the release of guidelines (2009–10), after the release of guidelines (2011–13) and over the whole of the study period (2009–13). These guidelines [11] aimed to specify indications, at the time, for the four available carbapenem molecules (doripenem has since been withdrawn from the French market) with the following rules of good clinical practice: carbapenem prescribing should be limited to nosocomial infections due to MDR Gram-negative bacteria, absence of a carbapenem-sparing alternative, empirical treatment with 48–72 h re-assessment and de-escalation using carbapenem-sparing regimen and limitation of ertapenem to ESBL-PE urinary tract infections treatment without alternative. We assumed that these guidelines, released in late 2010, were gradually implemented from 2011 within French HCFs through their antibiotic stewardship programs (ASPs) and driven by their ASP committee, especially the mandatory antibiotic advisor. To take into account the clustered structure of data (wards nested within HCFs), a random-effects logistic regression analysis was performed to determine factors associated with the reduction in carbapenem use. Indeed, traditional regression techniques, by ignoring this data structure and possible correlation of data, may lead to biased statistical inferences [17]. The binary outcome variable was the reduction in carbapenem use (yes/no) between 2009 and 2013. Independent variables were the following:

- ward characteristics;
- ward antibiotic use: initial antibiotic use (i.e., consumption of a given antibiotic in 2009), initial antibiotic prescribing profile (i.e., proportion in percent of a given antibiotic in the overall antibiotic consumption in 2009) and reduction in the use of a given antibiotic (binary variable: yes/no) between 2009 and 2013;
- regional ESBL-PE incidence rate in acute care settings in 2011, which was converted in binary data with the median as cut-off: a given ward was located in 'high-risk region' or in 'low-risk region' for ESBL-PE.

First, a univariable random-effects logistic regression analysis was carried out to assess crude relationship between the outcome variable and each independent variable. Second, to determine factors independently associated with the outcome, a multivariable random-effects logistic regression model was built by introducing all independent variables with a p value of less than 0.20 in univariable analysis except 'type of ward' and 'initial overall antibiotic use' that were forced into the model due to a strong presumption of confounding effect. A p value of less than 0.05 was considered as statistically significant. Analyses were conducted using the software package Stata, version 14.1 (Stata Corp., College Station, TX, USA).

Results

Ward characteristics

Data on participating wards are presented Table 1. A total of 493 wards from 259 HCFs (approximately 10% of French HCFs) were included in this study (85 ICUs, 227 medical wards and 181 surgical wards). These wards were from general hospitals at 78.8%, 61.2% and 52.5% for ICUs, medical and surgical wards, respectively.

Trends in antibiotic use

As the overall antibiotic consumption during the study period (2009–13), carbapenem consumption was higher in ICUs than in medical and surgical wards (Table 2): 73.4, 6.2 and 5.4 DDD/1000 PD, respectively. Additionally, in terms of initial carbapenem prescribing profile, data (medians) were the following: 3.8% (range, 0.2 to 14.6%) in ICUs, 0.5% (range, 0 to 6%) in medical wards and 0.4% (range, 0 to 4%) in surgical wards. Between 2009 and 2013, the overall antibiotic use slightly decreased in ICUs (from 1487 to 1479 DDD/1000 PD; – 0.52%) and in medical wards (from 622 to 616 DDD/1000 PD; – 0.89%), whereas it exhibited a moderate increase in surgical wards (from 592 to 625 DDD/1000 PD; + 5.68%). Regarding carbapenem use over the study period, relative changes showed an increase across the three types of wards (Fig. 1): ICUs (+ 5.65%), medical wards (+ 24.1%) and surgical wards (+ 25.1%). Interestingly, this increase did not affect 201 out of 493 (40.8%) wards included, in which we observed a reduction in carbapenem use: 38.8% (33/85) of ICUs, 41.9% (95/227) of medical wards and 40.3% (73/181) of surgical wards. Exploring temporal trends in carbapenem use before the release of guidelines (2009–10) revealed a statistically significant increase across the three types of wards (Fig. 1): ICUs (+ 7.5%), medical wards (+ 23.1%) and surgical wards (+ 17.8%). The time period after the release of guidelines (2011–13) was followed by, on the one hand, a trend reversal in carbapenem use in ICUs and medical wards (negative annual growth rate of consumption: – 2.9% and – 1.6%, respectively) and, on the other hand, a slowdown in this consumption in surgical wards (annual growth rate of consumption declined from + 17.8% to + 2.7%). We should also point out that the statistically significant decrease in carbapenem use after the release of guidelines within ICUs (– 4.9% [95% CI, – 6.4 to – 3.3]) and medical wards (– 4.6%

Table 1 Characteristics of participating hospital wards across France

Characteristic	ICU wards, $N = 85$	Medical wards, $N = 227$	Surgical wards, $N = 181$
No. of beds in 2013, median (interquartile range)	12 (9–16)	72 (36–150)	63 (44–99)
Type of HCF			
- University hospital	4 (4.7%)	4 (1.8%)	4 (2.2%)
- General hospital	67 (78.8%)	139 (61.2%)	95 (52.5%)
- Private hospital	9 (10.6%)	51 (22.5%)	71 (39.2%)
- Cancer centre	0	6 (2.6%)	6 (3.3%)
- Local hospital	0	17 (7.5%)	0
- Rehabilitation and long-term care facility	0	5 (2.2%)	0
- Military hospital	5 (5.9%)	5 (2.2%)	5 (2.8%)
Geographical area			
- North	30 (35.3%)	50 (22%)	45 (24.9%)
- West	9 (10.6%)	25 (11%)	17 (9.4%)
- East	14 (16.5%)	45 (19.8%)	36 (19.9%)
- South-east	12 (14.1%)	33 (14.5%)	31 (17.1%)
- South-west	20 (23.5%)	74 (32.6%)	52 (28.7%)

ICU intensive care unit; *HCF* type of healthcare facility from which the hospital ward included in the study was derived

[95% CI, – 5.8 to – 3.4]) was more marked in 2012. By contrast, the carbapenem use within surgical wards only displayed a downward trend (– 1.3% [95% CI, – 3.2 to + 0.7]) between 2011 and 2012, which did not reach statistical significance. As regards other antibiotic use (Table 2), in almost all cases where an upward trend was noted over the five-year study period, this increase was greater in surgical wards than in ICUs and medical wards (e.g., 3GC use). Conversely, in case of downward trend recorded, the decrease was absent or lesser in surgical wards than in other wards (e.g., fluoroquinolone use). It should also noteworthy that initial 3GC prescribing profile medians varied as follows: 13.3% (range, 6.2 to 28.2%) in ICUs, 8.7% (range, 1.4 to 30.4%) in medical wards and 4.8% (range, 0 to 19.3%) in surgical wards. Moreover, initial fluoroquinolone prescribing profile medians were: 13.7% (range, 2.6 to 33.3%) in ICUs, 16.6% (range, 5.7 to 32.5%) in medical wards and 13.1% (range, 2.8 to 33.4%) in surgical wards.

Factors associated with the reduction in carbapenem use

Statistical analysis results are reported in Table 3. Surprisingly, univariable analysis detected no significant difference in reducing carbapenem use according to ward characteristics. In contrast, as regards antibiotic use, wards

Table 2 Use of carbapenems and other antibiotic classes in hospital wards across France, 2009–2013

Antibiotic use, DDDs per 1000 patient-days (RC)[a]	ICU wards, $N = 85$	Medical wards, $N = 227$	Surgical wards, $N = 181$
All antibiotics	1487 (–0.52%)	615 (–0.89%)	607 (+ 5.68%)
Carbapenems	73.4 (+ 5.65%)	6.2 (+ 24.1%)	5.4 (+ 25.1%)
- Imipenem	62.1 (–0.74%)	5.3 (+ 13.9%)	4.2 (+ 27.5%)
- Meropenem	5.3 (+ 285%)	0.36 (+ 195%)	0.23 (+ 109%)
- Ertapenem	4.87 (–20.4%)	0.52 (+ 45.3%)	0.86 (– 13.3%)
- Doripenem	1.17 (–16.7%)	0.04 (+ 208%)	0.06 (+ 1125%)
Aminopenicillins ± β-lactamase inhibitors	417 (–2.86%)	318 (–1.65%)	268 (+ 0.94%)
Piperacillin/tazobactam	90.1 (+ 34.7%)	8.6 (+ 79%)	8 (+ 109%)
Third-generation cephalosporins	205.9 (+ 0.78%)	60.4 (+ 18.9%)	38.1 (+33.2%)
Fluoroquinolones	177.2 (–24.2%)	88.4 (– 21.3%)	75.1 (–13.1%)
Aminoglycosides	106.1 (+3.35%)	12.4 (–6.98%)	25.4 (+ 13.8%)
Glycopeptides	59.6 (–23.2%)	9.8 (–5.1%)	10.3 (+ 23.6%)
Imidazoles	61.9 (–3.93%)	20.2 (+ 20.6%)	39.6 (+ 9.96%)

DDD defined daily dose; *ICU* intensive care unit; *RC* relative change (%) between 2009 and 2013
[a]Pooled means in DDDs per 1000 patient-days and relative changes in percent

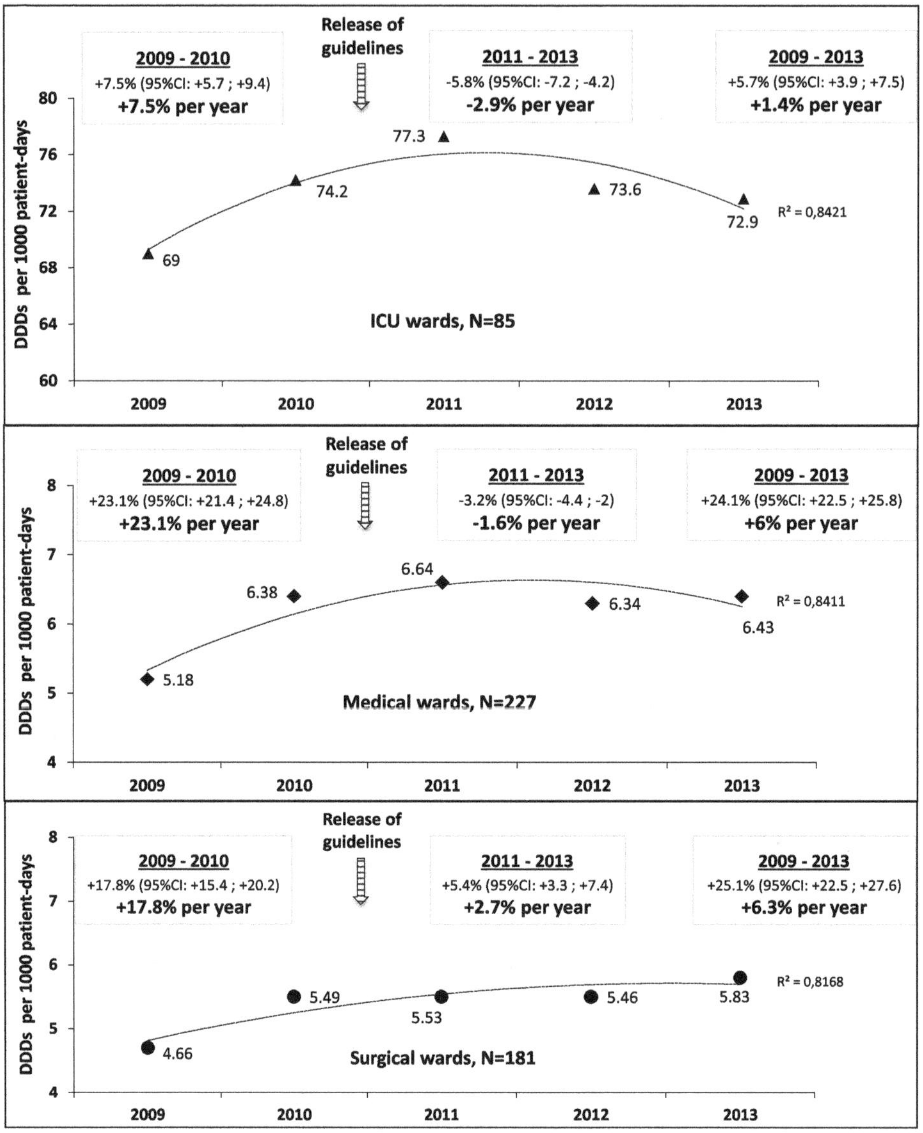

Fig. 1 Changes in carbapenem use in hospital wards across France from 2009 to 2013. For each time period (2009–10, 2011–13 and 2009–13), the relative change and the annual growth rate of carbapenem consumption (in bold) were computed. *CI*, confidence interval; *DDD* defined daily dose

that recorded a decline in their overall antibiotic use reduced more often their carbapenem use (univariable analysis, $p = 0.003$). In multivariable analysis (Table 3), the following factors were independently associated with a higher probability of reducing carbapenem use: a geographical location in Eastern France in comparison with South-eastern area of the country, a higher initial carbapenem prescribing profile and the reductions in consumption of fluoroquinolones, glycopeptides and piperacillin/tazobactam. Furthermore, other factors were independently associated with a lower probability of reducing carbapenem use: ICU wards (vs. medical wards), ward size increase, wards of cancer centres (vs. wards of general hospitals), a higher initial 3GC prescribing profile and location in a high-risk region for ESBL-PE.

Discussion

Antibiotic use and potential impact of guidelines on carbapenem use

In comparison with the meta-analysis of Bitterman et al. [18], our study showed that antibiotic consumption in ICUs and medical wards was lower in France than in other countries worldwide: for overall antibiotic use (1487 vs. 1563 DDD/1000 PD in ICUs and 615 vs. 677 DDD/1000 patient-days in medical wards), as well as for specific antibiotic classes, including carbapenems (73.4 vs. 109 DDD/1000 PD in ICUs and 6.2 vs. 16 DDD/1000 PD in medical wards). In the current study, the release of guidelines for carbapenems in late 2010 was followed by a significant decrease or a slowdown in their usage in French hospital wards. This finding suggests a potential

Table 3 Factors associated with the reduction in carbapenem use from random-effects logistic regression model

Variable	Univariable analysis		Multivariable analysis		
	OR	*p*	OR	*p*[a]	95% CI
Type of ward (reference: Medical)					
ICU	0.94	0.83	***0.07***	***0.005***	***0.01–0.46***
Surgical	0.95	0.81	0.66	0.19	0.35–1.23
Ward size in 2013, per increase of 50 beds	0.90	0.14	***0.79***	***0.02***	***0.64–0.97***
Type of HCF (reference: General hospital)					
University hospital	0.42	0.35	0.28	0.25	0.03–2.39
Private hospital	1.06	0.85	0.66	0.28	0.31–1.40
Cancer centre	0.37	0.29	***0.09***	***0.04***	***0.01–0.88***
Local hospital	2.33	0.18	1.19	0.83	0.25–5.54
Rehabilitation and long-term care facility	0.38	0.50	0.24	0.40	0.01–6.59
Military hospital	0.43	0.34	0.18	0.09	0.02–1.28
Geographical area (reference: South-east)					
North	1.42	0.42	2.33	0.09	0.88–6.16
West	1.15	0.80	1.09	0.90	0.30–3.94
East	1.93	0.15	***3.11***	***0.03***	***1.10–8.77***
South-west	1.78	0.17	1.57	0.36	0.60–4.12
Antibiotic use, DDDs per 1000 patients-days					
Initial CBP use[b]	1.01	0.01	0.97	0.08	0.95–1.00
Initial prescribing profile of CBPs[c]	1.22	0.002	***3.16***	***< 0.001***	***1.88–5.34***
Initial 3GC use[b]	1.00	0.79			
Initial prescribing profile of 3GCs[c]	0.97	0.16	***0.89***	***0.002***	***0.83–0.96***
Reduction in 3GC use[d]	1.34	0.23			
Initial FQ use[b]	1.00	0.25			
Initial prescribing profile of FQs[c]	1.02	0.29			
Reduction in FQ use[d]	2.21	0.004	***2.3***	***0.02***	***1.17–4.53***
Initial AG use[b]	1.00	0.50			
Initial prescribing profile of AGs[c]	0.97	0.44			
Reduction in AG use[d]	1.56	0.06	1.13	0.67	0.65–1.96
Initial AP ± BLI use[b]	1.00	0.83			
Initial prescribing profile of AP±BLIs[c]	1.00	0.99			
Reduction in AP ± BLI use[d]	1.10	0.68			
Initial Imidazole use[b]	1.00	0.98			
Initial prescribing profile of imidazoles[c]	0.97	0.45			
Reduction in imidazole use[d]	1.65	0.03	1.50	0.15	0.87–2.59
Initial GP use[b]	1.00	0.95			
Initial prescribing profile of GPs[c]	0.97	0.61			
Reduction in GP use[d]	1.83	0.01	***1.98***	***0.02***	***1.13–3.45***
Initial TZP use[b]	1.00	0.99			
Initial prescribing profile of TZP[c]	0.95	0.33			
Reduction in TZP use[d]	4.24	< 0.001	***4.02***	***< 0.001***	***1.99–8.14***
Initial use of other alternatives to CBPs[b]	1.00	0.88			
Initial prescribing profile of other alternatives to CBPs[c]	1.31	0.25			
Reduction in the use of other alternatives to CBPs[d]	1.07	0.79			

Table 3 Factors associated with the reduction in carbapenem use from random-effects logistic regression model *(Continued)*

Variable	Univariable analysis		Multivariable analysis		
	OR	p	OR	p^a	95% CI
Initial overall antibiotic use[b]	1.00	0.72	1.00	0.97	0.99–1.01
Reduction in the overall antibiotic use[d]	2.02	0.003	1.38	0.29	0.76–2.51
Region with high ESBL-PE incidence rate in acute care settings[e]	0.65	0.12	***0.40***	***0.01***	***0.19–0.82***

OR odds ratio, *CI* confidence interval, *ICU* intensive care unit, *HCF* healthcare facility, *DDD* defined daily dose, *CBP* carbapenem, *3GC* third-generation cephalosporin, *FQ* fluoroquinolone, *AG* aminoglycoside, *AP* ± *BLI* aminopenicillin ± β-lactamase inhibitor, *GP* glycopeptide, *TZP* piperacillin/tazobactam. *ESBL-PE* extended-spectrum β-lactamase-producing *Enterobacteriaceae*

[a]Significant associations ($p < 0.05$) from multivariable analysis are highlighted in bold italic

[b]Consumption of a given antibiotic in 2009

[c]Proportion (%) of a given antibiotic in the total antibiotic consumption in 2009

[d]Reduction in the consumption of a given antibiotic between 2009 and 2013

[e]Data from the French multidrug-resistant bacteria surveillance network; BMR-RAISIN, 2011

impact of these guidelines on reducing carbapenem use. Additionally, the magnitude of this impact appears more marked in ICUs and medical wards than in surgical wards. These guidelines fitted into the framework of the French national antibiotic action plans (initiated in 2001, the latest iteration being 2011–2016) [9] from the French Ministry of Health. The latter required from each HCF: (i) implementation of an ASP since 2002 and (ii) an annual public reporting of the compliance since 2007 with specific antimicrobial stewardship performance indicators, in order to enhance rational antibiotic use [19]. As with carbapenems, trends in the usage of other antibiotics suggest that efforts for curbing antibiotic overuse are more frequently successful in ICUs and medical wards than in surgical wards. This finding is consistent with a study carried out at the Zurich University Hospital, which reported a higher proportion of inappropriate therapeutic antibiotic use in surgical wards (49.3%), in comparison with ICU (32.4%) and medical wards (32.9%) [20]. Other studies [21, 22] showed in surgeons a poor adherence to ASP, sometimes even following an educational intervention program. Some factors specific to surgeons may explain this fact, such as lack of extensive training in infectious diseases and antibiotic usage of most surgical training programs [23]. Therefore, a special effort should be made for surgeons in ASP interventions that aim at reducing carbapenem use.

Factors modifying the probability of reducing ward-level carbapenem use

The multivariable analysis identified five factors positively associated with the reduction in carbapenem use. First, a geographical location in Eastern France was associated with a higher probability of reducing carbapenem use compared with a location in South-eastern of the country. This could be a result of specific local situations. We could cite as an example, the increasing spread of CPE, in a region previously hit by a major vancomycin-resistant enterococci outbreak [24], which may have prompted a better compliance with prudent carbapenem use to lower selection pressure. All other things being equal, including initial overall antibiotic use, a 1% increase in initial carbapenem prescribing profile was associated with more than threefold increase in the probability of reducing carbapenem use. Such an observation could be due to the fact that it is probably easier to reduce carbapenem use within wards with high proportions of carbapenems in the initial overall antibiotic use than within wards that use them sparingly. Indeed, in these wards with a high initial carbapenem prescribing profile, there was likely a greater room for improvement in terms of proper carbapenem use, notably through de-escalation strategies, which are still insufficiently implemented [25]. Lastly, wards, which reduced their consumptions of fluoroquinolones, glycopeptides and piperacillin/tazobactam, reduced more frequently their carbapenem use. Maybe this reflects what is covered by the positive and significant association between the reduction in overall antibiotic use and the reduction in carbapenem use in univariable analysis. This association was not significant in multivariable analysis. Furthermore, about the variable 'reduction in fluoroquinolone use', this could be also interpreted as a result of the involvement of fluoroquinolones in the occurrence of antibiotic-resistant bacteria [26], including ESBL-PE. Indeed, the reduction in fluoroquinolone use decreased the ESBL-PE risk and therefore the recourse to carbapenems. Moreover, this reduction in fluoroquinolone use is probably due to multiple ASP interventions within French HCFs and release of national guidelines, especially for urinary tract infections [27–29]. Clearly, the decrease in fluoroquinolone use over the study period has been partly achieved thanks to a shift of the antibiotic prescribing towards 3GCs and piperacillin/tazobactam, of which consumptions increased while overall antibiotic use remained almost stable. Besides, the positive association between the reduction in piperacillin/tazobactam use and the reduction in carbapenem use was surprising in view of the potential role of piperacillin/tazobactam as a carbapenem-sparing antibiotic. An optimistic explanation could be the 'virtous cycle' hypothesis, with a global improvement in prescribing, resulting in a decrease of all previously overprescribed antibiotics. In parallel, five other factors were negatively associated with reduction in carbapenem use. ICUs and wards of cancer centres had probabilities of reducing carbapenem use which were about 90% lower than those of medical wards and wards of general hospitals, respectively. Such a finding is consistent, given a higher severity and a more frequent previous antibiotic exposure in patients in these acute care settings, leading to a greater risk for developing severe infections with resistant Gram-negative bacteria [30]. Therefore, carbapenem prescribing can be less frequently avoidable. A 50-bed increase in ward size was associated with a 21% decrease in the probability of reducing carbapenem use. To explain this result, we assume that the number of doctors prescribing antibiotics increases with the ward size. It is likely that interventions conducted by ASP committees, which aim at promoting the proper use of carbapenems are harder to implement within larger wards, especially since the heterogeneity of antibiotic prescribing is possibly higher [31]. Lastly, a 1% increase in the initial prescribing profile of 3GCs was associated with 11% decrease in the probability of reducing carbapenem use, and this for the same level of initial overall antibiotic use. Likewise, wards located in high-risk regions for ESBL-PE exhibited a 60% decrease in the probability of reducing carbapenem use. The explanation for these two last findings is to be found in the ESBL-PE risk, which is promoted by 3GC use [26], and thus leads to more frequent carbapenem use. It should be recalled that 3GC use remained stable or increased between 2009 and 2013 across the three types of wards. Hence, the reduction in 3GC use appears as an essential factor in future ASPs aiming to reduce carbapenem prescribing. To a lesser extent, this is also the case for the reduction in fluoroquinolone use, which is already in progress and must be continued. For example, the retrospective multicentre study from Batard et al. [32], regarding emergency department patients treated for community-acquired pneumonia, revealed that use of 3GCs and fluoroquinolones was avoidable in 70% and 52% of cases, respectively. These antibiotics could be replaced with aminopenicillins ± β-lactamase inhibitors. Furthermore, recent applications of matrix-assisted laser desorption ionization–time of flight (MALDI-TOF) mass spectrometry (MS) for rapid detection of antibiotic resistance offer promising perspectives for optimizing antibiotic prescribing in clinical practice [33, 34]. In other terms, MALDI-TOF MS, in addition to being a technology for pathogen identification, could be a valuable tool for early therapeutic guidance by allowing for example an early de-escalation whenever possible. Nevertheless, in all cases, the issue of adherence to the guidelines is central to the success of such developments.

Limitations

This ward-level multicentre retrospective study is subject to various limitations. First, no patient-level confounding factor has been taken into account. Consequently, case-mix and potential ecological bias inherent to this type of study could not be controlled. Second, associations are suggestive and do not necessarily imply a cause-effect relationship. Therefore, these findings must be confirmed through randomized controlled intervention studies exploring joint effects of individual- and group-level factors. Third, we had no data regarding ASPs in HCFs enrolled in the study. As a result, we could not measure the implementation of carbapenem use guidelines. Fourth, DDD measurement presents biases mentioned elsewhere [35], including as a metric to study the impact of antibiotic stewardship. Fifth, no data was available regarding compliance with infection prevention and control measures. Indeed, hand hygiene, barrier precautions and carrier screening, by avoiding the spread of MDR bacteria, may influence carbapenem use. Additionally, none information on the occurrence of MDR bacteria outbreaks within HCFs was available in this study.

Conclusions

Despite these caveats, our study, carried out on a national scale, in a large number of hospital wards, suggests that a decrease in 3GC proportion in the overall antibiotic use, as well as the continuation of the reduction in fluoroquinolone use, could allow reducing ward-level carbapenem use. Thus, in their future interventions, ASPs should target not only wards with a higher carbapenem use, but also those with a higher 3GC prescription proportion to conduct actions focusing on both 3GCs and carbapenems to preserve the effectiveness of these antibiotics in French HCFs.

Abbreviations

3GC: Third-generation cephalosporin; 95% CI: Confidence interval; ASP: Antibiotic stewardship program; CPE: Carbapenemase-producing *Enterobacteriaceae*; DDD: Defined daily dose; ESBL-PE: Extended spectrum β-lactamase-producing *Enterobacteriaceae*; HCF: Healthcare facility; ICU: Intensive care unit; MALDI-TOF MS: Matrix-assisted laser desorption ionization–time of flight mass spectrometry; MDR: Multidrug-resistant; PD: Patient-day

Acknowledgements

The authors thank the French healthcare facilities that contributed to data collection within the framework of ATB-RAISIN and ATB-BMR networks.

ATB-RAISIN network steering committee:

Serge Alfandari, Anne Berger-Carbonne, Xavier Bertrand, Sandrine Boussat, Anne-Claude Crémieux, Catherine Dumartin, Pascal Fascia, Rémy Gauzit,

Marine Giard, Anne Ingels, François L Hériteau, Ludivine Lacavé, Patricia Le Gonidec, Anaïs Machut, Sylvie Maugat, Lory Mouchot, Muriel Péfau, Anne-Marie Rogues, Benoît Schlemmer, Hélène Sénéchal, Sophie Touratier.

Funding
The ATB-RAISIN network is partly funded by the French Institute for Public Health Surveillance (InVS – Santé Publique France).

Authors' contributions
CD, MP and HGH wrote the study project. CD and MP were responsible for collection and validation of data within the framework of the ATB-RAISIN network. AM, XB, AMR, MP, SA, RG, CD and HGH participated in the analysis and the interpretation of the data. AM and HGH prepared the first and revised draft of the manuscript. All authors read and approved the final version of the manuscript.

Consent for publication
Not applicable.

Competing interests
The authors declare that they have no competing interests.

Author details
[1]University Hospital of Besançon, Infection Control Department, F-25030 Besançon, France. [2]University Bourgogne-Franche-Comte, UMR 6249 Chrono-Environnement, F-25030 Besançon, France. [3]University Bordeaux, Inserm, Bordeaux Population Health Research Center, Team Pharmacoepidemiology, UMR 1219, F-33000 Bordeaux, France. [4]CHU Bordeaux, Southwestern Centre for Infection Prevention and Control, F-33000 Bordeaux, France. [5]Gustave Dron Hospital, Infectious Diseases Department, F-59208 Tourcoing, France. [6]AP-HP, Cochin University Hospital, Infectious Diseases Department, F-75014 Paris, France. [7]Service d'Hygiène Hospitalière, Centre Hospitalier Régional Universitaire, Hôpital Jean Minjoz, 3 Bd Fleming, 25030, Besançon, Cedex, France.

References
1. European Centre for Disease Prevention and Control. Surveillance of antimicrobial consumption in Europe 2012. Stockholm: ECDC; 2014.
2. Van Boeckel TP, Gandra S, Ashok A, Caudron Q, Grenfell BT, Levin SA, et al. Global antibiotic consumption 2000 to 2010: an analysis of national pharmaceutical sales data. Lancet Infect Dis. 2014;14(8):742–50.
3. Goel N, Wattal C, Oberoi JK, Raveendran R, Datta S, Prasad KJ. Trend analysis of antimicrobial consumption and development of resistance in non-fermenters in a tertiary care hospital in Delhi, India. J Antimicrob Chemother. 2011;66(7):1625–30.
4. European Centre for Disease Prevention and Control. Antimicrobial resistance surveillance in Europe 2015. In: Annual report of the European antimicrobial resistance surveillance network (EARS-net). Stockholm: ECDC. p. 2017.
5. Santé Publique France. Episodes impliquant des entérobactéries productrices de carbapénèmases en France. Situation épidémiologique du 4 septembre 2015. 2015. http://invs.santepubliquefrance.fr/Dossiers-thematiques/Maladies-infectieuses/Infections-associees-aux-soins/Surveillance-des-infections-associees-aux-soins-IAS/Enterobacteries-productrices-de-carbapenemases-EPC/. Accessed 02 Dec 2016.
6. Santé Publique France. Situation épidémiologique. Épisodes impliquant des entérobactéries productrices de carbapénémases (EPC) en France, 2004 à 2015. Données au 31 décembre 2015. 2017. http://invs.santepubliquefrance.fr/Dossiers-thematiques/Maladies-infectieuses/Infections-associees-aux-soins/Surveillance-des-infections-associees-aux-soins-IAS/Enterobacteries-productrices-de-carbapenemases-EPC/Episodes-impliquant-des-EPC-en-France.-Situation-epidemiologique-du-31-decembre-2015. Accessed 31 Mar 2017.
7. Albiger B, Glasner C, Struelens MJ, Grundmann H, Monnet DL. Carbapenemase-producing Enterobacteriaceae in Europe: assessment by national experts from 38 countries, may 2015. Euro Surveill. 2015;20(45)
8. Carlet J, Rambaud C, Pulcini C. Save antibiotics: a call for action of the world alliance against antibiotic resistance (WAAAR). BMC Infect Dis. 2014;14(436)
9. French Ministry of Health. National alert Plan on antibiotics, 2011–2016 [in French]. 2011. http://social-sante.gouv.fr/IMG/pdf/plan_antibiotiques_2011-2016_DEFINITIF.pdf. Accessed 02 Dec 2016.
10. Boucher HW, Talbot GH, Bradley JS, Edwards JE, Gilbert D, Rice LB, et al. Bad bugs, no drugs: no ESKAPE! An update from the Infectious Diseases Society of America. Clin Infect Dis. 2009;48(1):1–12.
11. Gauzit R, Gutmann L, Brun-Buisson C, Jarlier V, Fantin B. Recommandations de bon usage des carbapénèmes. Antibiotiques. 2010;12(4):183–9.
12. ANSM. L'évolution des consommations antibiotiques en France entre 2000 et 2013. ANSM: Saint Denis; 2014.
13. Santé Publique France. Surveillance de la consommation des antibiotiques, Réseau ATB-Raisin - Résultats 2015. 2017. http://invs.santepubliquefrance.fr/Publications-et-outils/Rapports-et-syntheses/Maladies-infectieuses/2017/Surveillance-de-la-consommation-des-antibiotiques. Accessed 12 Jun 2017.
14. WHO Collaborating Centre for Drug Statistics Methodology. Guidelines for ATC classification and DDD assignment. 2013. https://www.whocc.no/atc_ddd_index/. Accessed 02 Dec 2016.
15. Dumartin C, L'Heriteau F, Pefau M, Bertrand X, Jarno P, Boussat S, et al. Antibiotic use in 530 French hospitals: results from a surveillance network at hospital and ward levels in 2007. J Antimicrob Chemother. 2010;65(9):2028–36.
16. Fournier D, Chirouze C, Leroy J, Cholley P, Talon D, Plesiat P, et al. Alternatives to carbapenems in ESBL-producing Escherichia Coli infections. Med Mal Infect. 2013;43(2):62–6.
17. Goldstein H. Multilevel Statistical Models. 4th ed. London: Wiley; 2011.
18. Bitterman R, Hussein K, Leibovici L, Carmeli Y, Paul M. Systematic review of antibiotic consumption in acute care hospitals. Clin Microbiol Infect. 2016;22(6):561 e7–e19.
19. Trivedi KK, Dumartin C, Gilchrist M, Wade P, Howard P. Identifying best practices across three countries: hospital antimicrobial stewardship in the United Kingdom, France, and the United States. Clin Infect Dis. 2014;59(Suppl 3):S170–8.
20. Cusini A, Rampini SK, Bansal V, Ledergerber B, Kuster SP, Ruef C, et al. Different patterns of inappropriate antimicrobial use in surgical and medical units at a tertiary care hospital in Switzerland: a prevalence survey. PLoS One. 2010;5(11):e14011.
21. Knox MC, Edye M. Educational antimicrobial stewardship intervention ineffective in changing surgical prophylactic antibiotic prescribing. Surg Infect. 2016;17(2):224–8.
22. Rizan C, Phee J, Boardman C, Khera G. General surgeon's antibiotic stewardship: climbing the Rogers diffusion of innovation curve-prospective cohort study. Int J Surg. 2017;40:78–82.
23. Cakmakci M. Antibiotic Stewardship programmes and the surgeon's role. J Hosp Infect. 2015;89(4):264–6.
24. Henard S, Lozniewski A, Aissa N, Jouzeau N, Rabaud C. Evaluation of the duration of vanA vancomycin-resistant enterococcus faecium carriage and clearance during a large-scale outbreak in a region of eastern France. Am J Infect Control. 2011;39(2):169–71.
25. Gauzit R, Pean Y, Alfandari S, Bru JP, Bedos JP, Rabaud C, et al. Carbapenem use in French hospitals: a nationwide survey at the patient level. Int J Antimicrob Agents. 2015;46(6):707–12.
26. Gbaguidi-Haore H, Dumartin C, L'Heriteau F, Pefau M, Hocquet D, Rogues AM, et al. Antibiotics involved in the occurrence of antibiotic-resistant bacteria: a nationwide multilevel study suggests differences within antibiotic classes. J Antimicrob Chemother. 2013;68(2):461–70.
27. Doco-Lecompte T, Demore B, Henard S, Rughoo L, Burty C, Rondelot G, et al. Relevance of fluoroquinolone use in hospitals in the Lorraine region of France before and after corrective measures: an investigation by the Antibiolor network. Scand J Infect Dis. 2012;44(2):86–92.
28. Lafaurie M, Porcher R, Donay JL, Touratier S, Molina JM. Reduction of fluoroquinolone use is associated with a decrease in methicillin-resistant Staphylococcus Aureus and fluoroquinolone-resistant Pseudomonas Aeruginosa isolation rates: a 10 year study. J Antimicrob Chemother. 2012;67(4):1010–5.
29. Slekovec C, Leroy J, Vernaz-Hegi N, Faller JP, Sekri D, Hoen B, et al. Impact of a region wide antimicrobial stewardship guideline on urinary tract infection prescription patterns. Int J Clin Pharm. 2012;34(2):325–9.

30. Wilson AP, Livermore DM, Otter JA, Warren RE, Jenks P, Enoch DA, et al. Prevention and control of multi-drug-resistant gram-negative bacteria: recommendations from a joint working party. J Hosp Infect. 2016;92(Suppl 1):S1–44.
31. Cordoba G, Siersma V, Lopez-Valcarcel B, Bjerrum L, Llor C, Aabenhus R, et al. Prescribing style and variation in antibiotic prescriptions for sore throat: cross-sectional study across six countries. BMC Fam Pract. 2015;16(7)
32. Batard E, Lecadet N, Goffinet N, Hardouin JB, Lepelletier D, Potel G, et al. High variability among emergency departments in 3rd-generation cephalosporins and fluoroquinolones use for community-acquired pneumonia. Infection. 2015; 43(6):681–9.
33. Clark AE, Kaleta EJ, Arora A, Wolk DM. Matrix-assisted laser desorption ionization-time of flight mass spectrometry: a fundamental shift in the routine practice of clinical microbiology. Clin Microbiol Rev. 2013;26(3):547–603.
34. Jung JS, Popp C, Sparbier K, Lange C, Kostrzewa M, Schubert S. Evaluation of matrix-assisted laser desorption ionization-time of flight mass spectrometry for rapid detection of beta-lactam resistance in Enterobacteriaceae derived from blood cultures. J Clin Microbiol. 2014;52(3): 924–30.
35. Morris AM. Antimicrobial stewardship programs: appropriate measures and metrics to study their impact. Current treatment options in infectious diseases. 2014;6(2):101–12.

3

Prevalence and pattern of antibiotic resistance of *Staphylococcus aureus* isolated from door handles and other points of contact in public hospitals in Ghana

Courage Kosi Setsoafia Saba[1*], Jean Kwadwo Amenyona[2] and Stephen Wilson Kpordze[2]

Abstract

Background: Studies have implicated *Staphylococcus aureus* as the leading cause of septicemia in the Tamale metropolis of Ghana. The aim of this study was to determine the prevalence and antibiotic susceptibility of *S. aureus* and Methicillin Resistant *S. aureus* (MRSA) in the environments of three hospitals in Ghana.

Methods: A total of 120 swab samples were taken from door handles, stair railings and other points of contact at Tamale Teaching Hospital, Tamale Central Hospital and Tamale West Hospital. The swab samples were directly plated on Mannitol Salt and Baird Parker agar plates and incubated at 37 °C (± 2) for 18–24 h. An antibiotic susceptibility test was performed using the Clinical Laboratory Standard Institute's guidelines. Isolates resistant to both cefoxitin and oxacillin were considered to be MRSA.

Results: A total of 47 (39%) positive *S. aureus* samples were isolated from all three hospitals, of which, eight (17%) were putative MRSA isolates. One MRSA isolate was resistant to all the antibiotics used (cefoxitin, oxacillin, ciprofloxacin, erythromycin, tetracycline, ampicillin, streptomycin and sulfamethoxazole-trimethoprim). Five of the MRSA isolates were multi-drug resistant, whilst the other three were resistant to only two antibiotics. All the multi-drug resistant MRSA isolates were resistant to at least four antibiotics. The percentage of isolates resistant to oxacillin, ampicillin, ciprofloxacin, tetracycline, streptomycin, erythromycin, and sulfamethoxazole/trimethoprim were 17, 13, 9, 28, 89, 13 and 11% respectively.

Conclusion: The high multi-drug resistance of MRSA in hospital environments in Ghana reinforces the need for the effective and routine cleaning of door handles in hospitals. Further investigation is required to understand whether *S. aureus* from door handles could be the possible causes of nosocomial diseases in the hospitals.

Keywords: Healthcare associated infections, Methicillin resistant *Staphylococcus aureus*, Antibiotic resistance, Ghana

Background

Constant surveillance and adequate infection control measures for *Staphylococcus aureus* and Methicillin Resistant *Staphylococcus aureus* (MRSA) may reduce their roles in the incidence of nosocomial diseases and other infections in a clinical setting. However, there is a paucity of data *on S. aureus* prevalence and antibiotic susceptibility in low resource settings such as Ghana [1]. Most available data on *S. aureus* prevalence in Africa are patient-based, although the 'one health' concept (including environmental persistence) must be considered if this organism is to be effectively controlled. The ease of spread of resistant strains of *S. aureus* or MRSA cannot be overemphasized, especially in the Ghanaian context, where both environmental and personal hygiene are still rudimentary [2, 3]. *S. aureus* is known for its ability to develop resistance to almost all antibiotics, which makes it challenging to treat the range of infections it causes. There are reports of increasing resistance by MRSA and Methicillin Susceptible *S. aureus* (MSSA) to drugs of choice [4]. Very

* Correspondence: courageousgh@gmail.com
[1]Department of Biotechnology, Faculty of Agriculture, University for Development Studies, P. O Box TL 1882, Tamale, Ghana
Full list of author information is available at the end of the article

few published studies exist on investigating environmental samples as sources of possible nosocomial diseases in Ghana and in Africa in general. However, a study in the neonatal intensive care unit in Accra identified *S. aureus* as the predominant bacteria (44%) found in the hospital environment [5]. Similar work on swab samples in the hospital environment in Nigeria also recorded *S. aureus* as the most prevalent microbe (50.80%) in the hospital environment [6] and a study of door handles and bathtubs in the hospital environment in Benin implicated the Panton-Valentine Leukocidin (PVL) producing *S. aureus* as a cause of nosocomial diseases [7]. In the USA, current estimates indicate MRSA causes approximately 95,000 invasive infections and 19,000 mortality cases per year, which is higher than the mortality rates caused by AIDS/Human Immunodeficiency Virus, hepatitis, tuberculosis and influenza combined [8]. The prevalence of multi-drug resistant MRSA in clinical isolates has been reported to be very high in some African countries including Morocco, Kenya, Nigeria and Cameroon [9].

In the Tamale Metropolis of Ghana, *S. aureus* has been implicated in 60.9% of sepsis cases among children in the Tamale Teaching Hospital [10]. *S. aureus* was also reported to be the commonest contaminant found in donor blood in Tamale with the following resistance pattern: 71.5, 28.6, 71.5 and 10% to Ampicillin, Ciprofloxacin, Tetracycline and Erythromycin respectively [11]. In Ghana, *S. aureus* is the third most commonly isolated microbe from patients, after *E. coli* and *Pseudomonas* spp. [12], the second most prevalent bacteria among patients from teaching, regional and district hospitals with a multi-drug resistant rate of 42.3% [13], and the second most frequently isolated organism in bacteremia incidence in the Ashanti Region of Ghana [14].

The aim of this study was to determine the prevalence and antibiotic susceptibility of *S. aureus* and Methicillin Resistant *S. aureus* (MRSA) in the environments of three hospitals in Ghana. Specifically, the objectives of this study were to determine the prevalence of *S. aureus* and MRSA on the door handles, stair railings, tap handles and surgical room aprons in the environment of three hospitals, and to determine the antibiotic susceptibility levels of isolated *S. aureus* and MRSA.

Methods

The study was carried out at the three major government hospitals in the Tamale Metropolis of Ghana: Tamale Teaching Hospital (TTH), is a referral hospital for three regions of Ghana with 478 beds and over 2000 workers; Tamale Central Hospital (TCH), is a public tertiary healthcare facility with 156 beds and 442 staff, and Tamale West Hospital (TWH), which is also a public tertiary healthcare center with 126 beds and 370 staff. The sample collection started in February and ended in March 2015. Permission and ethical clearance was granted by all three hospitals to conduct this research.

Samples were randomly taken from 120 points of contact: 94 (78%) were taken from door handles, eight (7%) were from stair rails and 18 (15%) were from other points of contact (i.e. pipe taps, emergency beds, aprons in the theatre, and doors without handles) (Table 1). Out of the total 120 samples, 51 (43%) were taken from the TTH, 35 (29%) from TCH and 34 (28%) from TWH (Fig. 1). Individual sterile swabs (MEUS, Italy) moistened with sterile phosphate buffer saline (Oxoid, Hampshire, UK) were used to swab each points of contact. The samples were kept below 4 °C and transported to the laboratory for analysis within two hrs. All swab samples were then directly streaked onto Mannitol Salt agar (Oxoid) media and incubated at 37 °C for 24 h. Suspected *S. aureus* positive colonies were re-streaked on Baird Parker agar (BioMerieux S. A, Spain), and incubated at 37 °C for 24 h for confirmation. Pure cultures of *S. aureus* were plated onto nutrient agar (Oxoid,) prior to all susceptibility tests. Antibiotic susceptibility testing was performed and interpreted according to the Clinical and Laboratory Institute Standard (CLSI) guidelines [15]. The breakpoints were determined using National Committee for Clinical Laboratory Standards (NCCLS) document M31-A2 [16]. Oxacillin (1 μg), Ampicillin (25 μg), Ciprofloxacin (5 μg), Tetracycline (30 μg), Erythromycin (15 μg), Streptomycin (10 μg) and Sulphamethoxazole/Trimethoprim (25 μg) were used for the susceptibility tests (all anitbiotics obtained from BioMerieux). Cefoxitin disks were used to test only those isolates resistant to Oxacillin. Methicillin Resistant *S. aureus* strains were classified as those isolates resistant to Cefoxitin and Oxacillin. Multi-drug resistant isolates were classified as those resistant to three or more antibiotics. All isolates have been stored in 25% glycerol at −20 °C, and are available for future studies.

Results

Sources and isolation of *Staphylococcus aureus*

A total of 104 suspected small yellow colonies of *S. aureus* were isolated from Mannitol Salt agar plates, and of these 47 isolates *S aureus*, indicated by black colonies with clear zones, were confirmed on Baird Parker plates (Table 1).

Antibiotic susceptibility of *S. aureus* isolates

Antibiotic susceptibility tests were performed on the 47 (39%) positive *S. aureus* samples. Of the total 47 positive *S. aureus* isolates, the percentage of isolates resistant to Oxacillin (OX), Ampicillin (AMP), Ciprofloxacin (CIP), Tetracycline (TET), Streptomycin (SMN), Erythromycin, (ERY) and Sulfamethoxazole/Trimethoprim (SXT) was 17, 13, 9, 28, 89, 13 and 11% respectively. Twenty eight (60%) isolates were isolated from the TWH alone, with the following resistance pattern; OX (18%), AMP (14%),

Table 1 *S. aureus* prevalence at the various departments/wards at each hospital

Department/Hospital	TTH (%)	TCH (%)	TWH (%)	Total
Administration	1/9 (11%)	1/3 (33%)	3/3 (100%)	5/15 (33%)
OPD	2/12 (17%)	2/7 (29%)	11/12 (92%)	15/31 (48%)
Theatre	0/13 (0%)	1/5 (20%)	7/10 (58%)	8/28 (29%)
Laboratory	2/6 (33%)	2/3 (67%)	–	4/9 (44%)
Male ward	–	0/2 (0%)	5/5 (100%)	5/7 (71%)
Female ward	–	2/2 (100%)	0/2 (0%)	2/4 (50%)
Children's ward	0/2 (0%)	0/3 (0%)	–	0/5 (050
Child welfare centre	–	1/2 (50%)	–	1/2 (50%)
New born intensive care	–	0/2 (0%)	–	0/2 (0%)
Maternity	–	0/3 (0%)	–	0/3 (0%)
Festula department	–	2/3 (67%)	–	2/3 (67%)
X-ray	–	–	1/1 (100%)	1/1 (100%)
Aseptic ward	0/1 (0%)	–	–	0/1 (0%)
Male surgical ward	1/1 (100%)	–	–	1/1 (100%)
Elevator button	0/1 (0%)	–	–	0/1 (0%)
Stair rail	2/7 (29%)	–	1/1 (100%)	3/8 (38%)
Total	8/51 (16%)	11/35 (31%)	28/34 (82%)	47/120 (39%)

TTH Tamale Teaching Hospital, *TCH* Tamale Central Hospital, *TWH* Tamale West Hospital, *OPD* Out Patient Department

CIP (14%), TET (46%), SMN (89%), ERY, (21%) and SXT (14%). One MRSA isolate from TWH was resistant to all the antibiotics used. Eleven (23%) isolates were from the TCH with the following resistance pattern: OX (18%), AMP (9%), SMN (91%) and SXT (9%). There was no resistance to CIP, TET, and ERY at the TCH. Eight (17%) isolates were from the TTH with the following resistance pattern: OX (13%), AMP (13%) and SMN (87%). There was no resistance to CIP, TET, SXT and ERY at the TTH. The details of the susceptibility testing results can be found as an Additional file 1.

Multi-drug resistance pattern of the *S. aureus* isolates

From the 47 positive *S. aureus* isolates, nine (19%) were multi-drug resistant (resistant to three or more antibiotics), 11 (23%) were resistant to only two antibiotics, 23 (49%) were resistant to only one antibiotic and the remaining four (9%) showed no resistance to any of the antibiotics. Eight

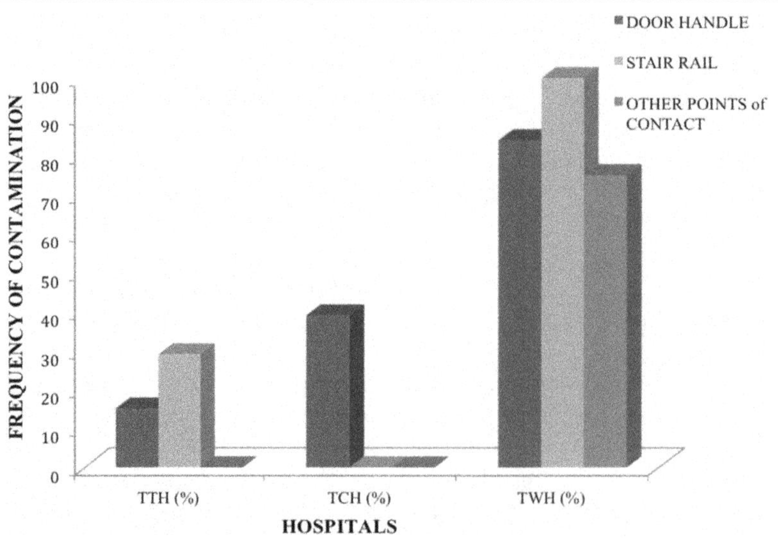

Fig. 1 *S. aureus* prevalence at the various hospitals. TTH, Tamale Teaching Hospital, TCH, Tamale Central Hospital, TWH, Tamale West Hospital

(89%) out of the nine multi- drug resistant *S. aureus* isolates were from TWH and one (11%) was from TCH. Nine (82%) of those resistant to only two antibiotics were from TWH while the remaining two (18%) were also from TTH. Ten (43%) of the isolates resistant to only one antibiotic were from TCH, eight (35%) were from TWH and five (22%) were from TTH. Out of the four that were not resistant to any antibiotic, three (75%) were from TWH and one (25%) was from TTH.

Antibiotic resistance pattern of the MRSA isolates

Of the total 47 (39%) positive *S. aureus* isolates, eight (17%) were Methicillin-resistant *S. aureus* (MRSA). The percentage resistance of the MRSA (eight isolates) to the antibiotics was OX (100%), AMP (38%), CIP (13%), TET (38%), SMN (87%), ERY, (25%), SXT (38%) and FOX (75%) (Fig. 2). Five (63%) of the MRSA isolates were multi-drug resistant and the other three (38%) were resistant to only two antibiotics. Seven of the MRSA isolates (87%) were from door handles and one (13%) was from a water tap in the TWH male ward. The MRSA resistant to all the antibiotics used was from a door handle from the TWH male's ward urinal.

Antibiotic resistance pattern of the MSSA isolates

Thirty-nine isolates (83%) of the total 47 positive *Staphylococcus* isolates were Methicillin-Susceptible *S. aureus* (MSSA). The rate of resistance of the 39 MSSA isolates to the antibiotics was: SMN (90%), TET (26%), ERY (10%), AMP (8%), CIP (8%) and SXT (5%) respectively (Fig. 2). Four (10%) of the MSSA were multi-drug resistant, nine (23%) were resistant to only two antibiotics, twenty-two (57%) were resistant to only one antibiotic and the remaining four (10%) were susceptible to all seven antibiotics. Of the four (10%) multi-drug resistant isolates, two (50%) were resistant to five antibiotics, one (25%) was resistant to four antibiotics and the remaining isolate (25%) was resistant to three antibiotics. Thirty-five of the MSSA isolates (90%) were resistant to Streptomycin (SMN). All the multi-drug resistant MSSA were from TWH. Three of the multi-drug resistant MSSA (75%) isolates were from door handles and the remaining isolate was from a theatre apron. Of the four multi-drug resistant MSSA isolates, the two that were resistant to five antibiotics were from the door handles of the theatre and the one resistant to four antibiotics was from the main entrance door handle of the male ward. The remaining isolate, resistant to three antibiotics, was from the door handle of the emergency ward at the OPD.

Discussion

MSSA and MRSA contamination of the hospital environment

This study was carried out to determine the prevalence and antibiotic resistance of *S. aureus* and MRSA isolates in the environments of three public hospitals in Ghana, and our results provide baseline information on *S. aureus* and MRSA prevalence in these hospital environments. Contamination of door handles with *S. aureus* occurred more at the administration blocks and OPD than the rest of the surfaces sampled; however, contamination recorded on the door handles and some of the surfaces in the operating theatres of these hospitals is clearly a concern. Although routine cleaning procedures are undertaken in these hospitals, they are not completely effective, and

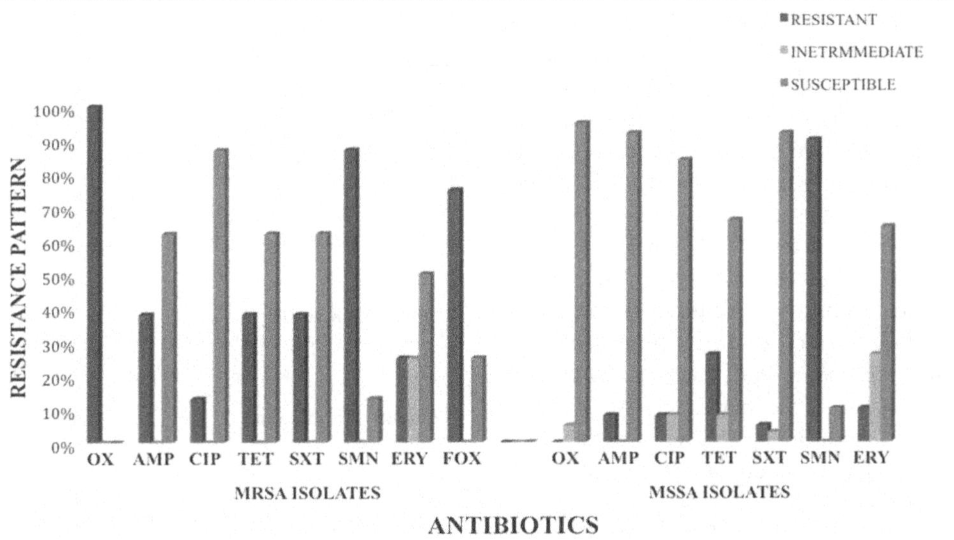

Fig. 2 Resistance rates of Methicillin Susceptible *S. aureus* versus Methicillin Resistant *S. aureus*. TTH, Tamale Teaching Hospital, TCH, Tamale Central Hospital, TWH, Tamale West Hospital. Cefoxitin (FOX), Oxacillin (OX), Ciprofloxacin (CIP), Erythromycin (ERY), Tetracycline (TET), Ampicillin (AMP), Streptomycin (SMN) and Sulfamethoxazole-trimethoprim (SXT)

improved methods of disinfecting these hospital environments are recommended [17]. During the course of this study, it was observed that more attention was paid to cleaning floors rather than door handles or knobs, which may have allowed a build-up of *S. aureus* on these surfaces. Subsequently, the high contamination rate of door handles and surfaces by *S. aureus* in hospitals is likely to be a contributing factor for these bacteria being implicated in blood stream infections in Tamale [9] and other parts of Ghana [11, 13].

Preventive measures such as improved personal hygiene and the regular cleaning and disinfection of hospital door handles, stair rails and other points of contact are highly recommended, especially in the TWH, which recorded the highest *S. aureus* contamination rate among the three hospitals. The results of this study are similar to those of Newman [5] for a hospital in Accra where the *S. aureus* prevalence was 44% on contact surfaces at neonatal unit, and that of Hammuel et al. [6] for a hospital in Nigeria. Our study reports higher MRSA prevalence (87%) than a similar study in Brazil, which recorded 33.3% prevalence of *S. aureus* on hospital ward surfaces (bedside tables, bed rails and door handles) [18]. In a similar study by Oie et al. [19], 27% (versus 39% in our study) of the door handles in a University hospital in Japan were contaminated with *S. aureus* of which 20.9% (versus 83% in our study) were MSSA and 8.7% (17% in our study) were MRSA.

Antibiotic resistance pattern

Antibiotic resistance has become a notorious health concern in the twenty-first Century. MRSA is an impediment to antimicrobial therapy, and the introduction of new classes of antimicrobial agents is usually followed by the emergence of resistant forms of this pathogen. The threat posed by MRSA was vividly demonstrated in this study, as one hospital isolate was resistant to all eight antibiotics used for the susceptibility test. Ghana is a place where poverty is prominent and people cannot afford to buy more expensive antibiotics, and the prevalence of MSRA on door handles, and particularly of theatre rooms, presents a significant threat to patients undergoing surgery.

Generally, the MSSA isolates in this study were more susceptible than the MRSA to antibiotics, but regular surveillance exercises should still be used to control the emergence of MRSA and other infectious diseases in hospitals. Resistance rates were fairly high for most of the antibiotics tested, although the pattern of resistance to Ciprofloxacin and Trimethoprim/sulfamethoxazole in MSRA isolates mean that these antibiotics can be recommended for the treatment of MRSA infections if antibiotics used in this study are the only available ones for treatment. These drugs also consistently demonstrate in vitro activity against *S. aureus* [4]. Hammuel et al. [6] also reported multi-drug resistance of *S. aureus* in the hospital environment in a similar study in Nigeria, but the multi-drug resistance of *S. aureus* in our study was lower (19% vs 31.30%).

Conclusions

This is the first study conducted on *S. aureus* on hospital door handles, stair rails and other points of contact in Ghana. There were high levels of contamination of *S. aureus* and MRSA on door handles in some of the hospitals. Isolates of *S. aureus* and MRSA had high rates of resistance to the antibiotics used in this study including one isolate that was resistant to all antibiotics. There is a need for periodic surveillance and monitoring of *S. aureus* and MRSA in the hospital environment as well as regular and effective cleaning of hospital door rails and contact surfaces in Ghanaian hospitals. This study provides preliminary information for the control of infections in the three hospitals studied. Further studies are needed, not only in Ghana, but across Africa, to understand the extent to which *S. aureus* isolated from contact surfaces in the hospital is contributing to nosocomial diseases.

Abbreviations

AMP: Ampicillin; CIP: Ciprofloxacin; ERY: Erythromycin; FOX: Cefoxitin; MRSA: Methicillin resistant *Staphylococcus aureus*; MSSA: Methicillin susceptible *Staphylococcus aureus*; OPD: Out patients department; OX: Oxacillin; SMN: Streptomycin; SXT: Sulfamethoxazole-trimethoprim; TCH: Tamale Central Hospital; TET: Tetracycline; TTH: Tamale Teaching Hospital; TWH: Tamale West Hospital

Acknowledgements

We are indebted to the University for Development Studies, Tamale, Ghana for permitting us to use the Spanish Laboratory Complex for this work. Our thanks also go to Bruno Gonzalez-Zorn from the Complutense University of Madrid for facilitating the purchase of materials for this research work. We appreciate very much the efforts of all the staff from the various hospitals that made this work a success.

Funding

This work was partly sponsored by the Government of Ghana from the research allowance grant and self-financed by the authors.

Authors'contributions

CKSS designed and wrote the manuscript. JKA and SWK were involved in the laboratory analysis. All authors read and approved the final manuscript.

Competing interests

The authors declare that they have no competing interests.

Consent for publication

Not applicable.

Author details

[1]Department of Biotechnology, Faculty of Agriculture, University for Development Studies, P. O Box TL 1882, Tamale, Ghana. [2]Department of Ecotourism and Environmental Management, Faculty of Renewable Natural Resources, University for Development Studies, P. O Box TL 1882, Tamale, Ghana.

References

1. Abdulgader SM, Shittu AO, Nicol MP, Kaba M. Molecular epidemiology of Methicillin-resistant *Staphylococcus aureus* in Africa: a systematic review. Front Microbiol. 2015;30(6):348.
2. Asare A, Enweronu-Laryea CC, Newman MJ. Hand hygiene practices in a neonatal intensive care unit in Ghana. J Infect Dev Ctries. 2009;5:352–6.
3. Owusu-Ofori A, Jennings R, Burgess J, Prasad PA, Acheampong F, Coffin SE. Assessing hand hygiene resources and practices at a large African teaching hospital. Infect Control Hosp Epidemiol. 2010;8:802–8.
4. Rayner C, Munckhof WJ. Antibiotics currently used in the treatment of infections caused by *Staphylococcus aureus*. Intern Med J. 2005;35(Suppl 2):S3–16.
5. Newman MJ. Neonatal intensive care unit: reservoirs of nosocomial pathogens. West Afr J Med. 2002;21(4):310–2.
6. Hammuel C, Jatau DE, Whong CMZ. Prevalence and antibiogram pattern of some nosocomial pathogens isolated from Hospital Environment in Zaria, Nigeria. Aceh Int J Sci Technol. 2014;3(3):131–9.
7. Ahoyo TA, Martin-Odoom A, Bankolé HS, Baba-Moussa L, Zonon N, Loko F, Prevost G, Sanni A, Dramane K. Epidemiology and prevention of nosocomial pneumonia associated with Panton-Valentine Leukocidin (PVL) producing *Staphylococcus aureus* in Departmental Hospital Centre of Zou Collines in Benin. Ghana Med J. 2012;46(4):234–40.
8. Hoyert DL, Xu JQ. Deaths: preliminary data for 2011. Natl Vital Stat Rep. 2012;61:1–52.
9. Kesah C, Ben Redjeb S, Odugbemi TO, Boye CS, et al. Prevalence of methicillin-resistant *Staphylococcus aureus* in eight African hospitals and Malta. Clin Microbiol Infect. 2003;9:153–6.
10. Acquah SE, Quaye L, Sagoe K, Ziem JB, Bromberger PI, Amponsem AA. Susceptibility of bacterial etiological agents to commonly-used antimicrobial agents in children with sepsis at the Tamale Teaching Hospital. BMC Infect Dis. 2013;18(13):89.
11. Opoku-Okrah C, Feglo P, Amidu N, Dakorah MP. Bacterial contamination of donor blood at the Tamale Teaching Hospital, Ghana. Afr Health Sci. 2009;9: 13–8.
12. Opintan JA, Newman MJ, Arhin RE, Donkor ES, Gyansa-Lutterodt M, Mills-Pappoe W. Laboratory-based nationwide surveillance of antimicrobial resistance in Ghana. Infect Drug Resist. 2015;8:379–89.
13. Newman MJ, Frimpong E, Donkor ES, Opintan JA, Asamoah-Adu A. Resistance to antimicrobial drugs in Ghana. Infect Drug Resist. 2011;4:215–20.
14. Nielsen MV, Sarpong N, Krumkamp R, Dekker D, Loag W, et al. Incidence and characteristics of bacteremia among children in Rural Ghana. PLoS One. 2012;7:e44063.
15. Clinical and Laboratory Standards Institute. Performance standards for antimicrobial susceptibility testing, 19th ed. Approved standard M100-S19. Wayne: Clinical and Laboratory Standards Institute; 2009.
16. National Committee for Clinical Laboratory Standards. Performance standards for antimicrobial disk and dilution susceptibility tests for bacteria isolated from animals-2nd edition: approved standard M31-A2. Wayne: National Committee for Clinical Laboratory Standards; 2002.
17. Boyce JM. Modern technologies for improving cleaning and disinfection of environmental surfaces in hospitals. Antimicrob Resist Infect Control. 2016;11(5):10.
18. Carvalho KS, Melo MC, Melo GB, Gontijo-Filho PP. Hospital surface contamination in wards occupied by patients infected with MRSA or MSSA in a Brazilian university hospital. J Basic Appl Pharm Sci. 2007;28(2):159–63.
19. Oie S, Hosokawa I, Kamiya A. Contamination of room door handles by methicillin-sensitive/methicillin-resistant *Staphylococcus aureus*. J Hosp Infect. 2002;51(2):140–3.

4

Resistance of *Staphylococcus aureus* to antimicrobial agents in Ethiopia

Serawit Deyno[1*], Sintayehu Fekadu[2] and Ayalew Astatkie[3]

Abstract

Background: Emergence of antimicrobial resistance by *Staphylococcus aureus* has limited treatment options against its infections. The purpose of this study was to determine the pooled prevalence of resistance to different antimicrobial agents by *S. aureus* in Ethiopia.

Methods: Web-based search was conducted in the databases of PubMed, Google Scholar, Hinari, Scopus and the Directory of Open Access Journals (DOAJ) to identify potentially eligible published studies. Required data were extracted and entered into Excel spread sheet. Statistical analyses were performed using Stata version 13.0. The *metaprop* Stata command was used to pool prevalence values. Twenty-one separate meta-analysis were done to estimate the pooled prevalence of the resistance of *S. aureus* to twenty-one different antimicrobial agents. Heterogeneity among the studies was assessed using the I^2 statistic and chi-square test. Publication bias was assessed using Egger's test. Because of significant heterogeneity amongst the studies, the random effects model was used to pool prevalence values.

Results: The electronic database search yielded 1317 studies among which 45 studies met our inclusion criteria. Our analyses demonstrated very high level of resistance to amoxicillin (77% [95% confidence interval (CI): 68%, 0.85%]), penicillin (76% [95% CI: 67%, 84%]), ampicillin (75% [95% CI: 65%, 85%]), tetracycline (62% [95% CI: 55%, 68%]), methicillin (47% [95% CI: 33%, 61%]), cotrimoxaziole (47% [95% CI: 40%, 55%]), doxycycline (43% [95% CI: 26%, 60%]), and erythromycin (41% [95% CI: 29%, 54%]). Relatively low prevalence of resistance was observed with kanamycin (14% [95% CI: 5%, 25%]) and ciprofloxacin (19% [95% CI: 13%, 26%]). The resistance level to vancomycin is 11% 995% CI: (4%, 20%). High heterogeneity was observed for each of the meta-analysis performed (I^2 ranging from 79.36% to 95.93%; all *p*-values ≤0.01). Eggers' test did not show a significant publication bias for all antimicrobial agents except for erythromycin and ampicillin.

Conclusions: *S. aureus* in Ethiopia has gotten notoriously resistant to almost to all of antimicrobial agents in use including, penicillin, cephalosporins, tetracyclines, chloramphenicol, methicillin, vancomycin and sulphonamides. The resistance level to vancomycin is bothersome and requires a due attention. Continued and multidimensional efforts of antimicrobial stewardship program promoting rational use of antibiotics, infection prevention and containment of AMR are urgently needed.

Keywords: Antimicrobial resistance, *Staphylococcus aureus*, Meta-analysis, Ethiopia

* Correspondence: dserawit@gmail.com
[1]Department of Pharmacology, School of Medicine, College of Medicine and Health Sciences, Hawassa University, P. O. Box 1560, Hawassa, Ethiopia
Full list of author information is available at the end of the article

Background

Staphylococcus aureus (*S. aureus*) infection is a major cause of skin, soft tissue, respiratory, bone, joint, and cardiovascular disorders [1]. *S. aureus* remains a versatile and dangerous pathogen in humans. The frequencies of both community-acquired and hospital-acquired staphylococcal infections have increased steadily. Treatment of these infections has become more difficult because of the emergence of multidrug-resistant strains [2].

Various mechanisms are responsible for *S. aureus* antimicrobial resistance (AMR). Penicillin is inactivated by β-lactamase. AMR to methicillin confers resistance to all β-lactamase-resistant penicillin's and cephalosporins which require the presence of the mec gene that encodes penicillin-binding protein [3]. The enterococcal plasmid-bearing gene for resistance to vancomycin has been transferred by conjugation to *S. aureus* in vitro [4]. Both increased cell-wall synthesis and alterations in the cell wall that prevent vancomycin from reaching sites of cell-wall synthesis have been suggested as mechanisms [4]. Increase in vancomycin use has led to the emergence of two types of glycopeptide-resistant *S. aureus*. The first one, designated vancomycin intermediate-resistant *S. aureus* (VISA), is associated with a thickened and poorly cross-linked cell wall is due to continuous exposure to glycopeptide. The second type, vancomycin-resistant *S. aureus* (VRSA), is due to acquisition from *Enterococcus* species of the *vanA* operon resulting in high-level resistance and is a rare phenomenon [5].

In Ethiopia the first published antimicrobial preliminary report on AMR was published by Plorde et al. in 1970 for different microbial agents [6]. Beginning from that time AMR report were made by different antimicrobial surveillances and studies, it showed rapid rise and spread of resistant strains.

Facilitating more appropriate choices of treatment, minimizing the morbidity and mortality due to resistant infections, and preserving the effectiveness of antimicrobials requires summarization and synthesis of the evidence regarding AMR in a country. Appropriately summarized and synthesized evidence is mandatory for updating national treatment guidelines. To our knowledge, no previous meta-analysis or systematic review has been conducted on *S. aureus* AMR to all antimicrobial commonly in use in Ethiopia. The purpose of this study was, therefore, to determine pooled prevalence of *S. aureus* resistance to common antimicrobial agents in Ethiopia based on the best available studies.

Methods

Study design

This study did a meta-analysis of prevalence of *S. aures* resistance to different antimicrobial agents in Ethiopia using the best available studies.

Literature search strategy

Web-based search using PubMed, Google Scholar, Hinari, Scopus and the Directory of Open Access Journals (DOAJ) was conducted in June 2016. Google search was used for unpublished works and government documents. Two of the authors (SD and SF) independently searched for relevant studies to be included in this meta-analysis. The PubMed search was carried out via the EndNote software. Relevant search results from Google scholar, Embase, Scopus and the DOAJ were individually downloaded and manually entered into EndNote. The reference lists of the identified studies were used to identify other relevant studies.

The search was done using various key words: Staphylococcus, antimicrobial resistance, antibiotic resistance, drug resistance, drug susceptibility, antibacterial resistance, Ethiopia. These key terms were used in various combinations using Boolean search technique. We did not limit the search by year or language of publication.

Study selection procedures and criteria

Study selection was performed in two stages independently by two of the authors (SD and SF). First, the titles and abstracts of all retrieved articles were reviewed and then grouped as "eligible for inclusion" if they did address the study question and "ineligible for inclusion" if they did not. Second, articles which were grouped under "eligible for inclusion" were reviewed in full detail for decision.

All available studies and data were included based on the following predefined inclusion criteria. 1) Studies that were original journal articles, short communications, or unpublished works; 2) Studies that did the antimicrobial susceptibility test according to the criteria of the Clinical Laboratory Standards Institute (CLSI) and defined antimicrobial resistance range according to CLSI manual [7], 3) Studies which used human infection sample.

Studies that 1) were duplicates, 2) were based on small number of isolates (1–10), 3) were conducted on non-human samples like on foods, food handlers' belongings, health workers belongings or health workers carriage and 4) which were based on non-infectious carriage were excluded from this meta-analysis.

Data extraction

Required data were extracted from eligible studies using Excel spreadsheet format prepared for this purpose by AA and SD. The data extracted from eligible studies include name of author(s), year of publication, place where the study was conducted, study design, total number of *S. aureus* isolate tested in the study, number of resistant *S. aureus* isolates, and isolate source. If the proportion of drug sensitive isolates (q) was reported, the number of resistant isolates was calculated by multiplying the number of isolates (n) by one minus the proportion of drug sensitive isolates (1-q) and if the proportion of drug resistant isolates was given the number of resistant isolates was found by multiplying the proportion (p) with total number of isolates (n).

Statistical analysis and reporting

Statistical analyses were performed using Stata version 13.0 (Statacorp, LP, college station, TX). The prevalence values from the different studies were pooled using the *metaprop* command in Stata [8]. We did twenty-one separate meta-analyses to estimate the pooled prevalence of the resistance of *S. aureus* to twenty one different antimicrobial agents. The number of studies included in each of the meta-analyses ranged from 4 to 39. Heterogeneity amongst the studies was assessed using the I^2 statistic. Because of significant heterogeneity amongst the studies the random-effects model (REM) was used to estimate the pooled prevalence and 95% CIs using the DerSimonian and Laird method [9]. The Freeman-Tukey double arcsine transformation was used so that studies reporting proportions near or at 0 and 1 would not be excluded from the meta-analysis. The possible presence of publication bias was checked using Egger's test [10].

For studies that appeared to report unusually higher prevalence of resistance compared to others, we did sensitivity analysis after dropping the study which we suspected of reporting a higher-than-usual result. If the point estimate of pooled prevalence after dropping a study lies within the 95% CI of the overall pooled estimate for all studies combined, we considered the given study as having non-significant influence on the overall pooled estimate. Otherwise, the study was considered as having significantly influencing the overall estimate.

Results of the current meta-analysis are reported as per the Preferred Reporting Items for Systematic Reviews and Meta-Analysis (PRISMA) guideline. The PRISMA checklist was used to ensure inclusion of relevant information (the filled checklist is included as Additional file 1: S1) [11].

Results

Included studies and characteristics

The electronic database search yielded 1317 from PubMed and 17,400 from Google scholar, Hinari, and Google search of which 16,083 articles remained after removing duplicate articles. Title and abstract screening reduced eligible articles to 76 for full text evaluation. After reading the full texts, 31 studies were excluded for various reasons. Thirteen studies were excluded as their report is based on small number of isolates (less than or equal to10) [12–24], four studies reported crude resistance for all bacterial pathogen isolated [25–28], eleven did not address our study question [29–36], six studies were based on samples taken from of healthy carriers [37–42], one study [43] was part of another study [44], and one study [45] suffered from environmental contamination of the samples during processing. Thus, 45 studies met our inclusion criteria (Fig. 1). Forty-one of the studies were journal articles, three were unpublished works [46–48] and one was an official government document from the Drug Administration and Control Authority (DACA) of Ethiopia [49].

S. aureus isolates from a total of 4570 patients were tested for their antimicrobial resistance. The isolates were from ear discharge [50–57], eye discharge [47, 58–60], blood [61–68], wound infection [69–74], surgical site infection [30, 73, 75–78], mixed samples [6, 46, 48, 49, 79–83], leprosy ulcer [84, 85], and urine sample [86, 87]. Twenty nine studies used primary data while nineteen studies used records from hospitals or regional laboratories (the characteristics of each included study is summarized Table 1).

Publication bias and heterogeneity

Evidence of high heterogeneity was observed for each of the meta-analyses performed (I^2 ranging from 79.36% to 95.93%; all p-values ≤ 0.01). Eggers' test did not suggest any significant publication bias except for erythromycin and ampicillin (see Additional file 2: S2).

Prevalence of *S. aureus* resistance to different antimicrobial agents

Summary of the pooled prevalence of *S. aureus* AMR prevalence for twenty-one different antimicrobial agents and the number of studies included in the meta-analysis for each agent are presented in Table 2. Prevalence of *S. aureus* resistance for each antimicrobial agent based on pharmacological classification of the agents is given below. As new anti-MRSA agents such as linezolid, daptomycin, tigecycline, telavancin and ceftaroline are rarely available in Ethiopia and no published studies available on resistance to this agents, our results do not cover such agents.

Prevalence of resistance to glycopeptides (vancomycin)

Nineteen studies were included for meta-analysis of vancomycin resistance prevalence. The pooled prevalence for *S. aureus* resistance to vancomycin in Ethiopia is 11% (95% confidence interval [CI]: 4%, 20%). The forest plot for vancomycin resistance is presented in Fig. 2. The results of sensitivity analysis after exclusion of the two studies that appeared to report outlier prevalence values separately and both together showed non-significant influence of the two studies on the overall estimate. The pooled prevalence of vancomycin resistance when Guta et al. and Desalegn et al. were removed

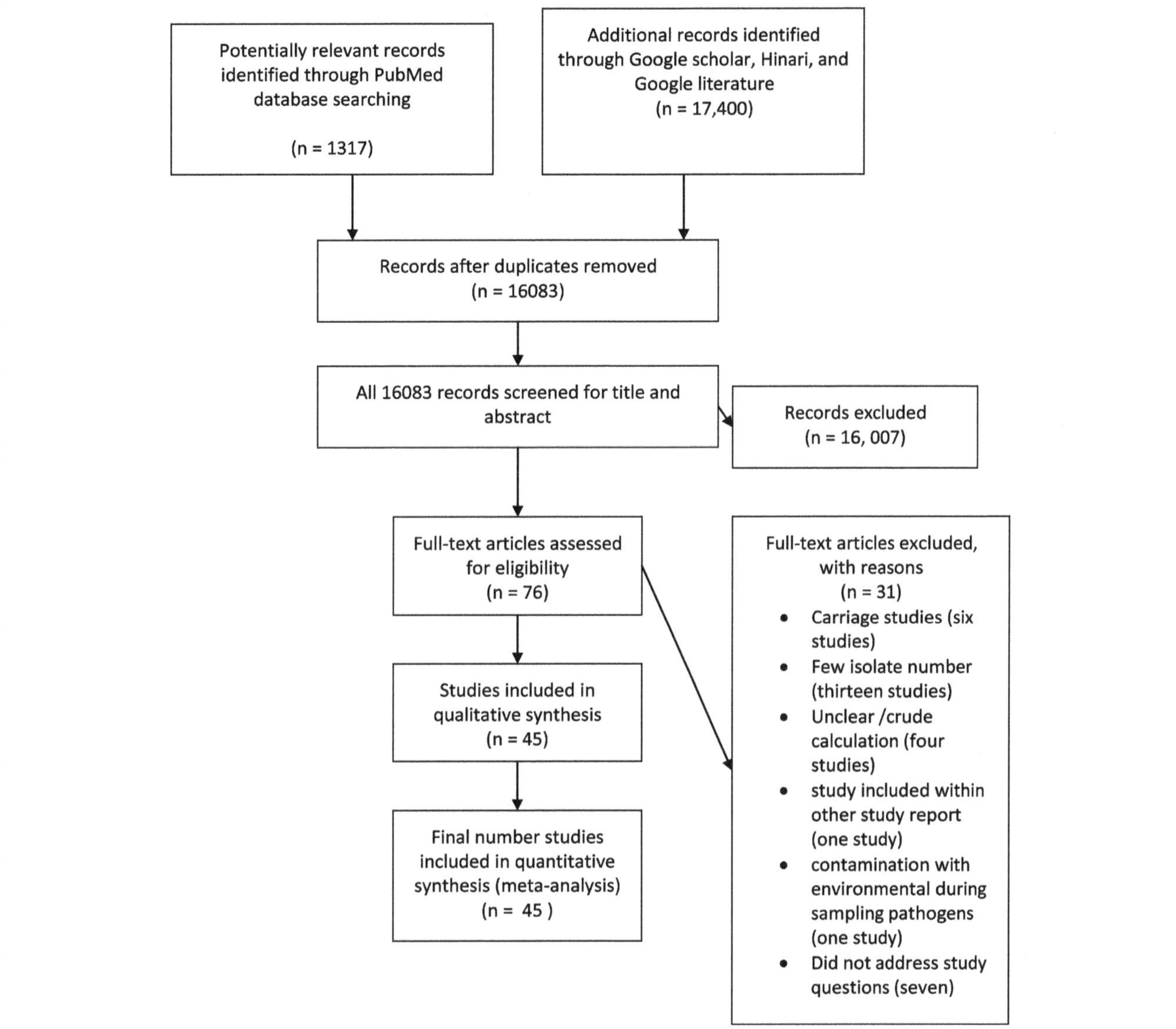

Fig. 1 Flow diagram of retrieval of studies: Number of studies screened, assessed for eligibility, and included in the meta-analysis with reasons

separately was 0.09, (95% CI: 0.03, 0.17). When, both Guta et al. and Desalegn et al. were excluded, vancomycin resistance was 0.07 (95% CI: 0.02, 0.14). All the three pooled values lie within the overall pooled estimate.

Prevalence of resistance to penicillin's

Here, the pooled prevalence of *S. aureus* resistance to penicillin G, amoxicillin, ampicillin, and amoxacilin-caluvanic acid was estimated. Resistance to penicillin G was estimated based on 33 studies, to amoxicillin based on 18 studies, to ampicillin based on 27 studies and to amoxacilin-caluvanic acid based on 12 studies. Pooled resistance rates were highest for β-lactamase-sensitive penicillin's. Resistance to amoxicillin was 77% (95% CI: 68%, 85%), to penicillin G 75% (95% CI: 65%, 85%) and to ampicillin 76% (95% CI: 67%, 84%). Resistance to carbencilin (β-lactam-sensitive antibiotic) was relatively lower than other β-lactam-antibiotics (34% [95% CI: 17%, 54%]).

Relatively lower resistance rate was observed to β-lactamase-resistant penicillin's: methicillin (47% [95% CI: 33%, 61%]) and amoxicillin-clavulanic acid (30% [95% CI: 19%, 43%]). The forest plots for methicillin and amoxacilin resistance are presented in Figs. 3 and 4, respectively while the forest plots for penicillin G, ampicillin, amoxicillin-clavulanic acid, and carbencillin resistance are presented in Additional file 3: S3, Additional file 4: S4, Additional file 5: S5 and Additional file 6: S6.

Prevalence of resistance to cephalosporins

Prevalence of the resistance of *S. aureus* to cephalosporins is similar to the prevalence of resistance to

Table 1 Characteristics of included studies

No	Study	Study period	Sample source	Data type	Sample size	No of *S. aureus* isolate
1.	Hailu et al., 2016	Jan.2013 -Apr. 2015.	Ear discharge	Secondary	368	78
2.	Abera et al., 2008	Apr -June 2006	Different clinical samples	Primary	221	142
3.	Abera et al., 2009	Sep. 2000 - Dec. 2008.	Ear discharge	Secondary	777	260
4.	Mama et al., 2014	May toSep. 2013.	wound infection	Primary	150	47
5.	Shiferaw et al., 2015	Feb.-May 2014	External ocular infections	Primary	160	21
6.	Sewunet, et al., 2013	Apr-July 2010	Burn patients wound	Primary	50	24
7.	Alebachew et al., 2012	March–May 2011	Wound burn patient's	Primary	114	66
8.	Biadglegne, et al., 2009	Sep. 2003-June 2008.	Urinary tract infections	Secondary	529	31
9.	Ferede et al., 2001	2001	Ear swabs	Primary	112	28
10.	Guta et al., 2014	Nov 2010-June 2011	surgical wounds	Primary	100	45
11.	Kahsay et al., 2014	Dec 2011-Mar 2012	surgical wounds	Primary	184	73
12.	Mengesha et al., 2014	Jan-June 2012	Surgical wounds	Primary	128	40
13.	Mulu et al., 2012	Oct 2010-Jan2011	post-operative wounds	Primary	294	11
14.	Denboba et al., 2016	2001–2011	Ear discharge	Secondary	1225	241
15.	Abera et al., 2011	2003–2011	Ear discharge	Secondary	897	207
16.	Kibret et al., 2010	2003 to 2010	Different clinical samples	Secondary	429	429
17.	Tenssay et al., 2002	May 1997-Aug1998	Different Clinical samples	Primary	545	61
18.	Wasihun et al., 2015	Nov 2014-June2015.	Ear discharege	Primary	162	46
19.	Worku et al., 2014	June-Oct 2013	Ear discharge	Primary	117	24
20.	Negussie et al., 2015	Oct 2011-Feb2012	Blood samples	Primary	201	13
21.	Gizachew et al., 2015	Sep-Feb2013/2014	Different Clinical samples	Secondary	4321	309
22.	Yismaw et al., 2008	Sep2001- Aug2005	Different Clinical samples	Secondary	-	616
23.	Ali et al., 2008	Mar2001-apr2005	Blood sample	Secondary	472	34
24.	Mulu et al., 2006	2005	wound infection	Secondary	151	51
25.	Azene et al., 2011	2003 to 2010	wound infection	Secondary	599	208
26.	Dessalegn et al., 2014	Nov2010 - Mar2011	post-surgical wound	Primary	194	66
27.	Gebrehiwot et al., 2012	July 2011–July 2012	Blood sample	Primary	181	17
28.	Lemma et al., 2012	Aug2006 – May 2007	leprosy ulcer	Primary	1827	68
29.	Shitaye et al., 2010	Oct 2006 -Mar2007	Blood samples	Primary	302	17
30.	Alebachew et al. 2016	March–May, 2013	Blood samples	Primary	100	13
31.	Dagnew, et al. 2013	Sept 2006 to Jan 2012	Blood sample	Secondary	390	17
32.	Endris, et al. 2014	Feb - May, 2012.	Blood samples	Primary	83	11
33.	Godebo et al., 2013	June-Dec., 2011	Wound	Primary	322	73
34.	Muluye et al., 2013	2009–2012	Ear discharge	Secondary	250	54
35.	Muluye et al., 2014	2009–2012	ocular infection	Secondary	102	13
36.	Wasihun et al., 2015	Nov 2014–2015	Blood culture	Primary	514	54
37.	Ramos et al., 2014	July–December, 2013	Sample from pus	Primary	68	15
38.	Dessie et al., 2016	Oct2013-Mar2014	Wound	Primary	107	19
39.	Plorde et al., 1970	Oct1969- Apr.1970	different clinical specimens	Primary	-	52
40.	Wolday et al., 1997	Jan1992–1994	Urine sample	Secondary	672	16
41.	Tesfaye 2013	Feb2012-Oct2012.	external ocular infection	Primary	198	42
42.	DACA 2009	2004 to 2008	Different clinical samples	Secondary	1422	722
43.	Tadesse 2014 (UP[a])	Dec 2013-Jun2014	Different clinical samples	Primary	188	79
44.	Neway et al., 2006(UP[a])	May-Aug. 2015	external ocular infection	Primary	288	63
45.	Endalafer 2008(UP[a])	Jun2007-Apr2008	Different clinical samples	Primary	215	14

[a]UP = unpublished work

Table 2 Pooled prevalence of *S. aureus* resistance to different antimicrobial agents in Ethiopia

	Agent	Number of studies	Total no of isolate tested	No of resistant isolate	Pooled AMR prevalence (95% CI)	I^2 (*p*-value)
1.	Vancomycin	19	1750	132	0.11 (0.04,0.20)	95.34 ($P \leq 0.01$)
2.	Methicilin	26	1179	843	0.47 (0.33,0.61)	96.82 ($P \leq 0.01$)
3.	Ciprofloxacin	31	2254	400	0.19 (0.13, 0.26)	93.06($P \leq 0.01$)
4.	Tetracycline	36	3019	1982	0.62 (0.55, 0.68)	92.06($P \leq 0.01$)
5.	Cotrimoxazole	35	2825	1364	0.47 (0.40, 0.55)	92.85($P \leq 0.01$)
6.	Chloramphenicol	34	2763	1128	0.37 (0.29,0.45)	94.28 ($P \leq 0.01$)
7.	Erythromycin	37	3828	2222	0.41 (0.29, 0.54)	98.28($P \leq 0.01$)
8.	Penicillin	33	2271	1627	0.76 (0.67, 0.84)	95.05($P \leq 0.01$)
9.	Clindamycin	14	1445	414	0.24 (0.12,0.37)	95.48($P \leq 0.01$)
10.	Carbencillin	6	398	184	0.34 (0.17,0.54)	86.89($P \leq 0.01$)
11.	Amoxicillin	18	870	660	0.77 (0.68,0.85)	87.44($P \leq 0.01$)
12.	Amoxicillin-clavulanic	12	524	166	0.30 (0.19,0.43)	88.64($P \leq 0.01$)
13.	Ampicillin	27	1814	1181	0.75 (0.65,0.85)	95.21($P \leq 0.01$)
14.	Gentamycin	39	3348	892	0.26 (0.18,0.34)	95.93($P \leq 0.01$)
15.	Ceftriaxone	28	2032	626	0.34 (0.25,0.43)	94.02($P \leq 0.01$)
16.	Cephalothin	15	2330	785	0.30 (0.18,0.43)	94.02($P \leq 0.01$)
17.	Cefoxitine	6	374	101	0.27 (0.06, 0.54)	95.74($P \leq 0.01$)
18.	Doxycline	14	541	239	0.43 (0.26,0.60)	93.32($P \leq 0.01$)
19.	Amikacin	4	211	62	0.23 (0.07,0.44)	90.42($P \leq 0.01$)
20.	Kanamycin	7	66	40	0.14 (0.05,0.25)	79.36($P \leq 0.01$)
21.	Norfloxacilin	11	751	186	0.25 (0.14,0.38)	92.79($P \leq 0.01$)

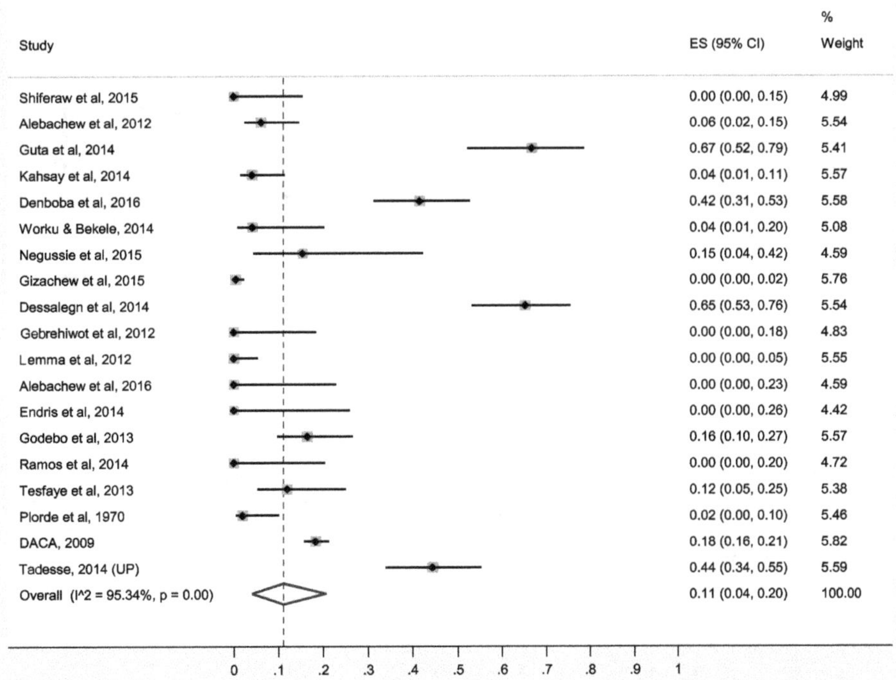

Fig. 2 Forest plot of the prevalence of *S. aureus* resistance to vancomycin

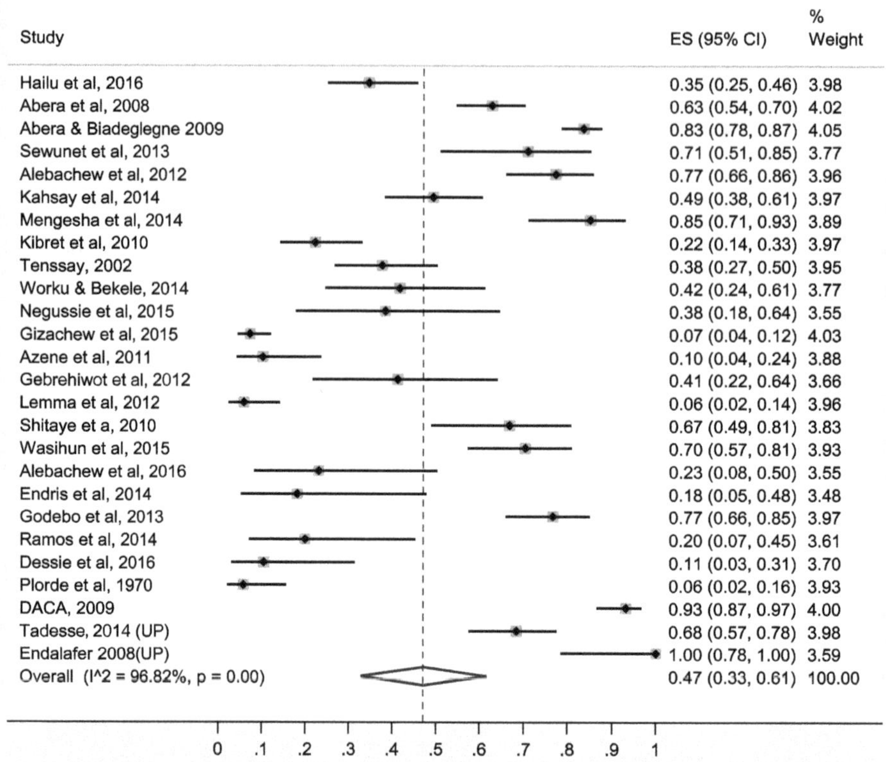

Fig. 3 Forest plot of the prevalence of *S. aureus* resistance to methicillin

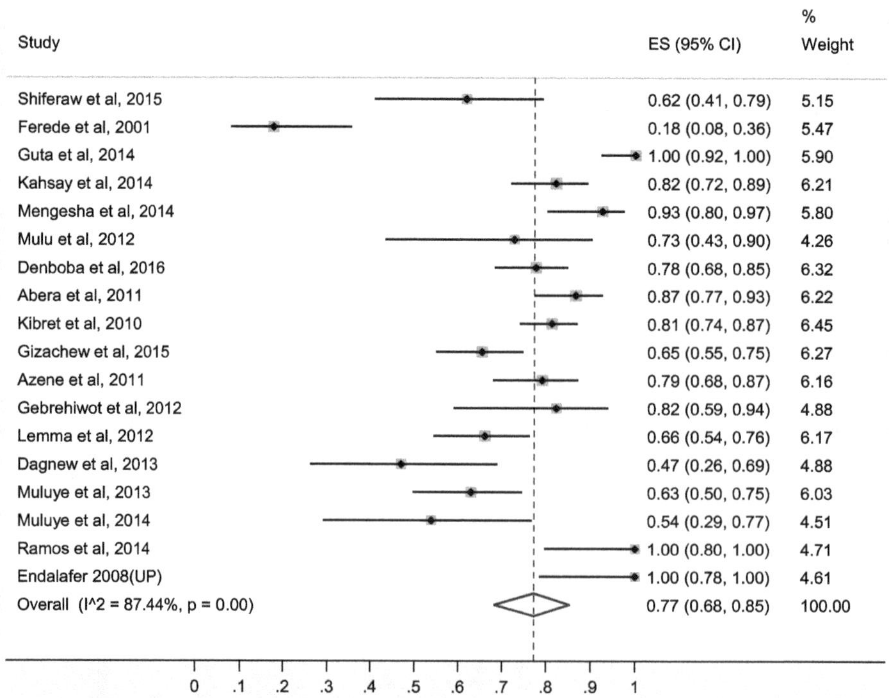

Fig. 4 Forest plot of the prevalence of *S. aureus* resistance to amoxicillin

β-lactamase-resistant penicillin's (amoxaclin-clavulanic acid). The prevalence of resistance to cephalothin is 30% (95% CI: 18%, 43%), to ceftriaxone 34% (95% CI: 25%, 43%) and to cefoxitine 27% (95% CI: 6%, 54%). The forest plot for ceftriaxone resistance is presented in Fig. 5 while the forest plots for cephalotine and cefoxitine resistance are presented respectively in Additional file 7: S7 and Additional file 8: S8.

Prevalence of resistance to floroquinolones

Two antimicrobial agents were tested from the floroquinolones: ciprofloxacin and norfloxacilin. Thirty one studies were used to estimate the prevalence of ciprofloxacin resistance and eleven studies were included for the estimation of norfloxacilin resistance. The pooled prevalence of *S. aureus* resistance to ciprofloxacin was 19% (95% CI: 13%, 26%) and to norfloxacillin 25% (95% CI: 14%, 38%). The forest plot for ciprofloxacin resistance is presented in Fig. 6 while the forest plot for norfloxacilin included as Additional file 9: S9.

Prevalence of resistance to protein synthesis inhibitors

Higher rates of resistance were observed with reversible inhibitors of protein synthesis compared to aminoglycosides (irreversible inhibitors of protein synthesis). Tetracycline showed the highest resistance rate (62% [95% CI: 55%, 68%]) followed by doxycycline 43% (95% CI: 26%, 60%), erythromycin (41% [95% CI: 29%, 54%]), and chloramphenicol (37% [95% CI: 29%, 54%]). Clindamycin and aminoglycosides showed relatively lower level of resistance (Table 2).

The prevalence of resistance to gentamycin is 26% (95% CI: 18%, 34%), to amikacin 23% (95% CI: 7%, 44%) and to kanamycin 14% (95% CI: 5%, 25%). The forest plot for gentamycin resistance is presented in Fig. 7 while the forest plots for erythromycin, chloramphenicol, doxycycline, amikacin, clindamycin, and kanamycin resistance are presented as the Additional file 10: S10, Additional file 11: S11, Additional file 12: S12, Additional file 13: S13, Additional file 14: S14 and Additional file 15: S15.

Prevalence of resistance to antimetabolites

Thirty five studies were included for estimation of pooled prevalence of *S. aureus* resistance to sulphametaxozole-trimethoprim and found to be 47% (95% CI: 40%, 55%). The forest plot for sulphametaxozole- trimethoprim resistance is presented in Fig. 8.

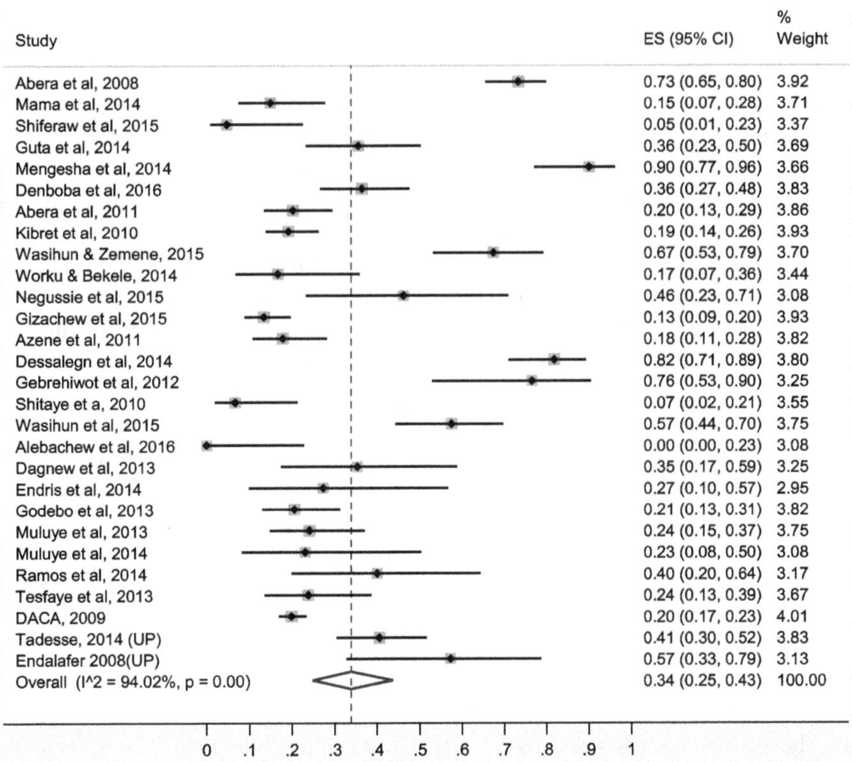

Fig. 5 Forest plot of the prevalence of *S. aureus* resistance to ceftriaxone

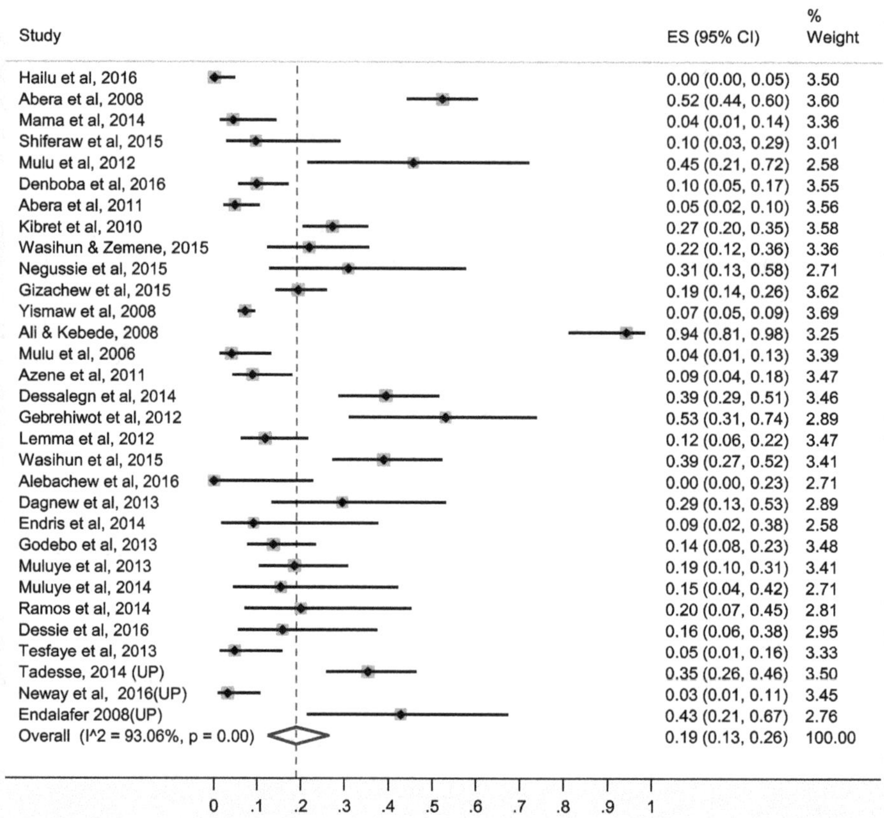

Fig. 6 Forest plot of the prevalence of *S. aureus* resistance to ciprofloxacin

Comparison of the prevalence of *S. aures* resistance to different antimicrobial agents

Comparison of the prevalence of *S. aures* resistance to different antimicrobial agents addressed by this meta-analysis is given in Fig. 9. It is found that the magnitude of *S.aureus* resistance to the different antimicrobial agents ranges from 11% to vancomycin to 77% to amoxicillin. Accordingly, invitro antimicrobial effectiveness in decreasing order believed to be vancomycin, kanamycin, ciprofloxacilin, amikacin, clindamycin, amoxacilin-clavulanic acid, cephalothin, carbencilin, ceftriaxone, cefoxitine, chloramphenicol, erythromycin, doxycycline, methicillin, cotrimoxazole, tetracycline, ampicillin, pencilin, and amoxacilin.

Discussion

In this meta-analysis, we estimated the pooled prevalence of *S. aureus* resistance to 21 different antimicrobial agents commonly used in Ethiopia. Generally 45 studies were included for the meta-analysis, however the number of studies included in each meta-analyses ranged from 4 to 39. Overall, the 45 studies provided evidence regarding the level of *S. aureus* resistance to different antimicrobial agents based on 4530 isolates. It was found that *S. aureus* resistance to commonly available antimicrobial agents in Ethiopia was alarmingly high ranging from 11% to vancomycin to 77% to amoxicillin.

The pooled estimate of the prevalence of *S. aureus* resistance particularly to methicillin (MRSA) in Ethiopia is similar to 2014 global surveillance reports of the World Health Organization (WHO) 2014 [88], which showed MRSA prevalence between 33% to 95% in Africa. The pooled prevalence of MRSA in Ethiopia 47% (95% CI: 33%–61%) is within the range of the global WHO report for Africa.

The pooled estimate in study for MRSA is in agreement with the pooled estimate of community acquired-MRSA prevalence in Asia, Europe, and North America which ranges from 23.1% to 47.4% [89]. However, the pooled estimate 47% (95% CI: 33%–61%) MRSA prevalence in Ethiopia is higher than pooled estimate of community acquired MRSA prevalence 30.2% based on 27 retrospective studies and 37.3% based on 5 prospective studies [90]. The higher prevalence in our study may be due to the inclusion of both community acquired and nosocomial infection in the original studies. Nosocomial infection are believed to have higher rate of resistance due to larger exposure rate to antimicrobial agents. Increasing resistance to antimicrobial agents in hospitals is

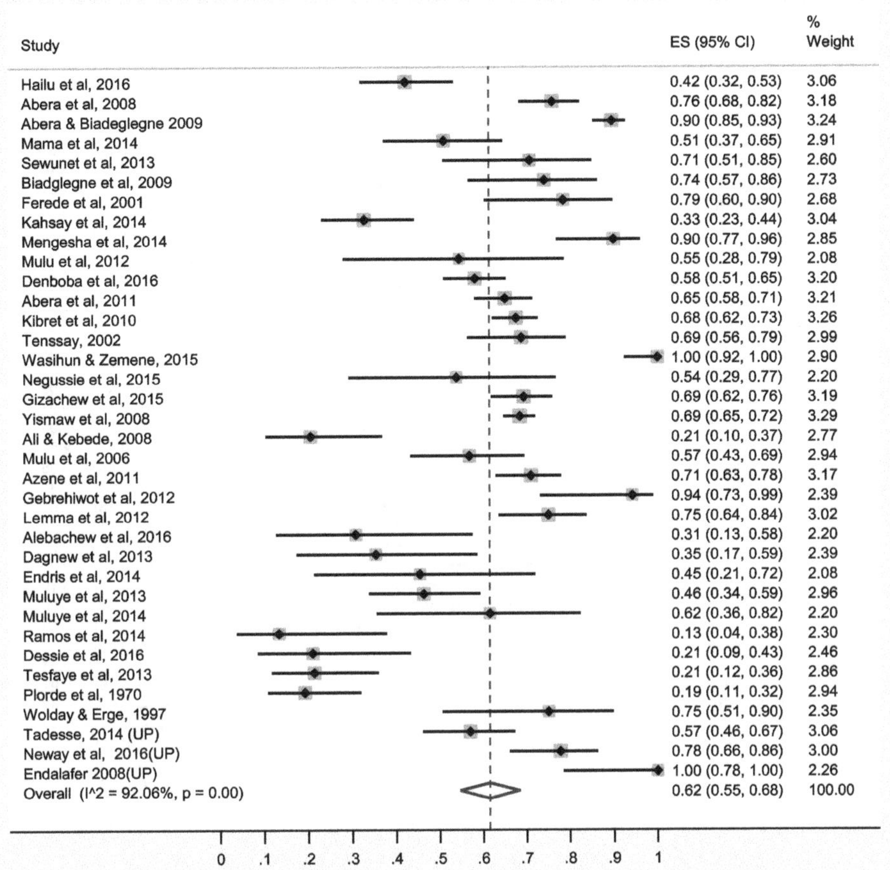

Fig. 7 Forest plot of the prevalence of *S. aureus* resistance to tetracycline

caused by transmission of resistant strains within hospitals by cross colonization of patients via hands of healthcare staff and direct patient to patient contact and subsequent spread [91].

Global pattern of AMR shows variation among different geographic, socioeconomic strata and among studies [49, 88, 92]. Variation may be to differences in time, place, design, and population involved in the study. This may be due to healthcare facilities conditions like implementation and monitoring of infection prevention policies and rational antibiotic usage which varies in different facilities. The most important reason is due to character of the study. Studies are conducted within a specified time and locality. It is reasonable to assume population under study might be infected by the same strains of agent at specified period of time and location. This could be a good reason why heterogeneity tests showed significant variability (p-value ≤0.01) among studies included in this meta-analysis for 2 1 antimicrobial agents.

S. aureus acquires resistance by various mechanisms: formation of alternative pathways for sulphonamides [93, 94], production of β-lactamase to β-lactam-sensitive antibiotics, increased efflux to tetracycline [95, 96], presence of acetyltransferase to chloramphenicol, decrease in accumulation to macrolide antibiotics [97], aminoglycoside-modifying enzymes production to aminoglycosides, altered topoisomerase IV and DNA gyrase expression for fluoroquinolones, and expression of mec gene altering penicillin binding protein to β-lactam antibiotics [98]. Since the AMR for β-lactam sensitive β-lactam antibiotics is very high, it can be speculated that most strains of *S. aureus* found in Ethiopia produce the β-lactamase enzyme. However, there is no molecular study conducted to identify the type of resistant strains and mechanism responsible for resistance in Ethiopia.

Lower rate of resistance was seen with β-lactamase-resistant antibiotics (amoxicillin-clavulanic acid, methicillin, ceftriaxone, cefoxtine, and cephalothin) compared to β-lactamase-sensitive penicillins. Unlike β-lactamase sensitive penicillin's, resistance to carbeniciln is significantly lower. The lower rate of resistance observed with carbencilin and clindamycin may be due to their infrequent use in Ethiopia [99].

Resistance to methicillin confers resistance to all β-lactamase-resistant penicillins and cephalosporins. This

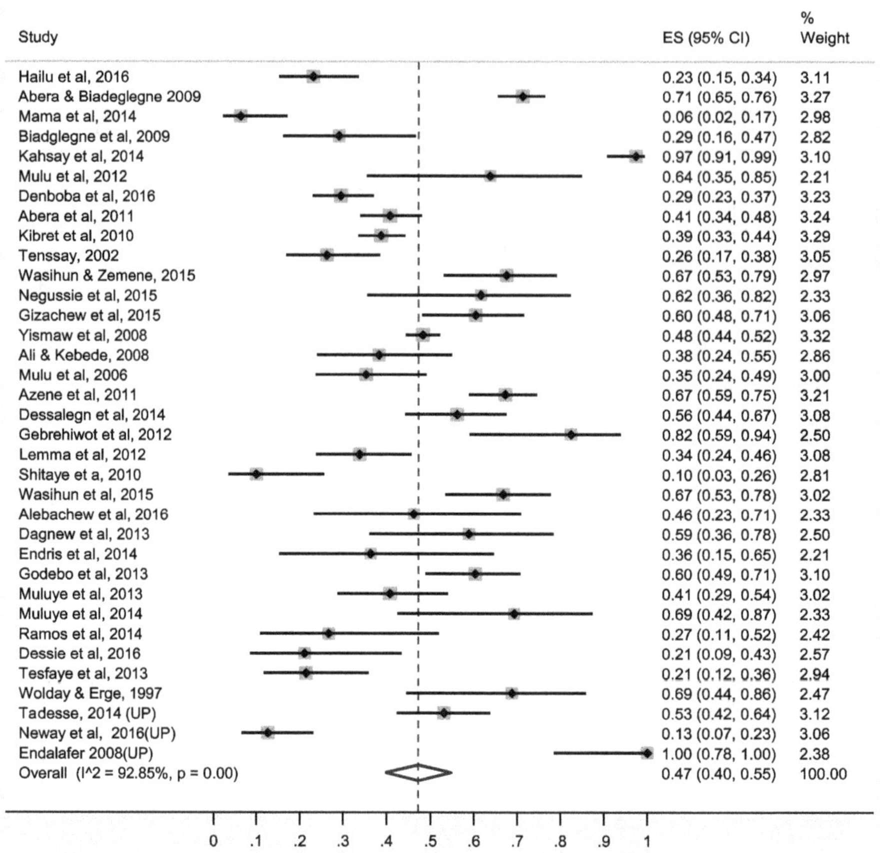

Fig. 8 Forest plot of the prevalence of *S. aureus* resistance to sulphametaxazole-trimethoprim

high level of resistance requires the presence of the mec gene that encodes penicillin-binding protein [98]. The implication of high prevalence of MRSA for suspected or verified *S. aureus* infections such as common skin and wound infections and surgical prophylaxis is that there is a need for better alternatives drugs. Alternative drugs needed to treat or prevent *S. aureus* infections are more expensive and, because of their adverse effects, monitoring during treatment is advisable which increases the costs even further.

The prevalence of resistance *S. aureus* to vancomycin 11% 995% CI: (4%, 20%) in this study is bothersome and higher compared to global prevalence estimate [100]. The prevalence of VISA was 2.05% before, 2.63% in 2006–2009, and 7.93% in 2010–2014. Vancomycin resistance is erasing all possible treatment options in Ethiopia for MRSA. The higher prevalence of vancomycin in Ethiopia compared to global estimate may be due to larger and irrational use of antimicrobial agents in Ethiopia,

The prevalence estimates of glycopeptides/vancomycin resistance from Guta et al., and Desalegn et al., were unusually high, however sensitivity analysis showed non-significant influence on the overall pooled prevalence estimate. The prevalence estimates from Guta et al. and Desalegn et al. were unusually high, however sensitivity analysis showed non-significant influence on the overall pooled prevalence estimate. Larger exposure probability to resistant strains due to larger use of vancomycin in hospital settings might have resulted in a relatively higher prevalence of vancomycin resistance in the two studies [73, 77].

In four of the twenty studies (published in 2014 and after) [48, 51, 73, 77], the prevalence of *S. aureus* resistance to vancomycin is higher than 40%. In contrast, in studies published before 2014 the prevalence of *S. aureus* resistance to vancomycin in Ethiopia is much lower (0% to 16%). This may indicate a rapid rise and spread of vancomycin resistant *S. aureus* strains in Ethiopia as the rate of vancomycin use and exposure in Ethiopia increases. This calls for inclusion for effective new anti-MRSA antimicrobial agents for treatment of staphylococcal infections in the national medicine list and effective antimicrobial stewardship programs for prevention and containment of antimicrobial resistance.

Staphylococcal infection in Ethiopia can be better treated by vancomycin, floroquinolones, and aminoglycosides

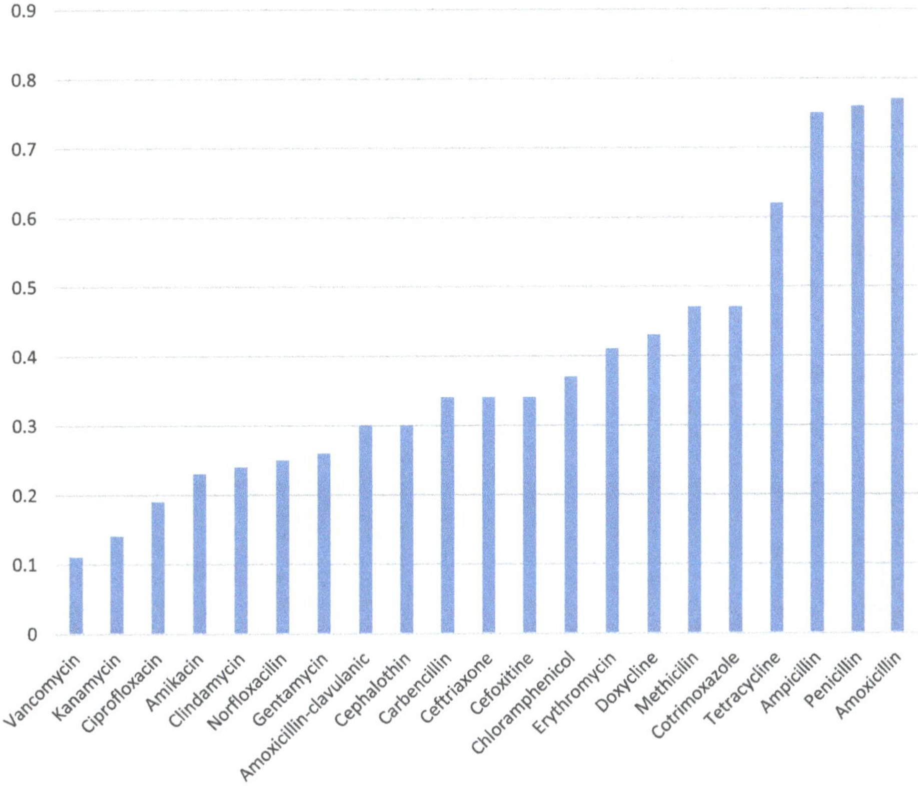

Fig. 9 Comparison of the prevalence of *S. aureus* resistance to different antimicrobial agents in Ethiopia

based on the finding of our invitro finding. However, clinical effectiveness study had not yet proved it. Resistance to vancomycin, the only choice for MRSA in Ethiopia, is of a great concern. It is bothersome due to lack of alternative agents in Ethiopia for the treatment of *S. aureus* infections. Making things worse, alternative new anti-MRSA agents (like linezolid, daptomycin, tigecycline, telavancin, and ceftaroline are rarely available in Ethiopia for treatment of vancomycin resistant *S. aureus.*

Many factors contribute to AMR. First, lack of infection prevention contributes to recurrent infection then to spread of resistant strains. Second, misuse of antimicrobials from prescription–dispensing-to patient use [101]. In Ethiopia, it is a common practice that antibiotics can be purchased without prescription, which leads to misuse of antibiotics by the public [102]. Third factor could be misuse of antibiotics by health professionals and non-standardized practice [101]. The fourth factor could be poor hospital hygienic conditions [103]. A last contributing factor could be lack of routine antimicrobial susceptibility testing which diverts to empiric therapy [49]. In line to strategies for prevention and containment of *S. aureus* there is a need for innovative way of halting AMR. Combination therapy and availability of new anti-MRSA agents will play vital role in fighting against AMR to *S. aureus*.

However, interpretation of the findings of this meta-analysis requires considering the limitations thereof. The limitations arise from the inherent characteristics of the included individual studies. First, this is invitro antimicrobial resistance testing and its direct translation to clinical effectiveness requires caution. Second, many studies involved very limited localities and were done mainly in teaching hospitals in bigger cities where patients with advanced, severe stages, recurrent infections are treated. Hence, the resistance level could have overestimated.

Conclusions

This meta-analysis demonstrates that *S. aureus* has gotten alarmingly resistant to many of common antimicrobials used in Ethiopia. It is highly resistant to penicillin, cephalosporin, tetracyclines, chloramphenicol, methicillin, sulphonamides, and vancomycin. Resistance to vancomycin is of a great concern and bothersome due to unavailability of treatment options for *S. aureus* infections in Ethiopia.

Continued and multidimensional efforts of antimicrobial stewardship programme promoting rational use of antimicrobials, infection prevention and containment of AMR are urgently needed. It is deemed necessary to include new anti-MRSA agents in national medicine list to treat resistant strains. Combination therapy, effective in battling AMR in many infectious diseases model, may prove significant advantage in battling resistance to *S. aureus*. Therapeutic options are urgently needed for patients infected with resistant *S. aureus*. Further researches focusing on clinical treatment outcome and identifying dynamics promoting resistance, high risk strains and molecular genetic basis of resistance are needed.

Additional files

Additional file 1: S1. RISMA Checklist.

Additional file 2: S2. Egger's test of publication bias.

Additional file 3: S3. Forest plot of the prevalence of *S. aureus* resistance to penicillin G.

Additional file 4: S4. Forest plot of the prevalence of *S. aureus* resistance to Ampicillin.

Additional file 5: S5. Forest plot of the prevalence of *S. aureus* resistance to amoxacilin-clavulanate.

Additional file 6: S6. Forest plot of the prevalence of *S. aureus* resistance to carbencilin.

Additional file 7: S7. Forest plot of the prevalence of *S. aureus* resistance to cephalothin.

Additional file 8: S8. Forest plot of the prevalence of *S. aureus* resistance to cefoxitine.

Additional file 9: S9. Forest plot of the prevalence of *S. aureus* resistance to norfloxacilin.

Additional file 10: S10. Forest plot of the prevalence of *S. aureus* resistance to erythromycin.

Additional file 11: S11. Forest plot of the prevalence of *S. aureus* resistance to chloramphenicol.

Additional file 12: S12. Forest plot of the prevalence of *S. aureus* resistance to doxycycline.

Additional file 13: S13. Forest plot of the prevalence of *S. aureus* resistance to amikacin.

Additional file 14: S14. Forest plot of the prevalence of *S. aureus* resistance to clindamycin.

Additional file 15: S15. Forest plot of the prevalence of *S. aureus* resistance to kanamycin.

Abbreviations
AMR: Antimicrobial resistance; MRSA: Methicillin resistant *Staphylococcus aureus*; NCCLs: National Committee for clinical Laboratory Standard; *S. aureus*: *Staphylococcus aureus*; VISA: Vancomycin intermediate *Staphylococcus aureus*; VRSA: Vancomycin resistant *Staphylococcus aureus*

Acknowledgements
Not applicable.

Funding
There was no funding support to conduct this meta-analysis.

Authors' contributions
SD, SF and AA conceptualized the research idea. SD and SF conducted literature search, selection and data extraction. AA performed the statistical analyses. SD prepared the draft manuscript. All authors revised, edited and approved the final manuscript.

Consent for publication
Not applicable.

Competing interests
The authors declare that they have no competing interests.

Author details
[1]Department of Pharmacology, School of Medicine, College of Medicine and Health Sciences, Hawassa University, P. O. Box 1560, Hawassa, Ethiopia. [2]Department of Microbiology, Faculty of Medicine, Shimane University, Shimane, Japan. [3]School of Public and Environmental Health, College of Medicine and Health Sciences, Hawassa University, Hawassa, Ethiopia.

References
1. Lowy FD. Staphylococcus aureus infections. N Engl J Med. 1998;339(8):520–32.
2. McGuinness WA, Malachowa N, FR DL. Vancomycin resistance in Staphylococcus Aureus. Yale J Biol Med. 2017;90(2):269–81.
3. Hiramatsu K. Mechanism of methicillin resistance and genetic background of Staphylococcus Aureus. Nihon Naika Gakkai Zasshi. 1992;81(10):1592–8.
4. Hiramatsu K, Hanaki H, Ino T, Yabuta K, Oguri T, Tenover FC. Methicillin-resistant Staphylococcus Aureus clinical strain with reduced vancomycin susceptibility. J Antimicrob Chemother. 1997;40:135–6.
5. Périchon B, Courvalin P. VanA-type vancomycin-resistant Staphylococcus Aureus. Antimicrob Agents Chemother. 2009;53(11):4580–7.
6. Plorde JJ, Eng SC, Wright LJ, Debesai A. Antibiotic sensitivities of common bacterial pathogens isolated in Addis Ababa; a preliminary report. Ethiop Med J. 1970;8(3):107–18.
7. Stephen J, Ronald J, Yvette S, José H, Ivonne D, Robert L, Susan E, Carol A: Manual of antimicrobial susceptibility testing. In. USA; 2005.
8. Nyaga VN, Arbyn M, Aerts M. Metaprop: a Stata command to perform meta-analysis of binomial data. Archives of Public Health. 2014;72:39.
9. DerSimonian R, Laird N. Meta-analysis in clinical trials. Control Clin Trials. 1986;7:177–88.
10. Egger M, Davey SG, Schneider M, Minder C. Bias in meta-analysis detected by a simple, graphical test. BMJ. 1997;315(7109):629–34.
11. Moher D, Liberati A, Tetzlaff J, Altman DG, The PRISMA Group. Perferred Reporting items for Systematic Review and Meta-analysis:The PRISMA statement. PLoS Med. 2009;6:e1000097.
12. Abrha A, Abdissa A, Beyene G, Getahun G, Girma T. Bacteraemia among severely malnourished children in jimma university hospital, ethiopia. Ethiopian journal of health sciences. 2011;21(3):175–82.
13. Alemu A, Moges F, Shiferaw Y, Tafess K, Kassu A, Anagaw B, Agegn A. Bacterial profile and drug susceptibility pattern of urinary tract infection in pregnant women at University of Gondar Teaching Hospital, Northwest Ethiopia. BMC research notes. 2012;5:197.
14. Beyene G, Tsegaye W. Bacterial uropathogens in urinary tract infection and antibiotic susceptibility pattern in jimma university specialized hospital, southwest ethiopia. Ethiopian journal of health sciences. 2011;21(2):141–6.
15. Demilie T, Beyene G, Melaku S, Tsegaye W. Urinary bacterial profile and antibiotic susceptibility pattern among pregnant women in north west ethiopia. Ethiopian journal of health sciences. 2012;22(2):121–8.
16. Tesfahunegn Z, Asrat D, Woldeamanuel Y, Estifanos K. Bacteriology of surgical site and catheter related urinary tract infections among patients admitted in Mekelle hospital, Mekelle, Tigray, Ethiopia. Ethiop Med J. 2009;47(2):117–27.
17. Assefa Y, Moges F, Endris M, Zereay B, Amare B, Bekele D, Tesfaye S, Mulu A, Belyhun Y. Bacteriological profile and drug susceptibility patterns in dacryocystitis patients attending Gondar University Teaching Hospital, Northwest Ethiopia. BMC Ophthalmol. 2015;15:34.
18. Gebremariam TT. Bacteriology and risk factors of bacterial keratitis in Jimma, Southwest Ethiopia. Ethiop Med J. 2015;53(4):191–7.
19. Kibret M, Abera B. Prevalence and antibiogram of bacterial isolates from urinary tract infections at Dessie Health Research Laboratory, Ethiopia. Asian Pac J Trop Biomed. 2014;4(2):164–8.
20. Tadesse E, Teshome M, Merid Y, Kibret B, Shimelis T. Asymptomatic urinary tract infection among pregnant women attending the antenatal clinic of Hawassa referral hospital, Southern Ethiopia. BMC research notes. 2014;7:155.
21. Wondimeneh Y, Muluye D, Alemu A, Atinafu A, Yitayew G, Gebrecherkos T, Damtie D, Ferede G. Urinary tract infection among obstetric fistula patients

at Gondar University Hospital, northwest Ethiopia. BMC Womens Health. 2014;14:12.
22. Yeshitela B, Gebre-Selassie S, Feleke Y. Asymptomatic bacteriuria and symptomatic urinary tract infections (UTI) in patients with diabetes mellitus in Tikur Anbessa specialized university hospital, Addis Ababa, Ethiopia. Ethiop Med J. 2012;50(3):239–49.
23. Gebre-Selassie S. Asymptomatic bacteriuria in pregnancy: epidemiological, clinical and microbiological approach. Ethiop Med J. 1998;36(3):185–92.
24. Derese B, Kedir H, Teklemariam Z, Weldegebreal F, Balakrishnan S. Bacterial profile of urinary tract infection and antimicrobial susceptibility pattern among pregnant women attending at antenatal Clinic in Dil Chora Referral Hospital, Dire Dawa, eastern Ethiopia. Ther Clin Risk Manag. 2016;12:251–60.
25. Moges AF, Genetu A, Mengistu G. Antibiotic sensitivities of common bacterial pathogens in urinary tract infections at Gondar hospital, Ethiopia. East Afr Med J. 2002;79(3):140–2.
26. Muluye D, Wondimeneh Y, Ferede G, Nega T, Adane K, Biadgo B, Tesfa H, Moges F. Bacterial isolates and their antibiotic susceptibility patterns among patients with pus and/or wound discharge at Gondar university hospital. BMC research notes. 2014;7:619.
27. Melaku S, Gebre-Selassie S, Damtie M, Alamrew K. Hospital acquired infections among surgical, gynaecology and obstetrics patients in Felege-Hiwot referral hospital, Bahir Dar, northwest Ethiopia. Ethiop Med J. 2012;50(2):135–44.
28. Kebede A, Adamu Y, Bejiga A. Bacteriological study of dacryocystitis among patients attending in Menelik II hospital, Addis Ababa, Ethiopia. Ethiop Med J. 2010;48(1):29–33.
29. Melaku S, Kibret M, Abera B, Gebre-Sellassie S. Antibiogram of nosocomial urinary tract infections in Felege Hiwot referral hospital, Ethiopia. Afr Health Sci. 2012;12(2):134–9.
30. Mulu W, Kibru G, Beyene G, Damtie M. Postoperative nosocomial infections and antimicrobial resistance pattern of bacteria isolates among patients admitted at Felege Hiwot referral hospital, Bahirdar, Ethiopia. Ethiopian journal of health sciences. 2012;22(1):7–18.
31. Seboxa T, Amogne W, Abebe W, Tsegaye T, Azazh A, Hailu W, Fufa K, Grude N, Henriksen TH. High mortality from blood stream infection in Addis Ababa, Ethiopia, is due to antimicrobial resistance. PLoS One. 2015;10(12):e0144944.
32. Tilahun B, Worku B, Tachbele E, Terefe S, Kloos H, Legesse W. High load of multi-drug resistant nosocomial neonatal pathogens carried by cockroaches in a neonatal intensive care unit at Tikur Anbessa specialized hospital, Addis Ababa, Ethiopia. Antimicrob Resist Infect Control. 2012;1:12.
33. Zenebe T, Kannan S, Yilma D, Beyene G. Invasive bacterial pathogens and their antibiotic susceptibility patterns in Jimma University specialized hospital, Jimma, Southwest Ethiopia. Ethiopian journal of health sciences. 2011;21(1):1–8.
34. Tibebu M, Embiyale W. Community acquired multi drug resistant Staphylococcus Aureus in a rural setting of north western Ethiopia: a tough challenge. Ethiop Med J. 2014;52(3):147–50.
35. Truneh M. Phage types and drug susceptibility patterns of Staphylococcus Aureus from two hospitals in northwest Ethiopia. Ethiop Med J. 1991;29(1):1–6.
36. Teshager L, Asrat D, Gebre-Selassie S, Tamiru S. Catheterized and non-catheterized urinary tract infections among patients attended at Jimma University teaching hospital, southwest, Ethiopia. Ethiop Med J. 2008;46(1):55–62.
37. Lemma MT, Zenebe Y, Tulu B, Mekonnen D, Mekonnen Z. Methicillin resistant Staphylococcus Aureus among HIV infected pediatric patients in Northwest Ethiopia: carriage rates and antibiotic co-resistance profiles. PLoS One. 2015;10(9):e0137254.
38. Kejela T, Bacha K. Prevalence and antibiotic susceptibility pattern of methicillin-resistant Staphylococcus Aureus (MRSA) among primary school children and prisoners in Jimma town, Southwest Ethiopia. Ann Clin Microbiol Antimicrob. 2013;12:11.
39. Gebreyesus A, Gebre-Selassie S, Mihert A. Nasal and hand carriage rate of methicillin resistant Staphylococcus Aureus (MRSA) among health care workers in Mekelle hospital, North Ethiopia. Ethiop Med J. 2013;51(1):41–7.
40. Dagnew M, Tiruneh M, Moges F, Tekeste Z. Survey of nasal carriage of Staphylococcus Aureus and intestinal parasites among food handlers working at Gondar University, Northwest Ethiopia. BMC Public Health. 2012;12(1):837.
41. Shibabaw A, Abebe T, Mihret A. Nasal carriage rate of methicillin resistant Staphylococcus Aureus among Dessie referral hospital health care workers; Dessie, Northeast Ethiopia. Antimicrob Resist Infect Control. 2013;2(1):25.
42. Shibabaw A, Abebe T, Mihret A. Antimicrobial susceptibility pattern of nasal Staphylococcus Aureus among Dessie referral hospital health care workers, Dessie, Northeast Ethiopia. Int J Infect Dis. 2014;25:22–5.
43. Yismaw G, Abay S, Asrat D, Yifru S, Kassu A. Bacteriological profile and resistant pattern of clinical isolates from pediatric patients, Gondar University teaching hospital, Gondar, Northwest Ethiopia. Ethiop Med J. 2010;48(4):293–300.
44. Yismaw G, Tiruneh M, Kassu A, Negeri C, Mulu A. A retrospective analysis of prevalence and antimicrobial susceptibility patterns of Staphylococcus Aureus in Gondar teaching hospital, 2001-2005. Ethiop Med J. 2008;46(2):143–8.
45. Asrat D, Amanuel YW. Prevalence and antibiotic susceptibility pattern of bacterial isolates from blood culture in Tikur Anbassa hospital, Addis Ababa, Ethiopia. Ethiop Med J. 2001;39(2):97–104.
46. Endalafer N. Bacterial nosocomial infections and their antimicrobial susceptibility patterns in surgical wards and surgical intensive care unit of Tikur Anbessa university hospital. Addis Ababa: Addis Ababa University; 2008.
47. Neway S, Desta K, Dessie W, Yeshitila B, Lema T. Bacterial profile and antimicrobial susceptibility pattern of external ocular infections with associated risk factors in Alert cente. Ethiopia: Addis Ababa; 2016.
48. Tadesse S. Antimicrobial resistance profile of *Staphylococcus aureus* isolated from clinical specimens and nasal swabs of patients at Tikur Anbessa specialized hospital. Addis Ababa: Addis Ababa University; 2014.
49. DACA. Antimicrobials use, resistance and containment baseline survey: syntheses of findings. Addis Ababa: DACA; 2009.
50. Hailu D, Mekonnen D, Derbie A, Mulu W, Abera B. Pathogenic bacteria profile and antimicrobial susceptibility patterns of ear infection at Bahir Dar regional Health Research Laboratory center Ethiopia. SpringerPlus. 2016;5:466.
51. Argaw-Denboba A, Abejew AA, Mekonnen AG. Antibiotic-resistant bacteria are major threats of otitis Media in Wollo Area, Northeastern Ethiopia: A Ten-Year Retrospective Analysis. Int J Microbiol. 2016;2016:8724671.
52. Muluye D, Wondimeneh Y, Ferede G, Moges F, Nega T. Bacterial isolates and drug susceptibility patterns of ear discharge from patients with ear infection at Gondar University Hospital, Northwest Ethiopia. BMC ear, nose, and throat disorders. 2013;13(1):10.
53. Wasihun AG, Zemene Y. Bacterial profile and antimicrobial susceptibility patterns of otitis media in Ayder Teaching and Referral Hospital, Mekelle University, Northern Ethiopia. SpringerPlus. 2015;4:701.
54. Abera B, Kibret M. Bacteriology and antimicrobial susceptibility of otitis Media at Dessie Regional Health Research Laboratory, Ethiopia. Ethiop J Health Dev. 2011;25(2):161–7.
55. Ferede D, Geyid A, Lulseged S, Melaku A. Drug susceptibility pattern of bacterial isolates from children with chronic suppurative otitis media. Ethiop J Health Dev. 2001;15(2):89–96.
56. Worku M, Bekele M. Bacterial isolate and antibacterial resistance pattern of ear infection among patients attending at Hawassa university referral hospital, Hawassa, Ethiopia. Indian J Otol. 2014;20:155–9.
57. Abera B, Biadeglegne F. Antimicrobial resistance patterns of Staphylococcus Aureus and Proteus spp. isolated from otitis media at Bahir Dar regional laboratory, north West Ethiopia. Ethiop Med J. 2009;47(4):271–6.
58. Shiferaw B, Gelaw B, Assefa A, Assefa Y, Addis Z. Bacterial isolates and their antimicrobial susceptibility pattern among patients with external ocular infections at Borumeda hospital, Northeast Ethiopia. BMC ophthalmology. 2015;15:103.
59. Muluye D, Wondimeneh Y, Moges F, Nega T, Ferede G. Types and drug susceptibility patterns of bacterial isolates from eye discharge samples at Gondar University Hospital, Northwest Ethiopia. BMC research notes. 2014;7:292.
60. Tesfaye T, Beyene T, Gelaw T, Bekele S, Saravanan M. Bacterial profile and antimicrobial susceptibility pattern of external ocular infections in Jimma University specialized hospital, Southwest Ethiopia. American Journal of Infectious Diseases and Microbiology. 2013;1(1):13–20.
61. Negussie A, Mulugeta G, Bedru A, Ali I, Shimeles D, Lema T, Aseffa A. Bacteriological profile and antimicrobial susceptibility pattern of blood culture isolates among septicemia suspected children in selected hospitals Addis Ababa, Ethiopia. Int J Biol Med Res. 2015;6(1):4709–17.
62. Alebachew G, Teka B, Endris M, Shiferaw Y, Tessema B. Etiologic Agents of Bacterial Sepsis and Their Antibiotic Susceptibility Patterns among Patients Living with Human Immunodeficiency Virus at Gondar University Teaching Hospital, Northwest Ethiopia. Biomed Res Int. 2016;2016:5371875.
63. Endris M, Takele Y, Woldeyohannes D, Tiruneh M, Mohammed R, Moges F, Lynen L, Jacobs J, van Griensven J, Diro E. Bacterial sepsis in patients with visceral leishmaniasis in Northwest Ethiopia. Biomed Res Int. 2014;2014: 361058.
64. Shitaye D, Asrat D, Woldeamanuel Y, Worku B. Risk factors and etiology of neonatal sepsis in Tikur Anbessa university hospital, Ethiopia. Ethiop Med J.

2010;48(1):11–21.

65. Wasihun AG, Wlekidan LN, Gebremariam SA, Dejene TA, Welderufael AL, Haile TD, Muthupandian S. Bacteriological profile and antimicrobial susceptibility patterns of blood culture isolates among febrile patients in Mekelle hospital, Northern Ethiopia. SpringerPlus. 2015;4:314.
66. Ali J, Kebede Y. Frequency of isolation and antimicrobial susceptibility pattern of bacterial isolates from blood culture, Gondar University teaching hospital, Northwest Ethiopia. Ethiop Med J. 2008;46(2):155–61.
67. Dagnew M, Yismaw G, Gizachew M, Gadisa A, Abebe T, Tadesse T, Alemu A, Mathewos B. Bacterial profile and antimicrobial susceptibility pattern in septicemia suspected patients attending Gondar University Hospital, Northwest Ethiopia. BMC research notes. 2013;6:283.
68. Gebrehiwot A, Lakew W, Moges F, Moges B, Anagaw B, Yismaw G, Nega T, Unakal C, Kassu A. Bacterial profile and drug susceptibility pattern of neonatal sepsis in Gondar University hospital, Gondar northwest Ethiopia. Pharm Lett. 2012;4(6):1811–6.
69. Alebachew T, Yismaw G, Derabe A, Sisay Z. Staphylococcus Aureus burn wound infection among patients attending yekatit 12 hospital burn unit, addis ababa, ethiopia. Ethiopian journal of health sciences. 2012;22(3):209–13.
70. Godebo G, Kibru G, Tassew H. Multidrug-resistant bacterial isolates in infected wounds at Jimma University Specialized Hospital, Ethiopia. Ann Clin Microbiol Antimicrob. 2013;12:17.
71. Azene MK, Beyene BA. Bacteriology and antibiogram of pathogens from wound infections at Dessie laboratory, north-east Ethiopia. Tanzania journal of health research. 2011;13(4):68–74.
72. Mulu A, Moges F, Tessema B, Kassu A. Pattern and multiple drug resistance of bacterial pathogens isolated from wound infection at University of Gondar Teaching Hospital, Northwest Ethiopia. Ethiop Med J. 2006;44(2):125–31.
73. Guta M, Aragaw K, Merid Y. Bacteria from infected surgical wounds and their antimicrobial resistance in Hawassa university referral teaching hospital, southern Ethiopia. Afr J Microbiol Res. 2014;8(11):1118–24.
74. Mama M, Alemseged A, Tsegaye S. Antimicrobial susceptibility pattern of bacterial isolates from wound infection and their sensitivity to alternative topical agents at Jimma University Specialized Hospital, South-West Ethiopia. Annals of Clinical Microbiology and Antimicrobials. 2014;13(1):14.
75. Kahsay A, Mihret A, Abebe T, Andualem T. Isolation and antimicrobial susceptibility pattern of *Staphylococcus aureus* in patients with surgical site infection at Debre Markos Referral Hospital, Amhara Region, Ethiopia. Arch Public Health. 2014;72(1):16.
76. Mengesha RE, Kasa BG, Saravanan M, Berhe DF, Wasihun AG. Aerobic bacteria in post surgical wound infections and pattern of their antimicrobial susceptibility in Ayder teaching and referral hospital, Mekelle, Ethiopia. BMC research notes. 2014;7:575.
77. Dessalegn L, Shimelis T, Tadesse E, Gebre-selassie S. Aerobic bacterial isolates from post-surgical wound and their antimicrobial susceptibility pattern: a hospital based cross-sectional study. Journal of Medical Research. 2014;3(2):18–23.
78. Dessie W, Mulugeta G, Fentaw S, Mihret A, Hassen M, Abebe E. Pattern of bacterial pathogens and their susceptibility isolated from surgical site infections at selected referral hospitals, Addis Ababa, Ethiopia. International journal of microbiology. 2016;2016:2418902.
79. Sewunet T, Demissie Y, Mihret A, Abebe T. Bacterial profile and antimicrobial susceptibility pattern of isolates among burn patients at Yekatit 12 hospital burn center, Addis Ababa, Ethiopia. Ethiopian journal of health sciences. 2013; 23(3):209–16.
80. Gizachew M, Abdella H, Tiruneh M. Antimicrobial Susceptibility Patterns of *Staphylococcus aureus* atthe University of Gondar Tertiary Hospital, Northwest Ethiopia: A Retrospective Cross Sectional Study. Bacteriology & Parasitology. 2015;6(3):1000228
81. Kibret M, Abera B. Antimicrobial resistance trend of bacteria from clinical isolates: an 8-year retrospective study at Dessie regional laboratory, Northeast Ethiopia. Ethiopian pharmaceutical journal. 2010;28:39–46.
82. Tenssay ZW. Multiple antimicrobial resistance in bacterial isolates from clinical and environmental sources of Jimma hospital, south West Ethiopia. Ethiopia Journal of Science. 2002;25(2):295–302.
83. Abera B, Alem A, Bezabih B. Methicillin-resistant strains of Staphylococcus Aureus and coagulase-negative staphylococus from clinical isolates at Felege Hiwot Refferal hospital, north West Ethiopia. Ethiop Med J. 2008; 46(2):149–54.
84. Lema T, Woldeamanuel Y, Asrat D, Hunegnaw M, Baraki A, Kebede Y, Yamuah L, Aseffa A. The pattern of bacterial isolates and drug sensitivities of infected ulcers in patients with leprosy in ALERT, Kuyera and Gambo hospitals, Ethiopia. Lepr Rev. 2012;83(1):40–51.
85. Ramos JM, Perez-Tanoira R, Garcia-Garcia C, Prieto-Perez L, Bellon MC, Mateos F, Tisisano G, Yohannes T, Reyes F, Gorgolas M. Leprosy ulcers in a rural hospital of Ethiopia: pattern of aerobic bacterial isolates and drug sensitivities. Ann Clin Microbiol Antimicrob. 2014;13:47.
86. Wolday D, Erge W. Increased incidence of resistance to antimicrobials by urinary pathogens isolated at Tikur Anbessa hospital. Ethiop Med J. 1997; 35(2):127–35.
87. Biadglegne F, Abera B. Antimicrobial resistance of bacterial isolates from urinary tract infections at Felge Hiwot referral hospital, Ethiopia. Ethiop J Health Dev. 2009;23(3):236–8.
88. WHO: Antimicrobial resistance: global report ton surveillance. France; 2014.
89. Li S, Li J, Qiao Y, Ning X, Zeng T, Shen X. Prevalence and invasiveness of community-acquired methicillin-resistant Staphylococcus Aureus: a meta-analysis. Indian J Pathol Microbiol. 2014;57(3):418–22.
90. Salgado CD, Farr BM, Calfee DP. Community-acquired methicillin-resistant Staphylococcus Aureus: a meta-analysis of prevalence and risk factors. Clin Infect Dis. 2003;36(2):131–9.
91. Struelens MJ. The epidemiology of antimicrobial resistance in hospital acquired infections: problems and possible solutions. BMJ. 1998;317(7159):652–4.
92. Falagas ME, Karageorgopoulos DE, Leptidis J, Korbila IP. MRSA in Africa: filling the global map of antimicrobial resistance. PLoS One. 2013;8(7):e68024.
93. Sevag MG, Green MN. The mechanism of resistance to sulfonamides: I. Factors controlling the formation of Arylamine from Tryptophane by Staphylococcus Aureus. J Bacteriol. 1944;48(6):615–22.
94. Steers E, Sevag MG. The mechanism of resistance to sulfonamides; a comparative study of the amino acid metabolism of Staphylococcus Aureus in relation to the mechanism of resistance. Arch Biochem. 1949;24(1):129–43.
95. Sompolinsky D, Zaidenzaig Y, Ziegler-Schlomowitz R, Abramova N. Mechanism of tetracycline resistance in Staphylococcus Aureus. J Gen Microbiol. 1970;62(3): 351–62.
96. Kono M, Sasatsu M, O'Hara K, Shiomi Y, Hayasaka T. Mechanism of resistance to some cephalosporins in Staphylococcus Aureus. Antimicrob Agents Chemother. 1983;23(6):938–40.
97. Yamagishi S, Nakajima Y, Inoue M, Oka Y. Decrease in accumulation of macrolide antibiotics as a mechanism of resistance in Staphylococcus Aureus. Japanese journal of microbiology. 1971;15(1):39–52.
98. Li XF, Fan XJ, Guo XJ, Feng P, Lu XJ, Gao YY, Xiong YL, Yu RJ, Ding X. A study on the mechanism of drug resistance in *Staphylococcus aureus*. Sichuan Da Xue Xue Bao Yi Xue Ban. 2006;37(3):365–8.
99. Stein M, Komerska J, Prizade M, Sheinberg B, Tasher D, Somekh E. Clindamycin resistance among Staphylococcus Aureus strains in Israel: implications for empirical treatment of skin and soft tissue infections. Int J Infect Dis. 2016;46: 18–21.
100. Zhang S, Sun X, Chang W, Dai Y, Ma X. Systematic review and meta-analysis of the epidemiology of vancomycin-intermediate and heterogeneous vancomycin-intermediate Staphylococcus Aureus isolates. PLoS One. 2015; 10(8):e0136082.
101. Yadesa TM, Gudina EK, Angamo MT. Antimicrobial use-related problems and predictors among hospitalized medical in-patients in Southwest Ethiopia: prospective observational study. PLoS One. 2015;10(12):e0138385.
102. Gebretekle GB, Serbessa MK. Exploration of over the counter sales of antibiotics in community pharmacies of Addis Ababa, Ethiopia: pharmacy professionals' perspective. Antimicrobial resistance and infection control. 2016;5:2.
103. Abera B, Kibret M, Mulu W. Knowledge and beliefs on antimicrobial resistance among physicians and nurses in hospitals in Amhara region, Ethiopia. BMC pharmacology & toxicology. 2014;15:26.

5

Phenotypic and genotypic characterization of antibiotic resistance of methicillin-resistant *Staphylococcus aureus* isolated from hospital food

Farhad Safarpoor Dehkordi[1], Hasan Gandomi[1*], Afshin Akhondzadeh Basti[1*], Ali Misaghi[1] and Ebrahim Rahimi[2]

Abstract

Background: Pathogenic biotypes of the Methicillin-resistant *Staphylococcus aureus* (MRSA) strains are considered to be one of the major cause of food-borne diseases in hospitals. The present investigation was done to study the pattern of antibiotic resistance and prevalence of antibiotic resistance genes of different biotypes of the MRSA strains isolated from various types of hospital food samples.

Methods: Four-hundred and eighty-five raw and cooked hospital food samples were cultured and MRSA strains were identified using the oxacillin and cefoxitin disk diffusion tests and *mecA*-based PCR amplification. Isolated strains were subjected to biotyping and their antibiotic resistance patterns were analyzed using the disk diffusion and PCR methods.

Results: Prevalence of *S. aureus* and MRSA were 9.69 and 7.62%, respectively. Meat and chicken barbecues had the highest prevalence of MRSA. Prevalence of bovine, ovine, poultry and human-based biotypes in the MRSA strains were 8.10, 8.10, 32.43 and 48.64%, respectively. All of the MRSA strains recovered from soup, salad and rice samples were related to human-based biotypes. MRSA strains harbored the highest prevalence of resistance against penicillin (100%), ceftaroline (100%), tetracycline (100%), erythromycin (89.18%) and trimethoprim-sulfamethoxazole (83.78%). *TetK* (72.97%), *ermA* (72.97%), *msrA* (64.86%) and *aacA-D* (62.16%) were the most commonly detected antibiotic resistance genes.

Conclusions: Pattern of antibiotic resistance and also distribution of antibiotic resistance genes were related to the biotype of MRSA strains. Presence of multi-drug resistance and also simultaneous presence of several antibiotic resistance genes in some MRSA isolates showed an important public health issue Further researches are required to found additional epidemiological aspects of the MRSA strains in hospital food samples.

Keywords: Methicillin-resistant *Staphylococcus aureus*, Biotypes, Antimicrobial resistance, Hospital food

Background

Consumption of contaminated food is one of the most common cause of outbreak of food-borne diseases in hospitals [1]. Based on the general weakness of the hospitalized patients and also the possibility of occurrence of suppression in their immune system, hospital foodstuffs should have a high quality and safety [1].

The most cases of food-borne outbreaks in hospitals are occurred due to the consumption of food contaminated with *Staphylococcus aureus* (*S. aureus*) [2, 3]. *Staphylococcus aureus* is commonly found in nose and respiratory system and on the skin [2, 3]. It is responsible for the occurrence of nosocomial and community-acquired infections, food-borne diseases and food poisoning [2, 3]. Occurrence of different types of gastrointestinal diseases which are known by vomiting, nausea, abdominal cramps, weakness and diarrhea and also toxic shock syndrome are attributed to the *S. aureus* strains [2, 3].

* Correspondence: Aakhond@ut.ac.ir; Gandomih@ut.ac.ir
[1]Department of Food Hygiene and Quality Control, Faculty of Veterinary Medicine, University of Tehran, Tehran, Iran
Full list of author information is available at the end of the article

One of the most interesting questions about the contamination of foods with *S. aureus* concerns the source of these contamination organisms [4–6]. When foods or some of their ingredients are of animal origin it can be of importance to determine whether the strains of *S. aureus* isolated originate from animals or from humans [4–6]. *S. aureus* can be disseminated in the host's environment. Presence of several biotypes in the *S. aureus* strains (bovine, ovine, poultry and human) with different microbiological characters has increased the importance of the issue [4–6]. Identification of *S. aureus* biotypes is a practical approach to determine the exact routes of food contamination and also find their microbiological and epidemiological similarities and differences [4–6]. Biotyping of *S. aureus* strains isolated from hospital food samples is essential to trace their origin and their public health significance, to investigate the relationship of the strains, and to determine their diversity within and between samples [4–6].

Food-borne *S. aureus* strains are usually resistant against several types of antibiotics [7–9]. Nowadays, methicillin-resistant *S. aureus* (MRSA) has become a serious problem in hospitals [7–9]. Documented data revealed that about 50-70% of the *S. aureus* strains isolated from the hospital environment were MRSA [7–9]. MRSA strains are responsible for about 100,000 cases of infections with around 20% mortality rate each year in the United States [7]. High pathogenicity of MRSA strains [9], its high resistance to several types of antibiotics [9] and its food-borne aspects [9] have increased the importance of isolation of MRSA in hospital food samples. Staphylococcal food poisoning is an intoxication that results from the consumption of foods containing sufficient amounts of one (or more) preformed enterotoxin [2, 3]. Therefore, the risk of MRSA contaminated food might be due to the important factors like cross-contamination [2, 3, 7].

MRSA strains of both animal and human origins are believed to serve as important reservoirs of antimicrobial resistance genes which can transfer and integrate into the MRSA genome leading to the emergence of new and potentially more resistant strains [10–13]. Documented data revealed that presence of certain antibiotic resistance genes is responsible for occurrence of severe antibiotic resistance [10–13]. Reports showed that high presence of *mecA*, *aacA-D*, *tetK* and *tetM*, *ermA* and *ermC*, *msrA*, *linA* and *vatA*, *vatB* and *vatC* antibiotic resistance genes in the *S. aureus* strains isolated of foodstuffs caused severe occurrence of resistance against methicillin, aminoglycosides, tetracyclines, macrolide–lincosamide-streptogramin B, macrolides, lincosamides and streptogramin A groups of antibiotics, respectively [10–13].

Reports of methicillin-resistant strains are challenging due to the large proportion of methicillin-resistant strains and increasing numbers of isolates reinforcing the need to revise their importance to food safety [10–14]. Therefore, screening of these elements is important for public health and despite the importance of such a screen, limited data are available for MRSA at the species level among the hospital food samples.

MRSA strains have been tested in hospital food samples to assess microbiological safety, sanitation conditions during processing, and storage quality of products. High pathogenicity of MRSA strains and general weakness of hospitalized patients make it necessary to assess the presence of MRSA strains in hospital food samples. The current research was done to study the prevalence rate and antimicrobial resistance properties of the MRSA biotypes isolated from various types of raw and cooked hospital food samples in Iran.

Methods

Samples

From June 2015 to June 2016, a total of 485 various types of raw and cooked hospital food samples including raw meat (n = 38), raw chicken (n = 37), raw fish (n = 9), meat barbecue (n = 31), chicken barbecue (n = 82), grilled fish (n = 19), soup (n = 94), salad (n = 56) and cooked rice (n = 119) were randomly collected from the big hospitals of the Isfahan province, Iran. Samples were immediately transferred to the Food Hygiene Research Center of the Islamic Azad University of Shahrekord in cooler with ice-packs. All food samples showed normal physical characters including odor, color and consolidation.

Isolation and identification of *S. aureus*

Each sample was aseptically weighed in an analytical balance and 25 g were transferred into a sterile plastic bag. Then, 225 mL of buffered peptone water (Merck, Germany) was added and homogenized in a Stomacher Bagmixer 400 W (Interscience, Saint-Nom, France) for 2 min. Five milliliter aliquot of the enriched homogenate was transferred into 50 mL Trypticase Soy Broth (TSB, Merck, Germany) supplemented with 10% NaCl and 1% sodium pyruvate. After incubation at 35 °C for 18 h, a loopful of the culture was plated onto Baird-Parker agar supplemented with egg yolk tellurite emulsion (Merck, Germany) and incubated overnight at 37 °C. Black shiny colonies surrounded by 2 to 5-mm clear zones were further identified on the basis of Gram staining, hemolytic activity on sheep blood agar (Merck, Germany), catalase activity, coagulated test (rabbit plasma), oxidase test, glucose O/F test, resistance to bacitracin (0.04 U), mannitol fermentation on Mannitol salt agar (Merck, Germany), urease activity, nitrate reduction, phosphatase, deoxyribonuclease (DNase, Merck, Germany) test, voges-proskaver (Merck, Germany) test and carbohydrate (xylose, sucrose, trehalose and maltose, fructose, lactose, mannose) fermentation tests [11].

Identification of Methicillin-resistant *Staphylococcus aureus* strains

Cefoxitin (30 µg) and oxacillin (1 µg) susceptibility tests were used to distinguish the MRSA strains from *S. aureus* isolates of hospital food samples. All tests were performed using the guidelines of the Clinical and Laboratory Standards Institute (CLSI) [15].

MRSA isolates were identified another time using the PCR-based amplification of *mecA* gene. MRSA strains were sub-cultured on TSB media (Merck, Germany) and further incubated for 48 h at 37 °C. Genomic DNA was extracted from bacterial colonies using the DNA extraction kit (Fermentas, Germany) according to manufacturer's instruction.

The PCR reactions were performed in a total volume of 25 µL, including 1.5 mM MgCl2, 50 mM KCl, 10 mM Tris-HCl (pH 9.0), 0.1% Triton X-100, 200 µM dNTPs each (Fermentas, Germany), 2.5 µL PCR buffer (10×), 2.5 mM of each primer *mecA1* (5′-ACGAGTAG ATGCTCAATATAA-3′) and *mecA2* (5′-CTTAGTT CTTTAGCGATTGC-3′) (Gen Bank Accession Number NC_003923M), 1.5 U of Taq DNA polymerase (Fermentas, Germany) and 5 µL of the extracted DNA template of the MRSA isolates. The PCR cycling conditions were as follows: initial denaturation at 94 °C for 3 min, followed by 30 cycles of 94 °C for 30 s, 60 °C for 30 s, and 72 °C for 30 s, followed by an extra cycle of annealing at 60 °C for 30 s, and a final extension at 72 °C for 5 min.

Biotyping of the MRSA strains

Biotyping of the MRSA strains was done according to the method described by Devriese (1984) [16] with minor modifications. MRSA isolates were examined for production of staphylokinase and β-hemolysin, coagulation of bovine plasma and ability to growth on crystal violet agar. Staphylokinase production of the MRSA isolates were studied by incubating on bovine fibrin plates with or without dog serum as a plasminogen source. Staphylokinase production is determined by observation of lear zones on the bovine fibrin plates with dog serum. MRSA isolates were also cultured on 5% sheep blood agar media for determination of production of Beta-haemolysin. Development of broad discolored zones with sharp edges clearing at 4 °C is a marker for production of Beta-haemolysin. Coagulation of bovine plasma is studied by adding 0.1 mL of an overnight culture of the MRSA isolates in Brain Heart Infusion broth (Merck, Germany) to tubes with diluted (1:3) bovine plasma. Occurrence of big clots within 6 h were considered as positive reaction. MRSA strains were also streaked into the crystal violet agar media and appearance of A (crystal violet spots with a bright or pale yellow color and yellow spots with blue margins), C (blue or violet growth spots with or without an orange tint) and E (white spots or white growth with a blue hue) types were studied.

Antibiotic susceptibility test of MRSA strains

Patterns of antimicrobial resistance of the MRSA strains were studied using the simple disk diffusion technique. The Mueller–Hinton agar (Merck, Germany) medium was used for this purpose. Susceptibility of MRSA isolates were tested against several types of antibiotic groups including Penicillins (penicillin (10 µg/disk)), Cephems (ceftaroline (30 µg/disk),), Aminoglycosides (gentamicin (10 µg/disk), amikacin (30 µg/disk), kanamycin (30 µg/disk)), Macrolides (azithromycin (15 µg/disk) and erythromycin (15 µg/disk)), Tetracyclines (tetracycline (30 µg/disk), doxycycline (30 µg/disk)), Fluoroquinolones (ciprofloxacin (5 µg/disk) and levofloxacin (5 µg/disk)), Lincosamides (clindamycin (2 µg/disk)), Folate pathway inhibitors (trimethoprim-sulfamethoxazole (25 µg/disk)), Phenicols (chloramphenicol (30 µg/disk)) and Ansamycins (rifampin (5 µg/disk)) antibiotic agents (Oxoid, UK) using the instruction of Clinical and Laboratory Standards Institute [17]. The plates containing the discs were allowed to stand for at least 30 min before incubated at 37 °C for 24 h. The diameter of the zone of inhibition produced by each antibiotic disc was measured and interpreted using the CLSI zone diameter interpretative standards [17]. *Staphylococcus aureus* ATCC 25923 was used as quality control organism in antimicrobial susceptibility determination.

PCR-based amplification of antibiotic resistance genes

Table 1 represents the list of primers and PCR conditions used for amplification of antibiotic resistance genes in the MRSA strains isolated from various types of hospital food samples [18, 19]. A programmable DNA thermo-cycler (Eppendorf Mastercycler 5330, Eppendorf-Nethel-Hinz GmbH, Hamburg, Germany) was used in all PCR reactions.

Statistical analysis

Statistical analysis was done using the SPSS 21.0 statistical software (SPSS Inc., Chicago, IL, USA). Chi-square test and Fisher's exact two-tailed test were used to assess any significant relationship between prevalence of MRSA strains, their biotypes, antibiotic resistance genes and antibiotic resistance pattern. P value <0.05 was considered as statistical significant level.

Results

In this study, the prevalence of *S. aureus* strains in various types of raw and cooked hospital food samples were investigated and the results are shown in Table 2. Forty-

Table 1 Target genes, oligonucleotide primers and PCR conditions used for detection of antibiotic resistance genes in the MRSA strains isolated from various types of hospital food samples

Target gene	Primer sequence (5′-3′)	PCR product (bp)	PCR programs	PCR volume (50 μL)
AacA-D	F: TAATCCAAGAGCAATAAGGGC R: GCCACACTATCATAACCACTA	227	1 cycle: 94 ^{oC} ———— 5 min. 25 cycle: 94 ^{oC} ———— 60 s 55 ^{oC} ———— 70 s 72 ^{oC} ———— 60 s 1 cycle: 72 ^{oC} ———— 10 min	5 μL PCR buffer 10X 1.5 mM Mgcl$_2$ 200 μM dNTP (Fermentas) 0.5 μM of each primers F & R 1.25 U Taq DNA polymerase (Fermentas) 2.5 μL DNA template
ermA	F: AAGCGGTAAACCCCTCTGA R: TTCGCAAATCCCTTCTCAAC	190		
ermC	F: AATCGTCAATTCCTGCATGT R: TAATCGTGGAATACGGGTTTG	299		
tetK	F: GTAGCGACAATAGGTAATAGT R: GTAGTGACAATAAACCTCCTA	360		
vatC	F: AAAATCGATGGTAAAGGTTGGC R: AGTTCTGCAGTACCGGATTTGC	467		
tetM	F: AGTGGAGCGATTACAGAA R: CATATGTCCTGGCGTGTCTA	158	1 cycle: 94 ^{oC} ———— 6 min. 34 cycle: 95 ^{oC} ———— 50 s 55 ^{oC} ———— 70 s 72 ^{oC} ———— 60 s 1 cycle: 72 ^{oC} ———— 8 min	5 μL PCR buffer 10X 2 mM Mgcl$_2$ 200 μM dNTP (Fermentas) 0.5 μM of each primers F & R 1.5 U Taq DNA polymerase (Fermentas) 5 μL DNA template
vatA	F: TGGTCCCGGAACAACATTTAT R: TCCACCGACAATAGAATAGGG	268		
msrA	F: GGCACAATAAGAGTGTTTAAAGG R: AAGTTATATCATGAATAGATTGTCCTGTT	940	1 cycle: 94 ^{oC} ———— 6 min. 34 cycle: 95 ^{oC} ———— 60 s 50 ^{oC} ———— 70 s 72 ^{oC} ———— 70 s 1 cycle: 72 ^{oC} ———— 8 min	5 μL PCR buffer 10X 2 mM Mgcl$_2$ 150 μM dNTP (Fermentas) 0.75 μM of each primers F & R 1.5 U Taq DNA polymerase (Fermentas) 3 μL DNA template
vatB	F: GCTGCGAATTCAGTTGTTACA R: CTGACCAATCCCACCATTTTA	136	1 cycle: 94 ^{oC} ———— 6 min. 35 cycle: 95 ^{oC} ———— 50 s 55 ^{oC} ———— 70 s 72 ^{oC} ———— 80 s 1 cycle: 72 ^{oC} ———— 10 min	5 μL PCR buffer 10X 2 mM Mgcl$_2$ 150 μM dNTP (Fermentas) 0.75 μM of each primers F & R 1.5 U Taq DNA polymerase (Fermentas) 3 μL DNA template
linA	F: GGTGGCTGGGGGGTAGATGTATTAACTGG R: GCTTCTTTTGAAATACATGGTATTTTTCGA	323	1 cycle: 94 ^{oC} ———— 6 min. 30 cycle: 95 ^{oC} ———— 60 s 57 ^{oC} ———— 60 s 72 ^{oC} ———— 60 s 1 cycle: 72 ^{oC} ———— 10 min	5 μL PCR buffer 10X 2 mM Mgcl$_2$ 150 μM dNTP (Fermentas) 0.75 μM of each primers F & R 1.5 U Taq DNA polymerase (Fermentas) 3 μL DNA template

seven out of 485 hospital food samples (9.69%) were positive for *S. aureus*. Furthermore, the prevalence of *S. aureus* in raw food samples with animal origin, cooked food samples with animal origin and cooked food samples without animal origin were 23.80, 9.09 and 4.08%, respectively. Chicken meat samples had the highest prevalence of *S. aureus* (27.02%) among all studied raw food samples. Meat barbecue samples had the highest prevalence of *S. aureus* (26.31%) among all studied cooked food samples with animal origin. Salad samples had the highest prevalence of *S. aureus* (7.41%) among all studied cooked food samples without animal origin. None of the raw and cooked fish samples were *S. aureus* positive. Statistically significant difference was seen in the prevalence of *S. aureus* between different types of food samples ($P < 0.05$). Moreover, a statistically significant difference was found in the prevalence of *S. aureus* between raw and cooked food samples.

Thirty–seven out of 47 *S. aureus* isolates (78.72%) were recognized as MRSA. The prevalence of MRSA strains in raw foods with animal origin, cooked foods with animal origin and cooked foods without animal origin were 16.66, 9.09 and 4.08%, respectively. All of the *S. aureus* isolates of meat barbecue, chicken barbecue, soup and salad samples had complete resistance against methicillin. Rice had the lowest prevalence of MRSA strains (20%). Statistically significant difference was seen in the prevalence of MRSA between different

Table 2 Prevalence of *S. aureus* and MRSA strains isolated from various types of hospital food samples

Types of samples			No samples collected	N (%) of *S. aureus* positive samples	N (%) of MRSA positive samples
Raw foods	With animal origin	Meat	38	10 (26.31)	6 (50)
		Chicken	37	10 (27.02)	8 (80)
		Fish	9	–	–
		Total	84	20 (23.80)	14 (70)
Cooked foods	With animal origin	Meat barbecue	31	5 (16.12)	5 (100)
		Chicken barbecue	82	7 (8.53)	7 (100)
		Grilled fish	19	–	–
		Total	132	12 (9.09)	12 (100)
	Without animal origin	Soup	94	6 (6.38)	6 (100)
		Salad	56	4 (7.14)	4 (100)
		Rice	119	5 (4.20)	1 (20)
		Total	269	15 (5.57)	11 (73.33)
Total			485	47 (9.69%)	37 (78.72)

types of food samples ($P < 0.05$). Statistically significant difference was also found in the prevalence of *S. aureus* between raw and cooked food samples ($P < 0.05$).

Table 3 represents the prevalence of different biotypes among the MRSA strains isolated from various types of hospital food samples. The prevalence of bovine, ovine, poultry and human-based biotypes in the MRSA strains isolated from various types of hospital food samples were 8.10, 8.10, 32.43 and 48.64%, respectively. The biotypes of the 2.70% of MRSA strains were determined as unknown. All of the MRSA strains recovered from soup, salad and rice samples were related to human-based biotypes. Statistically significant difference was seen in the prevalence of different biotypes between different types of food samples ($P < 0.05$).

Antibiotic resistance pattern of the MRSA strains isolated from animal, human and unknown origins is presented in Table 4. We found that MRSA strains harbored a high prevalence of resistance against penicillin (100%), ceftaroline (100%), tetracycline (100%), erythromycin (86.48%), trimethoprim-sulfamethoxazole (83.78%), doxycycline (81.08%) and gentamicin (81.08%) antibiotic agents. MRSA strains showed low prevalence of resistance against chloramphenicol (29.72%), rifampin (35.13%), levofloxacin (43.24%), kanamycin (43.24%), clindamycin (48.64%), and ciprofloxacin (48.64%) antibiotic agents. Statistically significant difference was seen in the prevalence of antibiotic resistance between various studied biotypes ($P < 0.05$).

Distribution of antibiotic resistance genes in the MRSA strains isolated from animal, human and unknown origins is presented in Table 5. The most frequently detected antibiotic resistance genes among the MRSA strains were *tetK* (72.97%), *ermA* (72.97%), *msrA* (64.86%) and *aacA-D* (62.16%). Prevalence of *vatC*, *vatB*, *ermC* and *tetM* antibiotic resistance genes were 5.40, 18.91, 27.02 and 27.02%, respectively. The most commonly detected antibiotic resistance gene in the MRSA strains of animal,

Table 3 Prevalence of different biotypes among the MRSA strains isolated from various types of hospital food samples

Types of samples (N of MRSA positive samples)	N (%) of positive samples for each biotype				
	Bovine	Ovine	Poultry	Human	Unknown
Meat (6)	1 (16.66)	3 (50)	1 (16.66)	1 (16.66)	–
Chicken (8)	–	–	5 (62.50)	2 (25)	1 (12.50)
Meat barbecue (5)	2 (40)	–	1 (20)	2 (40)	–
Chicken barbecue (7)	–	–	5 (71.42)	2 (28.57)	–
Soup (6)	–	–	–	6 (100)	–
Salad (4)	–	–	–	4 (100)	–
Rice (1)	–	–	–	1 (100)	–
Total (37)	3 (8.10)	3 (8.10)	12 (32.43)	18 (48.64)	1 (2.70)

Table 4 Antibiotic resistance pattern of the MRSA strains isolated from animal, human and unknown origins

Origins (N of MRSA strains)		N (%) isolates resistant to each antibiotic														
		Penicillins	Cephems	Aminoglycosides			Macrolides		Tetracyclines		Fluoroquinolones		Lincosamides	Folate inhibitors	Phenicols	Ansamycins
		P10[a]	Cft	Gen	Amk	Kan	Azi	Ert	Tet	Dox	Cip	Lev	Clin	Tr-Sul	C30	Rif
Animal origins	Meat (5)	5 (100)	5 (100)	5 (100)	2 (40)	1 (20)	1 (20)	5 (100)	5 (100)	4 (80)	1 (20)	1 (20)	1 (20)	4 (80)	2 (40)	1 (20)
	Chicken (5)	5 (100)	5 (100)	4 (80)	3 (60)	2 (40)	2 (40)	4 (80)	5 (100)	4 (80)	2 (40)	2 (40)	2 (40)	4 (80)	2 (40)	1 (20)
	Meat barbecue (3)	3 (100)	3 (100)	2 (66.66)	2 (66.66)	1 (33.33)	–	2 (66.66)	3 (100)	2 (66.66)	–	–	2 (66.66)	3 (100)	1 (33.33)	–
	Chicken barbecue (5)	5 (100)	5 (100)	4 (80)	3 (60)	2 (40)	3 (60)	4 (80)	5 (100)	4 (80)	3 (60)	3 (60)	3 (60)	4 (80)	2 (40)	1 (20)
	Total (18)	18 (100)	18 (100)	15 (83.33)	10 (55.55)	6 (33.33)	6 (33.33)	15 (83.33)	18 (100)	14 (77.77)	6 (33.33)	6 (33.33)	8 (44.44)	15 (83.33)	7 (38.88)	3 (16.66)
Human origins	Meat (1)	1 (100)	1 (100)	1 (100)	1 (100)	1 (100)	1 (100)	1 (100)	1 (100)	1 (100)	1 (100)	1 (100)	1 (100)	1 (100)	–	1 (100)
	Chicken (2)	2 (100)	2 (100)	2 (100)	2 (100)	1 (50)	2 (100)	2 (100)	2 (100)	2 (100)	1 (50)	1 (50)	1 (50)	1 (50)	1 (50)	1 (50)
	Meat barbecue (2)	2 (100)	2 (100)	1 (50)	2 (100)	1 (50)	2 (100)	2 (100)	2 (100)	2 (100)	1 (50)	1 (50)	1 (50)	2 (100)	–	1 (50)
	Chicken barbecue (2)	2 (100)	2 (100)	2 (100)	2 (100)	1 (50)	2 (100)	2 (100)	2 (100)	2 (100)	1 (50)	1 (50)	1 (50)	2 (100)	1 (50)	1 (50)
	Soup (6)	6 (100)	6 (100)	5 (83.33)	4 (66.66)	3 (50)	5 (83.33)	5 (83.33)	6 (100)	4 (66.66)	4 (66.66)	3 (50)	3 (50)	5 (83.33)	1 (16.66)	3 (50)
	Salad (4)	4 (100)	4 (100)	3 (75)	3 (75)	2 (50)	3 (75)	3 (75)	4 (100)	3 (75)	3 (75)	2 (50)	2 (50)	3 (75)	1 (25)	2 (50)
	Rice (1)	1 (100)	1 (100)	–	1 (100)	1 (100)	1 (100)	1 (100)	1 (100)	1 (100)	1 (100)	1 (100)	1 (100)	1 (100)	–	1 (100)
	Total (19)	19 (100)	19 (100)	15 (78.94)	16 (84.21)	10 (52.63)	16 (84.21)	17 (89.47)	19 (100)	16 (84.21)	12 (63.15)	10 (52.63)	10 (52.63)	16 (84.21)	4 (21.05)	10 (52.63)
Unknown origin	Chicken (3)	1 (100)	1 (100)	1 (100)	1 (100)	–	–	1 (100)	1 (100)	1 (100)	–	–	–	1 (100)	–	–
Total (37)		37 (100)	37 (100)	30 (81.08)	26 (70.27)	16 (43.24)	22 (59.45)	32 (86.48)	37 (100)	30 (81.08)	18 (48.64)	16 (43.24)	18 (48.64)	31 (83.78)	11 (29.72)	13 (35.13)

[a] *P10* penicillin (10 μg/disk), *Cft* ceftaroline (30 μg/disk), *Gen* gentamicin (10 μg/disk), *Amk* amikacin (30 μg/disk), *Kan* kanamycin (30 μg/disk), *Azi* azithromycin (15 μg/disk), *Ert* erythromycin (15 μg/disk), *Tet* tetracycline (30 μg/disk), *Do* doxycycline (30 μg/disk), *Cip* ciprofloxacin (5 μg/disk), *Lev* levofloxacin (5 μg/disk), *Clin* clindamycin (2 μg/disk), *Tr-Sul* trimethoprim-sulfamethoxazole (25 μg/disk), *C30* chloramphenicol (30 μg/disk), *Rif* rifampin (5 μg/disk)

Table 5 Distribution of antibiotic resistance genes in the MRSA strains isolated from animal, human and unknown origins

Origins (N of MRSA strains)		N (%) of isolates harbor each gene									
		aacA-D	*tetK*	*tetM*	*msrA*	*ermA*	*ermC*	*vatA*	*vatB*	*vatC*	*LinA*
Animal origins	Meat (5)	4 (80)	5 (100)	2 (40)	4 (80)	4 (80)	1 (20)	3 (60)	1 (20)	–	1 (20)
	Chicken (5)	3 (60)	3 (60)	1 (20)	2 (40)	3 (60)	1 (20)	2 (40)	1 (20)	1 (20)	2 (40)
	Meat barbecue (3)	2 (66.66)	3 (100)	1 (33.33)	2 (66.66)	3 (100)	1 (33.33)	2 (66.66)	1 (33.33)	–	2 (66.66)
	Chicken barbecue (5)	2 (40)	3 (60)	2 (40)	3 (60)	4 (80)	1 (20)	2 (40)	1 (20)	–	2 (40)
	Total (18)	11 (61.11)	14 (77.77)	6 (33.33)	11 (61.11)	14 (77.77)	4 (22.22)	9 (50)	4 (22.22)	1 (5.55)	7 (38.88)
Human origins	Meat (1)	1 (100)	1 (100)	–	1 (100)	1 (100)	–	1 (100)	–	–	1 (100)
	Chicken (2)	2 (100)	2 (100)	1 (50)	2 (100)	1 (50)	1 (50)	1 (50)	1 (50)	–	1 (50)
	Meat barbecue (2)	2 (100)	2 (100)	–	2 (100)	2 (100)	1 (50)	1 (50)	–	–	1 (50)
	Chicken barbecue (2)	2 (100)	2 (100)	1 (50)	2 (100)	2 (100)	1 (50)	1 (50)	1 (50)	–	1 (50)
	Soup (6)	2 (33.33)	2 (33.33)	1 (16.66)	3 (50)	3 (50)	2 (33.33)	2 (33.33)	1 (16.66)	1 (16.66)	2 (33.33)
	Salad (4)	2 (50)	2 (50)	1 (25)	2 (50)	2 (50)	1 (25)	1 (25)	–	–	2 (50)
	Rice (1)	1 (100)	1 (100)	–	1 (100)	1 (100)	–	1 (100)	–	–	1 (100)
	Total (19)	12 (63.15)	12 (63.15)	4 (21.05)	13 (68.42)	12 (63.15)	6 (31.57)	8 (42.10)	3 (15.78)	1 (5.26)	9 (47.36)
Unknown origin	Chicken (1)	–	1 (100)	–	–	1 (100)	–	–	–	–	–
Total (37)		23 (62.16)	27 (72.97)	10 (27.02)	24 (64.86)	27 (72.97)	10 (27.02)	17 (45.94)	7 (18.91)	2 (5.40)	16 (43.24)

human and unknown origins were *tetK* (77.77%) and *ermA* (77.77%), *msrA* (68.42%) and *tetK* (100%) and *ermA* (100%), respectively. MRSA strains with unknown origin were only positive for *tetK* and *ermA* antibiotic resistance genes. Statistically significant difference was seen in the prevalence of antibiotic resistance genes between different biotypes ($P < 0.05$).

Discussion

S. aureus is considered as one of the most common causes of nosocomial infections, as well as the cause of most cases of food poisoning in hospitals [4, 20]. Hospital meals are an indispensable portion of patient care. Safe and complete meals can encourage patients to eat well and giving them the nutrients they need to recover from surgery or illness.

Foodstuff contamination with *S. aureus* may occur directly from infected food-producing animals or may result from poor hygiene during production processes, or the retail and storage of food, since humans may also harbor microorganisms. The current research is the first report of the biotyping and molecular characterization of antibiotic resistance in the MRSA strains isolated from various types of raw and cooked hospital food samples. Findings obtained from this research revealed that the prevalence of *S. aureus* in different types of hospital food samples was 9.69%. The prevalence rate of the *S. aureus* in hospital food samples of our research was higher than that of Spain (6.10%) [21] and Iran (6.42%) [22], Portugal (11.10%) [23] and Brazil (50%) [24].

Investigations conducted in the U.S. as well as numerous other countries, including Canada, Taiwan, China, Denmark, South Korea, Austria, France, Belgium, Italy, and The Netherlands, have isolated MRSA mainly from different types of foods [4, 20]. Costa et al. (2015) [25] revealed that 28.10% of hospital food samples harbored MRSA strains. They showed that the prevalence of MRSA strains in beef, chicken, pork and fish samples were 23.30, 23.30, 37.50 and 30%, respectively which was higher than that found in our study.

Biotyping is a simple method used to trace the origin of *S. aureus* strains isolated from food samples. The results of our study showed that all of the MRSA strains isolated from rice, salad and soup samples were derived from humans. Furthermore, 48.64% of MRSA isolates of hospital food samples had human origin. Generally, the results revealed the role of infected humans in the dissemination and also transmission of MRSA strains to hospital food samples. The role of food handlers in transmission of MRSA strains into the food samples has also been reported by Castro et al. (2016) [23], Ferreira et al. (2014) [24], Costa et al. (2015) [25] and Ayçiçek et al. (2004) [26]. A study which was conducted by Kitai et al. (2005) [27] supported the high prevalence of poultry-based biotypes found in our investigation (71.42%). They reported that about 80% of all *S. aureus* isolates of foodstuffs belonged to the poultry-based biotypes, while prevalence of human-based biotypes was 22.10%. Normanno et al. (2007) [28] revealed that the prevalence of human, ovine, not-host-specific, bovine and poultry-based biotypes of the *S. aureus* isolates of Italian food samples were 50.40, 23.20, 17.60, 7.20 and 1.60%, respectively.

S. aureus causes food intoxication and doesn't lead to food infection [2, 3]. Therefore, the risk of MRSA contaminated hospital food might be due to the cross-contamination. High prevalence of MRSA strains in cooked food samples may be due to the cross-contamination of cooked foods through food handlers and kitchen equipment.

Our results showed that the antibiotic resistance pattern and prevalence of the antibiotic resistance genes were highly dependent to the biotypes of the MRSA strains. The human-based biotypes of the MRSA strains harbored higher prevalence of resistance against human-based antibiotics including ceftaroline, amikacin, kanamycin, azithromycin, doxycycline, ciprofloxacin, levofloxacin, clindamycin and rifampin. Furthermore, animal-based biotypes harbored higher prevalence of resistance against animal-based antibiotics or those which are routine in veterinary medicine including penicillin, gentamicin, erythromycin, tetracycline, trimethoprim-sulfamethoxazole and chloramphenicol. Poultry-based biotypes of the MRSA strains had a higher prevalence of resistance against chloramphenicol ($P < 0.05$). It may be due to the higher prescription of chloramphenicol in aviculture. MRSA strains of our study harbored the highest prevalence of resistance against antibiotics of the penicillins, cephems and tetracyclines groups. There were no previously published data about the relations between biotypes and prevalence of antibiotic resistance in the MRSA strains. Similar antibiotic resistance patterns of the MRSA strains isolated from different types of food and clinical samples have also been reported against aminoglycosides [29–33], cephems [29, 31–33], penicillins [29, 31–33], macrolides [29–33], tetracyclines [29, 31, 32], fluoroquinolones [29–33], lincosamides [29–32], folate inhibitors [29–33], phenicols [29, 31, 32] and ansamycins [29, 31, 32] groups of antibiotics. Fowoyo and Ogunbanwo (2017) [34] reported that the *S. aureus* strains isolated from ready to eat foodstuffs exhibited the high prevalence of resistance against ampicillin (86.70%), trimethoprim–sulfamethoxazole (74.90%), amoxicillin–clavulanic acid (52.50%), cefotaxime (3.50%), oxacillin (35.70%), ciprofloxacin (23.90%), erythromycin (15.70%), gentamicin (11.40%) and ofloxacin (7.10%). Rong et al. (2017) [35] reported that the prevalence of antibiotic resistance in the *S. aureus* strains isolated from different types of food samples against ampicillin, penicillin, amoxicillin–clavulanic acid, cefoxitin, ceftazidime, cefepime, kanamycin, streptomycin, amikacin, gentamicin, norfloxacin, ciprofloxacin, erythromycin, tetracycline, clindamycin, chloramphenicol, trimethoprim-sulfamethoxazole, vancomycin and rifampicin were 88.20, 88.20, 73.90, 8.40, 10.90, 8.40, 22.70, 14.30, 1.70, 4.20, 6.70, 5.00, 53.80, 26.90, 12.60, 7.507.50, 0 and 2.50%, respectively. MRSA strains should resist completely against all types of beta-lactams and penicillins [17], but it is surprising that some studies show that the MRSA strains isolated from food and also clinical samples don't have complete resistance against several types of beta-lactams and also penicillins [36, 37].

Most of the tetracycline-resistant MRSA strains harbored *tetK* and *tetM* genes. Prevalence of *aacA-D* gene was high among gentamicin, amikacin and kanamycin-resistant MRSA strains. Prevalence of *msrA*, *ermA* and *ermC* and *linA* were also significant among the macrolide, erythromycin and clindamycin-resistant MRSA strains. Therefore, the pattern of the antibiotic resistance of the MRSA strains of hospital food samples was confirmed by the PCR amplification of the specific antibiotic resistance genes. MRSA strains of our study had considerable prevalence of resistance against clindamycin (48.64%). The most imperative mechanism involving resistance against clindamycin is modulated by methylase enzyme which often encoded by *ermA* and *ermC* genes [38]. Prevalence of *ermA* and *ermC* antibiotic resistance genes among the MRSA strains of our research were 72.97 and 27.02%, respectively. Majority of our isolates carried two tetracyclines, two erythromycins, one macrolide and several streptogramin resistance determinants reveals a great diffusion of these types of resistance. *TetK*, *ermA*, *msrA* and *aacA-D* which encode resistance against tetracycline, erythromycin, macrolides and aminoglycosides were the most commonly detected antibiotic resistance genes in the MRSA strains isolated of hospital food samples. The literature survey did not indicate any report on the prevalence of *vatA*, *vatB*, *vatC*, *msrA*, *ermA*, *ermC*, *linA*, *aacA-D*, *tetK* and *tetM* genes among the MRSA strains of hospital food samples. Kumar et al. (2010) [39] reported that the most commonly identified antibiotic resistance genes among the *S. aureus* isolates of food samples were *linA* (51.60%), *msrB* (46.10%), *tetK* (34.40%), *tetM* (34.40%), *msrA* (26.60%) and *aacA-D* (26.60%). Karataş et al. (2017) [40] revealed the higher prevalence of *ermA* than *ermc* antibiotic resistance genes among the clindamycin, erythromycin and telithromycin-resistant and also higher prevalence of *tetM* than *tetK* antibiotic resistance genes among the tetracycline-resistant MRSA strains which were similar to our findings. Our results were also similar with those of the previous research which was conducted by Simeoni et al. (2008) [41]. They reported that the prevalence of *tetM*, *tetO*, *tetK*, *ermA*, *ermB*, *ermC*, *aac*, *blaZ* and *mecA* antibiotic resistance genes amongst the *S. aureus* strains isolated from meat samples were 100, 0, 91.66, 16.66, 33.33, 58.33, 0, 100 and 58.33%, respectively. High prevalence of *tetK* and *tetM* antibiotic resistance genes in the MRSA isolates can be clarified by their usual genetic locations. Presence of *tetK* gene on small multicopy plasmids and *tetM* on conjugative transposons contributes to the spread of these determinants [42]. Some of the MRSA strains harbored *ermC* gene. This gene is often located on small multicopy plasmids which are present in many different staphylococcal species [42]. The *ermA* gene is usually carried by transposons which could explain its high prevalence amongst the MRSA strains. Resistance to aminoglycosides (43.24 to 81.08%) which encode by the *aacA-D* gene (62.16%) is more prevalent amongst the human-based biotypes. It is because of this gene is usually more diffused in staphylococci of human origin [42]. Johler et al. (2011) [42] reported that prevalence of *ermC*, *tetK* and *tetM* antibiotic resistance genes among the *S. aureus* strains isolated from cases of food poisoning, milk and pork were 25, 4.87 and 0%, 50, 0 and 12.82 and 0%, 12.19, and 53.84%, respectively. Podkowik et al. (2012) [43] reported that the prevalence of tetracycline resistance genes (*tetO*, *tetK* and *tetM*) and erythromycin resistance methylase gene (*ermA*, *ermB* and *ermC*) among the *S. aureus* strains isolated from ready to eat meat products were 44 and 60%, respectively.

Conclusions

The present investigation is the first report of the biotyping and study the antimicrobial resistance properties of MRSA strains isolated from raw and cooked hospital food samples. In this study, a total prevalence of 7.62% of MRSA as well as high prevalence of human and poultry-based biotypes was seen in hospital food samples. Considerable prevalence of resistance against penicillin, ceftaroline, tetracycline, erythromycin, trimethoprim-sulfamethoxazole, doxycycline and gentamicin antibiotic agents and high distribution of *tetK*, *ermA*, *msrA* and *aacA-D* antibiotic resistance genes may pose a potential public health threat. Our findings exhibited that the pattern of antibiotic resistance and also distribution of antibiotic resistance genes were dependent on the biotype of MRSA strains. Human-based biotypes had a higher prevalence of resistance against human-based antibiotics and their corresponding resistance genes. Raw food samples with animal origin had the lower prevalence of human-based biotypes, while cooked food samples had a higher prevalence of human-based biotypes. Presence of multi-drug resistance and also simultaneous presence of several antibiotic resistance genes in some MRSA isolates must be considered as serious health hazard. Cooking food thoroughly is important, but preventing cross-contamination is the most effective ways to prevent occurrence of MRSA in hospital food. Further researches are required to understand higher epidemiological aspects of the MRSA strains in hospital food samples.

Abbreviations

MRSA: Methicillin-resistant *Staphylococcus aureus*; PCR: Polymerase chain reaction; *S. aureus*: *Staphylococcus aureus*; SPSS: Statistical package for the social sciences

Acknowledgements

The authors would like to thank Ms. Zeinab Torki Baghbaderani and Ms. Shohreh Habibian Dehkordi for their assistance in sample collection. Authors would also thank from Mr. Manouchehr Momeni Shahraki, Mr. Mohammad Rabiei Faradonbeh, Dr. Ali Zamen Salehifard Jouneghani and Dr. Mohammad Sakhaei Shahreza for their important assistance in the laboratory based examinations. The authors would also thank from Prof. Pezhvak Khaki, Prof. Taghi Zahraei Salehi and Prof. Hesam-aldin Akbarein for their important roles in the research project. Authors also would like to thank from the Iran National Science Foundation-Science Deputy of Presidency Project N 91003935 for its financial supports. We would like to thank from the Faculty of Veterinary Medicine, University of Tehran, Tehran, Iran for its financial supports.

Funding

This work was supported by the Faculty of Veterinary Medicine, University of Tehran, Tehran, Iran (grant no. 7507001/6/36) and also Iran National Science Foundation-Science Deputy of Presidency Project (grant no. 91003935).

Authors' contributions

FSD designed the study and carried out the culture-based identification, biotyping and PCR genetic alignment. AAB and HG supported the study and carried out the samples collection, disk diffusion and statistical analysis. ER and AM carried out the writing and drafting of the manuscript. All authors read and approved the final manuscript.

Consent for publication

There was no consent for publication.

Competing interests

The authors declare that they have no competing interests.

Author details

[1]Department of Food Hygiene and Quality Control, Faculty of Veterinary Medicine, University of Tehran, Tehran, Iran. [2]Department of Food Hygiene and Public Health, Faculty of Veterinary Medicine, Shahrekord Branch, Islamic Azad University, Shahrekord, Iran.

References

1. Ranjbar R, Masoudimanesh M, Dehkordi FS, Jonaidi-Jafari N, Rahimi E. Shiga (Vero)-toxin producing *Escherichia coli* isolated from the hospital foods; virulence factors, o-serogroups and antimicrobial resistance properties. Antimicrob Resist Infect Control. 2017;6:4.
2. Parsaeimehr M, Akhondzadeh Basti A, Radmehr B, Misaghi A, Abbasifar A, Karim G, et al. Effect of *Zataria multiflora* Boiss. Essential oil, nisin, and their combination on the production of enterotoxin C and α-hemolysin by *Staphylococcus aureus*. Foodborne Pathog Dise. 2010;7:299–305.
3. Azizkhani M, Misaghi A, Basti AA, Gandomi H, Hosseini H. Effects of *Zataria multiflora* Boiss. Essential oil on growth and gene expression of enterotoxins a, C and E in *Staphylococcus aureus* ATCC 29213. Int J Food Microbiol. 2013; 163:159–65.
4. Wendlandt S, Schwarz S, Silley P. Methicillin-resistant *Staphylococcus aureus*: a food-borne pathogen? Annu Rev Food Sci Technol. 2013;4:117–39.
5. Capita R, Alonso-Calleja C, García-Fernández MC, Moreno B. Characterization of *Staphylococcus aureus* isolated from poultry meat in Spain. Poult Sci. 2002;81:414–21.
6. Blaiotta G, Fusco V, Eiff CV, Villani F, Becker K. Biotyping of enterotoxigenic *Staphylococcus aureus* by enterotoxin gene cluster (*egc*) polymorphism and *spa* typing analyses. Appl Environ Microbiol. 2006;72:6117–23.
7. Klevens RM, Morrison MA, Nadle J, Petit S, Gershman K, Ray S, et al. Invasive methicillin-resistant *Staphylococcus aureus* infections in the United States. JAMA. 2007;298:1763–71.
8. Baumgartner A, Niederhauser I, Johler S. Virulence and resistance gene profiles of *Staphylococcus aureus* strains isolated from ready-to-eat foods. J Food Prot. 2014;77:1232–6.
9. Hasanpour Dehkordi A, Khaji L, Sakhaei Shahreza MH, Mashak Z, Safarpoor Dehkordi F, Safaree Y, et al. One-year prevalence of antimicrobial susceptibility pattern of methicillin-resistant *Staphylococcus aureus* recovered from raw meat. Trop Biomed. 2017;34:396–404.
10. Osman K, Badr J, Al-Maary KS, Moussa IM, Hessain AM, Girah ZM, et al. Prevalence of the antibiotic resistance genes in coagulase-positive-and negative-staphylococcus in chicken meat retailed to consumers. Front Microbiol. 2016;7:1846.
11. Fijałkowski K, Peitler D, Karakulska J. Staphylococci isolated from ready-to-eat meat - identification, antibiotic resistance and toxin gene profile. Int J Food Microbiol. 2016;238:113–20.
12. Osman KM, Abd El-Razik KA, Marie HSH, Arafa A. Coagulase-negative staphylococci collected from bovine milk: species and antimicrobial gene diversity. J Food Saf. 2016;36:89–99.
13. Osman KM, Amer AM, Badr JM, Helmy NM, Elhelw RA, Orabi A, et al. Antimicrobial resistance, biofilm formation and mecA characterization of methicillin-susceptible *S. aureus* and non-*S. aureus* of beef meat origin in Egypt. Front Microbiol. 2016;7:222.
14. Bhargava K, Zhang Y. Characterization of methicillin-resistant coagulase-negative staphylococci (MRCoNS) in retail meat. Food Microbiol. 2014;42:56–60.
15. Clinical and Laboratory Standards Institute (CLSI). Performance standards for antimicrobial susceptibility testing; 17th informational supplement. CLSI document M100-S17. Wayne: Clinical and Laboratory Standards Institute; 2007.
16. Devriese LA. A simplified system of biotyping *Staphylococcus aureus* strains isolated from different animal species. J Appl Bacteriol. 1984;56:215–20.
17. Clinical and Laboratory Standards Institute (CLSI). Performance standards for antimicrobial susceptibility testing; twenty-fifth informational supplement. CLSI document M100-S25. Wayne: Clinical and Laboratory Standards Institute; 2015.
18. Lina G, Quaglia A, Reverdy M, Leclercq R, Vandenesch F, Etienne J. Distribution of genes encoding resistance to macrolides, lincosamides, and streptogramins among staphylococci. Antimicrob Agent Chemother. 1999;43:1062–6.
19. Strommenger B, Kettlitz C, Werner G, Witte W. Multiplex PCR assay for simultaneous detection of nine clinically relevant antibiotic resistance genes in *Staphylococcus aureus*. J Clin Microbiol. 2003;41:4089–94.
20. Sergelidis D, Angelidis AS. Methicillin-resistant *Staphylococcus aureus*: a controversial food-borne pathogen. Lett Appl Microbiol. 2017;64:409–18.
21. Gutiérrez D, Delgado S, Vázquez-Sánchez D, Martínez B, Cabo ML, Rodríguez A, et al. Incidence of *Staphylococcus aureus* and analysis of associated bacterial communities on food industry surfaces. Appl Environ Microbiol. 2012;78:8547–54.
22. Madahi H, Rostami F, Rahimi E, Dehkordi FS. Prevalence of enterotoxigenic *Staphylococcus aureus* isolated from chicken nugget in Iran. Jundishapur J Microbiol. 2014;7:e10237.
23. Castro A, Santos C, Meireles H, Silva J, Teixeira P. Food handlers as potential sources of dissemination of virulent strains of *Staphylococcus aureus* in the community. J Infect Publ Health. 2016;9:153–60.
24. Ferreira J, Costa W, Cerqueira E, Carvalho J, Oliveira L, Almeida R. Food handler-associated methicillin-resistant *Staphylococcus aureus* in public hospitals in Salvador, Brazil. Food Control. 2014;37:395–400.
25. Costa WLR, Ferreira JS, Carvalho JS, Cerqueira ES, Oliveira LC, Almeida RCDC. Methicillin-resistant *Staphylococcus aureus* in raw meats and prepared foods in public hospitals in Salvador, Bahia, Brazil. J Food Sci. 2015;80:M147–M50.
26. Ayçiçek H, Aydoğan H, Küçükkaraaslan A, Baysallar M, Başustaoğlu AC. Assessment of the bacterial contamination on hands of hospital food handlers. Food Control. 2004;15:253–9.
27. Kitai S, Shimizu A, Kawano J, Sato E, Nakano C, Kitagawa H, et al. Prevalence and characterization of *Staphylococcus aureus* and enterotoxigenic *Staphylococcus aureus* in retail raw chicken meat throughout Japan. J Vet Med Sci. 2005;67:269–74.

28. Normanno G, La Salandra G, Dambrosio A, Quaglia N, Corrente M, Parisi A, et al. Occurrence, characterization and antimicrobial resistance of enterotoxigenic *Staphylococcus aureus* isolated from meat and dairy products. Int J Food Microbiol. 2007;115:290–6.
29. Momtaz H, Dehkordi FS, Rahimi E, Asgarifar A, Momeni M. Virulence genes and antimicrobial resistance profiles of *Staphylococcus aureus* isolated from chicken meat in Isfahan province, Iran. J Appl Poult Res. 2013;22:913.
30. Paludi D, Vergara A, Festino AR, Di Ciccio P, Costanzo C, Conter M, et al. Antimicrobial resistance pattern of methicillin-resistant *Staphylococcus aureus* in the food industry. J Biol Regul Homeost Agents. 2011;25:671–7.
31. Sallam KI, Abd-Elghany SM, Elhadidy M, Tamura T. Molecular characterization and antimicrobial resistance profile of methicillin-resistant *Staphylococcus aureus* in retail chicken. J Food Prot. 2015;78:1879–84.
32. Jackson CR, Davis JA, Barrett JB. Prevalence and characterization of methicillin-resistant *Staphylococcus aureus* isolates from retail meat and humans in Georgia. J Clin Microbiol. 2013;51:1199–207.
33. Daka D, G/Silassie S, Yihdego D. Antibiotic-resistance *Staphylococcus aureus* isolated from cow's milk in the Hawassa area, South Ethiopia. Ann Clin Microbiol Antimicrob. 2012;11:26.
34. Fowoyo PT, Ogunbanwo ST. Antimicrobial resistance in coagulase-negative staphylococci from Nigerian traditional fermented foods. Ann Clin Microbiol Antimicrob. 2017;16:4.
35. Rong D, Wu Q, Xu M, Zhang J, Yu S. Prevalence, virulence genes, antimicrobial susceptibility, and genetic diversity of *Staphylococcus aureus* from retail aquatic products in China. Front Microbiol. 2017;8:714.
36. Kejela T, Bacha K. Prevalence and antibiotic susceptibility pattern of methicillin-resistant *Staphylococcus aureus* (MRSA) among primary school children and prisoners in Jimma town, Southwest Ethiopia. Ann Clin Microbiol Antimicrob. 2013;12:11.
37. Eko KE, Forshey BM, Carrel M, Schweizer ML, Perencevich EN, Smith TC. Molecular characterization of methicillin-resistant *Staphylococcus aureus* (MRSA) nasal colonization and infection isolates in a veterans affairs hospital. Antimicrob Resist Infect Control. 2015;4:10.
38. Zelazny AM, Ferraro MJ, Glennen A, Hindler JF, Mann LM, Munro S, et al. Selection of strains for quality assessment of the disk induction method for detection of inducible clindamycin resistance in staphylococci: a CLSI collaborative study. J Clin Microbiol. 2005;43:2613–5.
39. Kumar R, Yadav BR, Singh RS. Genetic determinants of antibiotic resistance in *Staphylococcus aureus* isolates from milk of mastitic crossbred cattle. Curr Microbiol. 2010;60:379–86.
40. Karataş E, Ekşi F, Zer Y. Investigation of antibiotic resistance genes and panton-valentine leucocidin in *Staphylococcus aureus* strains isolated from various clinical samples. Acta Medica Mediterr. 2017;33:341.
41. Simeoni D, Rizzotti L, Cocconcelli P, Gazzola S, Dellaglio F, Torriani S. Antibiotic resistance genes and identification of staphylococci collected from the production chain of swine meat commodities. Food Microbiol. 2008;25:196–201.
42. Johler S, Layer F, Stephan R. Comparison of virulence and antibiotic resistance genes of food poisoning outbreak isolates of *Staphylococcus aureus* with isolates obtained from bovine mastitis milk and pig carcasses. J Food Prot. 2011;74:1852–9.
43. Podkowik M, Bystroń J, Bania J. Prevalence of antibiotic resistance genes in staphylococci isolated from ready-to-eat meat products. Pol J Vet Sci. 2012; 15:233–7.

6

Behaviour change interventions to influence antimicrobial prescribing: a cross-sectional analysis of reports from UK state-of-the-art scientific conferences

T. M. Rawson[1*], L. S. P. Moore[1,3], A. M. Tivey[2], A. Tsao[2], M. Gilchrist[3], E. Charani[1] and A. H. Holmes[1,3]

Abstract

Background: To improve the quality of antimicrobial stewardship (AMS) interventions the application of behavioural sciences supported by multidisciplinary collaboration has been recommended. We analysed major UK scientific research conferences to investigate AMS behaviour change intervention reporting.

Methods: Leading UK 2015 scientific conference abstracts for 30 clinical specialties were identified and interrogated. All AMS and/or antimicrobial resistance(AMR) abstracts were identified using validated search criteria. Abstracts were independently reviewed by four researchers with reported behavioural interventions classified using a behaviour change taxonomy.

Results: Conferences ran for 110 days with >57,000 delegates. 311/12,313(2.5%) AMS-AMR abstracts (oral and poster) were identified. 118/311(40%) were presented at the UK's infectious diseases/microbiology conference. 56/311(18%) AMS-AMR abstracts described behaviour change interventions. These were identified across 12/30(40%) conferences. The commonest abstract reporting behaviour change interventions were quality improvement projects [44/56 (79%)]. In total 71 unique behaviour change functions were identified. Policy categories; "guidelines" (16/71) and "service provision" (11/71) were the most frequently reported. Intervention functions; "education" (6/71), "persuasion" (7/71), and "enablement" (9/71) were also common. Only infection and primary care conferences reported studies that contained multiple behaviour change interventions. The remaining 10 specialties tended to report a narrow range of interventions focusing on "guidelines" and "enablement".

Conclusion: Despite the benefits of behaviour change interventions on antimicrobial prescribing, very few AMS-AMR studies reported implementing them in 2015. AMS interventions must focus on promoting behaviour change towards antimicrobial prescribing. Greater focus must be placed on non-infection specialties to engage with the issue of behaviour change towards antimicrobial use.

Keywords: Antimicrobial Resistance, Stewardship, Quality improvement, Cross-specialty, Infection

* Correspondence: tmr07@ic.ac.uk; timothy.rawson07@imperial.ac.uk
[1]National Institute for Health Research Health Protection Research Unit in Healthcare Associated Infections and Antimicrobial Resistance, Imperial College London, Hammersmith Campus, Du Cane Road, London W12 0NN, UK
Full list of author information is available at the end of the article

Background

In the United Kingdom (UK), about one third of all hospital inpatients receive antimicrobials during their admission with a significant proportion of these identified as inappropriate [1–3]. This accounts for a large amount of unnecessary antimicrobial exposure. Antimicrobial resistance (AMR) is a leading patient safety issue that requires urgent interventions to curb its exponential growth. One target of interventions to address the problem of AMR is the promotion of the appropriate use of antimicrobials in humans, which is thought to be a leading driver for the growth of AMR [4].

To address this and promote the appropriate use of antimicrobial agents a number of national and international antimicrobial stewardship (AMS) initiatives have been implemented [5–8]. A key facet of these interventions targets improving and sustaining individual prescribing behaviours. Implementation of AMS programmes have been demonstrated to reduce rates of AMR and improve health and economic outcomes [9–11]. However, despite these positive steps forward, several challenges appear to remain in promoting the sustainable use of antimicrobials across clinical practice [12].

Firstly, there is a growing body of evidence to describe the cultural and social factors that influence antimicrobial prescribing across healthcare settings as well as qualitative data that supports the role of behaviour change interventions in improving antimicrobial prescribing [13–16]. Despite this, very little evidence exists to describe the current landscape of behaviour change interventions being implemented within this field [12, 13, 15–20]. Secondly, despite evidence to support engagement of infection specialists with the AMS-AMR agenda, there appears to be poorer engagement across other clinical specialties in terms of formal training and awareness at state-of-the-art scientific conferences [21–23]. Finally, although there are described frameworks and taxonomy's available from which to begin mapping behaviour change methods [24, 25], very little data is currently available to describe the appropriateness of these specifically for AMS interventions.

In this cross-sectional study we aimed to explore antimicrobial stewardship interventions reported at major cross specialty UK state-of-the-art scientific conferences in 2015, which contained behaviour change interventions. We aimed to determine the number and type of behaviour change interventions reported by different specialties and compare these to currently available behaviour change taxonomies to identify potential gaps and highlight potential targets for future interventions.

Methods

Abstract identification & screening

All major medical specialties recognised by the Royal College of Physicians, London, UK, were identified and included alongside major surgical specialties identified by the intercollegiate surgical curriculum programme. Psychiatric, paediatric, and obstetrics and gynaecology specialties were also included. UK specialists (specialist trainees or consultants) in each of the defined fields were consulted by email to determine the largest clinical scientific/research conference within the UK in 2015. Two specialists from each field, who were based in the North West London area were contacted for their opinions. Where there was disagreement, the authors opted for the conference with the largest attendance. Educational, continuing professional development and sub-specialty conferences were not considered for inclusion given their often focused agendas, which may have biased our findings.

Each major conference per specialty was identified and abstract booklets extracted and interrogated. Conference characteristics collated included; location, conference dates, estimated attendance and total number of abstracts accepted (either as oral, poster or publication only). Accepted conference abstracts (invited, oral, poster and publication only) were then identified and interrogated using a previously validated search criterion to identify all abstracts relating to AMS and AMR. [21, 22] All identified oral, poster, or published only abstracts from the search were then anonymously reviewed by two out of three authors (TMR, AMT, & AT). Abstracts were included if they were deemed to be describing an aspect of AMS [26] or AMR [27] in terms of direct effect on patients. In vitro studies with no translational benefit to individual patients were excluded. For the purpose of our investigation we focused on bacterial resistance and stewardship, abstracts relating solely to antiviral, antifungal, antiprotozoal or antimycobacterial resistance were excluded. This focus was selected given that anti-bacterial agents make up over 93% of all antimicrobials prescribed for systemic use [28]. Furthermore, the large variation in prescribing of other antimicrobial classes across different specialties may have influenced our results. When there was disparity between the opinions of reviewers' a fourth independent reviewer (LSPM) was consulted to reach consensus.

Characterising behaviour change interventions

Once all AMS-AMR abstracts had been identified the rates of AMS-AMR coverage between specialty conferences was assessed. Abstracts were then re-read by at least two of four researchers (TMR, AMT, AT, & LSPM) and categorised into types of intervention reported in the abstracts. To categorise the types of interventions reported a modified version of intervention and policy framework definitions provided by Michie and colleagues for the construction of their behaviour change wheel were used (Additional file 1: Table S1) [25]. In the original behaviour change wheel, three layers (policy, intervention, and behaviour systems are described). Within the classification used in this study, behaviour systems were not included (capability, opportunity, motivation, and behaviour; COM-B) as reported interventions were focused on the two levels of the framework above this, which aim to directly influence COM-B [25]. Researchers attempted, where possible, to categorise reported behaviour change interventions into one or more of the sixteen functions (split into policies and interventions) described within this framework. Although the framework is designed to provide flexibility and accommodate multiple interventions/policy combinations, researchers attempted to strictly categorise reported interventions into the fewest number of categories possible. When there was discrepancy the group discussed these issues until consensus was reached. Descriptive statistics was performed in SPSS 22.0 (IBM, Chicago, IL) with Chi-squared with Yates correction. Ethics approval was not required for this observational study.

Results

AMS-AMR coverage at UK state-of-the-art scientific conferences in 2015

Thirty specialty state-of-the-art scientific conferences abstract booklets were identified and extracted for analysis. These conferences ran over >110 days with >57,000 delegates estimated to of attended them in 2015 (Table 1). In total, 12,313 abstracts were extracted for analysis with 311

Table 1 UK state-of-the-art scientific conference summary

Speciality	City	Date commenced	No Days	No delegates	No abstracts accepted
Anaesthetics [44]	Edinburgh	23/09/2015	3	800	161
Breast Surgery [45]	Bournemouth	15/06/2015	2	870	221
Cardiology [46]	Manchester	08/06/2015	3	2448	235
Dermatology [47]	Manchester	06/07/2015	4	1200	372
Emergency Medicine [34]	Manchester	28/09/2015	3	650	69
Endocrinology [37]	Edinburgh	02/11/2015	3	1000	526
Gastroenterology [48]	London	22/06/2015	4	4500	1240
Primary Care [38]	Glasgow	01/10/2015	3	1600	450
General Surgery [49]	Manchester	22/04/2015	3	1500	1065
Surgery (ASiT) [50]	Glasgow	27/02/2015	3	700	602
Genitourinary Medicine [30]	Glasgow	01/06/2015	3	500	299
Geriatrics [36]	Brighton	14/10/2015	3	500	76
Haematology [51]	Edinburgh	20/04/2015	3	1000	257
Infection/Microbiology [29]	Glasgow	21/11/2015	3	1000	375
Intensive Care [52]	London	07/12/2015	3	1250	154
Nephrology [43]	London	28/05/2015	4	8190	1945
Neuro surgery [53]	York	09/09/2015	3	200	139
Neurology [33]	Harrogate	20/05/2015	3	600	194
Obstetrics & Gynaecology [54]	Brisbane	12/04/2015	4	2300	770
Ophthalmology [55]	Liverpool	18/05/2015	4	1700	228
Orthopaedics [31]	Liverpool	15/09/2015	4	1600	96
Paediatric surgery [56]	Cardiff	22/07/2015	3	346	83
Paediatrics [57]	Birmingham	28/04/2015	3	2000	546
Plastic surgery [32]	Birmingham	25/11/2015	3	400	78
Psychiatry [35]	Birmingham	29/06/2015	4	2500	79
Respiratory [58]	London	02/12/2015	3	2200	460
Rheumatology [59]	Manchester	28/04/2015	3	2000	677
Transplant surgery [60]	Bournemouth	11/03/2015	3	700	382
Urology [61]	Manchester	15/06/2015	4	1200	161
Vascular surgery [62]	Bournemouth	11/11/2015	3	800	373

(2.5%) identified as related to AMS-AMR (Fig. 1). Of these, 118/311 (38%) were presented at the UK's infectious diseases/microbiology conference [29]. This made up 38% (144/375) of all conference abstracts reported at this conference. Genitourinary medicine [30] had the second highest coverage with 9% (26/299), orthopaedics [31] third and plastic surgery [32] fourth with 8% of abstracts related to AMS-AMR each (8/96 & 6/78, respectively). All other specialty's had <5% AMS-AMR coverage with neurology [33], emergency medicine [34], psychiatry [35], geriatrics [36], and endocrinology [37] not having any AMS-AMR related coverage at their 2015 conferences. Compared to published data on conference coverage in the UK in 2014 [21] there was no significant difference in the level of AMS-AMR reporting (311/12,313, 2.5%, in 2015 & 221/7843, 2.8%, in 2014; $p = 0.22$). Infection/microbiology had a significantly larger proportion of AMS-AMR abstracts compared to all other specialties reviewed within this study ($p < 0.01$).

Reported behaviour change interventions for antimicrobial prescribing

Of the 311 AMS-AMR abstracts identified 56 (18%) described behaviour change interventions (Table 2). Of these, 28/56 (50%) were reported at the infection/microbiology conference with general surgery conferences reporting the second largest proportion with 7/56 (13%). In total, behaviour change interventions were reported across 12/30 (40%) specialty state-of-the-art conferences with infection/microbiology reporting a significantly greater amount that all other conferences ($p < 0.01$). The commonest abstracts reporting behaviour change interventions were quality improvement projects accounting for 44/56 (79%) of all reported behaviour change interventions. However, this represented a minority of all AMS-AMR quality improvement projects identified with 80/124 (65%) either not reporting any intervention or not reporting a specific behaviour change intervention. The remainder of behaviour change interventions included were found to be reported within observational studies (12/56; 21%). This also represented a minority of observational studies reporting AMS-AMR topics across clinical specialties (12/54; 22%).

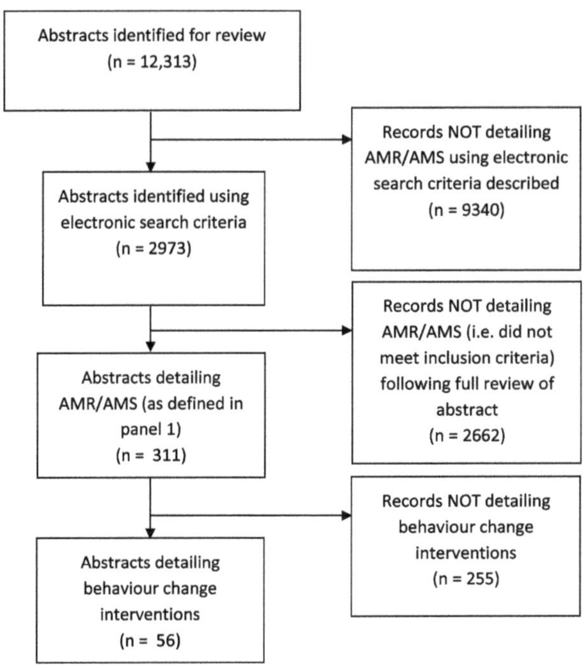

Fig. 1 Selection method to identify antimicrobial stewardship/antimicrobial resistance abstracts among state-of-the-art conferences in 2015

In total, 71 unique behaviour change functions were identified across the 56 abstracts reported behaviour change interventions (Table 2). Eight abstracts were deemed to describe multiple behaviour change interventions with six of these being reported at the infectious diseases/microbiology conference [29] and two at the primary care conference [38]. Policy categories; "guidelines" (16/71) and "service provision" (11/71) were the most frequently reported. Intervention functions; "education" (6/71), "persuasion" (7/71), "enablement" (9/71), and environmental restructuring (9/71) were also common. Intervention categories "incentivisation" and "coercion" and policy categories "fiscal" and "legislation" were not reported in any interventions. However, only infection/microbiology and primary care tended to report a broad variety of interventions, with the majority of interventions reported in the remaining ten specialties tending to focus on enablement (intervention) and guidelines or service provision (policy). The types of functions reported in abstracts that described multiple behaviour change interventions (8/56; 14%) are highlighted in Table 3. In abstracts reporting multiple behaviour change intervention functions there was a mix of policy and intervention targets with guidelines featuring in 6/8 (75%), environmental restructuring, education and persuasion all featuring in 4/8 (50%), and service provision in 3/8 (38%) of the abstracts.

Discussion

Clinical state-of-the-art conferences provide an opportunity for medical professionals to participate in research and reporting. They also allow us to gain an insight into different levels of research being undertaken within the field; from small scale research undertaken at the local level, to large scale studies being performed by key opinion leaders and organisations. This provides a window into the activities within specialties that is less influenced by publication bias than can often be observed through systematically reviewing peer-reviewed

Table 2 Outline of behavioural interventions reported per UK specialty

	Education	Persuasion	Incentivise	Coercion	Training	Restriction	Environmental restructure	Modelling	Enablement	Communication	Guidelines	Fiscal	Regulation	Legislation	Environmental	Service provision
Endocrinology																
Geriatrics																
Psychiatry																
Emergency Medicine																
Neurology																
Cardiology																
Ophthalmology																
Paediatric surgery																
Paediatrics											1					
Anaesthetics																
Breast Surgery																
Vascular surgery																
Obstetrics & Gynaecology																
Intensive Care											1					
Neurosurgery								1								
Transplant Surgery																
Dermatology																1
Haematology																
Urology											1					1
Plastic Surgery																
Gastroenterology											1					
Respiratory																
Orthopaedics								1			1					
Rheumatology																
General Surgery (ASiT)	1						1		1				1			
Primary Care	2[a]	2[a]					1[a]	1	1		2[a]					
Nephrology									1		1					
Genitourinary Medicine																
General Surgery							2		1		2		1			1
Infection/ Microbiology	3[a]	5[a]			1	1	5[a]		5	2[a]	6[a]		1		2[a]	8[a]

Legend: [a]Interventions may have been part of a bundle of interventions reported in one abstract
NB. One behaviour change intervention has been excluded as the full nature of the intervention was not clearly defined

Table 3 Outline of intervention functions reported in abstracts reporting multiple behaviour change interventions

Primary Care	1.	Guideline, persuasion, & modelling
	2.	Education, persuasion & environmental restructuring
Infection/Microbiology	3.	Guideline, persuasion & environmental
	4.	Guideline, persuasion & service provision
	5.	Guideline, environmental restructuring, education, communication
	6.	Guideline, education, service provision, environmental restructure
	7.	Guideline & service provision
	8.	Education & environmental restructuring

publications. Within this study, we observed a low rate of behaviour change intervention reporting across the majority of specialty state-of-the-art conferences in 2015. Infection specialties reported a significantly greater number and broader variety of AMS-AMR interventions with the majority of interventions reported by non-infection specialties falling into a narrow band of intervention and policy based functions.

These observations are concerning given the recent focus placed upon the need for cross-specialty engagement with AMS-AMR and behaviour change interventions. This has been supported broadly in the literature [4, 13, 16, 21, 22, 39]; by national organisations including Public Health England (PHE) [18], the British Society for Antimicrobial Chemotherapy (BSAC), and government [40]; and major international governments and organisations [6, 7]. These findings highlight the need to broaden the focus of AMS campaigns beyond infection specialties to promote leadership from within cohorts, which can drive behaviour change towards antimicrobial use.

This must be supported by clear and defined tools to help specialties engage and design AMS-AMR behaviour change interventions and assess the impact of these on patient outcomes. Whilst the use of behaviour change taxonomies allows content of interventions to be coded and categorised, facilitating the analysis of behaviour change interventions [24, 41], they are not appropriate for determining the effectiveness of interventions. Furthermore, for the field of AMS-AMR there remains no definition on what an appropriate behaviour change intervention is. This makes evaluating behaviour change challenging as certain functions of any framework used may be irrelevant or actually have a negative impact on behaviours within this context. [24, 41, 42] Kok and colleagues argue that as behavioural determinants are often specific to behaviours, populations, and contexts characterisations should thus be individualised and tailored for such [24, 41]. This will require engagement and drive from within clinical specialties to review current practices, define the context in which AMS-AMR interventions need to be implemented, and then tailor behaviour change interventions to optimise their effect within their local environment.

Finally, in a previous study "high risk" specialties were identified that currently use large amounts of antimicrobials and also experience high levels of healthcare associated infections [21]. This study reported that certain "high risk" specialties such as infection and intensive care had relatively high levels of engagement with AMS-AMR, whilst other specialties such as haematology and nephology tended to have a low apparent engagement at scientific conferences [21]. Within this study, we have observed an overall low rate of behaviour change interventions across all high risk specialties reported previously with only infection [29] and nephrology [43] reporting any behaviour change interventions in 2015. Furthermore, specialties with relatively high coverage of AMS-AMR at scientific conferences, such as Genitourinary Medicine, failed to report on behaviour change interventions despite having 9% coverage of AMS-AMR topics in 2015. This highlights the need for greater pan-specialty promotion of behaviour change interventions for AMS-AMR given the significant lack of focus on reporting such interventions currently.

There are several limitations to this study. Firstly, we only selected one leading state-of-the-art conference for each major clinical specialty in the UK. This makes our findings difficult to generalise across other countries and also may have introduced bias through excluding smaller, conferences and meetings, where specialties may have had more of an AMS-AMR focus. However, this method was selected as we aimed to generate a representative picture of current behaviour change interventions and the importance placed upon this by different specialties. By selecting leading state-of-the-art conferences we hoped that this would reflect the current overall importance of this subject within the specialty as well as allow for a more representative view of work being undertaken in the field. Secondly, we did not review invited talks and seminars provided by conferences given that they often were not presenting original data or results. Furthermore, as the taxonomy used to describe behaviour change does not allow for evaluation of the effectiveness of interventions it is not possible to evaluate whether interventions described were "appropriate" for the context in which they were described. Finally, as only a relatively small number of specialists from a specific geographical area were contacted to seek opinions on defining the largest UK conference in their field this may have introduced bias in our conference selection. To address this we ensured that two specialists from each field were contacted for their opinions. When there was discrepancy in responses from the individuals, conference attendance size was considered as the determinant with the conference with the largest attendance selected.

Conclusion

In conclusion, despite evidence to support the role of behaviour change interventions for improving antimicrobial prescribing, very few studies reported implementing them at UK state-of-the-art conferences in 2015. Future research must focus on providing appropriate frameworks and mechanisms to allow clinical specialties to engage with AMS-AMR and design and evaluate the impact of behaviour change interventions within their specific contexts.

Acknowledgements
The authors would like to thank members of Imperial College NHS Healthcare Trust who participated in the study. The authors would also like to acknowledge the National Institute of Health Research Imperial Biomedical Research Centre and the National Institute for Health Research Health Protection Research Unit (NIHR HPRU) in Healthcare Associated Infection and Antimicrobial Resistance at Imperial College London in partnership with Public Health England and the NIHR Imperial Patient Safety Translational Research Centre. The views expressed in this publication are those of the authors and not necessarily those of the NHS, the National Institute for Health Research or the UK Department of Health.

Funding
This report is independent research funded by the National Institute for Health Research Invention for Innovation (i4i) programme, Enhanced, Personalized and Integrated Care for Infection Management at Point of Care (EPIC IMPOC), II-LA-0214-20008.

Authors' contributions
TMR, LSPM, & AH conceived the study design. TMR, EC, ANT, AT, & LSMP extracted and analysed the data. TMR drafted the initial manuscript. All authors (TMR, LSPM, EC, AT, ANT, MG, & AH) reviewed and contributed significantly to revision of the manuscript, agreeing on the final format for submission to ARIC.

Competing interests
The authors declare that they have no competing interests.

Consent for publication
Not applicable.

Author details
[1]National Institute for Health Research Health Protection Research Unit in Healthcare Associated Infections and Antimicrobial Resistance, Imperial College London, Hammersmith Campus, Du Cane Road, London W12 0NN, UK. [2]Imperial College School of Medicine, Imperial College London, South Kensington Campus, London SW7 2AZ, UK. [3]Imperial College Healthcare NHS Trust, Hammersmith Hospital, Du Cane Road, London W12 0HS, UK.

References

1. English surveillance programme for antimicrobial utilisation and resistance (ESPAUR). 2014. Available at: https://www.gov.uk/government/uploads/system/uploads/attachment_data/file/362374/ESPAUR_Report_2014__3_.pdf. Accessed 3 Oct 2016.
2. ESPAUR. English surveillance programme for antimicrobial utilisation and resistance (ESPAUR) 2010 to 2014 Report 2015 About Public Health England. 2015.
3. Raveh D, Levy Y, Schlesinger Y, Greenberg A, Rudensky B, Yinnon AM. Longitudinal surveillance of antibiotic use in the hospital. QJM. 2001; 94:141–52.
4. Holmes AH, Moore LSP, Sundsfjord A, et al. Understanding the mechanisms and drivers of antimicrobial resistance. Lancet. 2015;6736: Available at: http://linkinghub.elsevier.com/retrieve/pii/S0140673615004730.
5. Dellit TH, Owens RC, McGowan JE, et al. Infectious Diseases Society of America and the Society for Healthcare Epidemiology of America Guidelines for Developing an Institutional Program to Enhance Antimicrobial Stewardship. Clin Infect Dis. 2007;44:159–77.
6. Cruickshank M. Antimicrobial stewardship in Australian hospitals. 2011. Available at: http://www.safetyandquality.gov.au/wp-content/uploads/2011/01/Antimicrobial-stewardship-in-Australian-Hospitals-2011.pdf.
7. Core Elements of Hospital Antibiotic Stewardship Programs. 2014: 1–25. Available at: http://www.cdc.gov/getsmart/healthcare/implementation/core-elements.html. Accessed 3 Oct 2016.
8. ESPAUR SSTF Implementation subgroup. Start Smart - Then Focus Antimicrobial Stewardship Toolkit for English Hospitals. 2015. Available at: https://www.gov.uk/government/uploads/system/uploads/attachment_data/file/417032/Start_Smart_Then_Focus_FINAL.PDF.
9. Macdougall C, Polk RE, Campus V. Antimicrobial Stewardship Programs in Health Care Systems. Clin Microbiol Rev. 2005;18:638–56.
10. Roberts RR, Hota B, Ahmad I, et al. Hospital and societal costs of antimicrobial-resistant infections in a Chicago teaching hospital: implications for antibiotic stewardship. Clin Infect Dis. 2009;49:1175–84.
11. Raymond DP, Pelletier SJ, Crabtree TD, et al. Impact of a rotating empiric antibiotic schedule on infectious mortality in an intensive care unit. Crit Care Med. 2001;29:1101–8.
12. Charani E, Cooke J, Holmes A. Antibiotic stewardship programmes-what's missing? J Antimicrob Chemother. 2010;65:2275–7.
13. Charani E, Edwards R, Sevdalis N, et al. Behavior change strategies to influence antimicrobial prescribing in acute care: a systematic review. Clin Infect Dis. 2011;53:651–62.
14. Rawson TM, Charani E, Moore LSP, et al. Mapping the decision pathways of acute infection management in secondary care among UK medical physicians: A qualitative study. BMC Med. 2016;14:1–10.
15. Charani E, Castro-Sanchez E, Sevdalis N, et al. Understanding the determinants of antimicrobial prescribing within hospitals: The role of 'prescribing etiquette'. Clin Infect Dis. 2013;57:188–96.
16. Davey P, Brown E, Charani E, et al. Interventions to improve antibiotic prescribing practices for hospital inpatients. Cochrane Database Syst Rev. 2013. Available at: http://onlinelibrary.wiley.com/doi/10.1002/14651858.CD003543.pub3/full .
17. Skodvin B, Aase K, Charani E, Holmes A, Smith I. An antimicrobial stewardship program initiative: a qualitative study on prescribing practices among hospital doctors. Antimicrob Resist Infect Control. 2015;4:24. Available at: http://dx.doi.org/10.1186/s13756-015-0065-4.
18. Public Health England, Department of Health. Behaviour change and antibiotic prescribing in healthcare settings Literature review and behavioural analysis. 2015. Available at: https://www.gov.uk/government/uploads/system/uploads/attachment_data/file/405031/Behaviour_Change_for_Antibiotic_Prescribing_-_FINAL.pdf.
19. Teixeira Rodrigues A, Roque F, Falcão A, Figueiras A, Herdeiro MT. Understanding physician antibiotic prescribing behaviour: A systematic review of qualitative studies. Int J Antimicrob Agents. 2013;41:203–12.
20. Teixeira Rodrigues A, Ferreira M, Piñeiro-Lamas M, Falcão A, Figueiras A, Herdeiro MT. Determinants of physician antibiotic prescribing behaviour: a 3-year cohort study in Portugal. Curr Med Res Opin. 2016;7995:1–24.
21. Rawson TM, Moore LSP, Gilchrist MJ, Holmes AH. Antimicrobial stewardship: are we failing in cross-specialty clinical engagement? J Antimicrob Chemother. 2015;dkv337: Available at: http://www.jac.oxfordjournals.org/lookup/doi/10.1093/jac/dkv337.
22. Rawson TM, Butters TP, Moore LSP, Castro-Sánchez E, Cooke FJ, Holmes AH. Exploring the coverage of antimicrobial stewardship across UK clinical postgraduate training curricula. J Antimicrob Chemother. 2016;dkw280: Available at: http://www.jac.oxfordjournals.org/lookup/doi/10.1093/jac/dkw280.
23. Castro-Sánchez E, Drumright LN, Gharbi M, Farrell S, Holmes AH. Mapping antimicrobial stewardship in undergraduate medical, dental, pharmacy, nursing and veterinary education in the United Kingdom. PLoS One. 2016;11:1–10.

24. Kok G, Gottlieb NH, Peters G-JY, et al. A Taxonomy of Behavior Change Methods; an Intervention Mapping Approach. Health Psychol Rev. 2015;31:1–32.
25. Michie S, van Stralen MM, West R. The behaviour change wheel: a new method for characterising and designing behaviour change interventions. Implement Sci. 2011;6:42. Available at: http://www.pubmedcentral.nih.gov/articlerender.fcgi?artid=3096582&tool=pmcentrez&rendertype=abstract.
26. Pope SD, Dellit TH, Owens RC, Hooton TM. Results of survey on implementation of Infectious Diseases Society of America and Society for Healthcare Epidemiology of America guidelines for developing an institutional program to enhance antimicrobial stewardship. Infect Control Hosp Epidemiol. 2009;30:97–8.
27. WHO. Antimicrobial Resistance Global Report on Surveillance 2014. World Heal Organ 2014. Available at: http://www.who.int/drugresistance/documents/surveillancereport/en/.
28. European Surveillence of Antimicrobial Consumption. Report on Point Prevalence Survey of Antimicrobial Prescription in European Hospitals, 2009. 2009. Available at: http://ecdc.europa.eu/en/activities/surveillance/ESAC-Net/publications/Documents/report_survey_antimicrobial_prescriptions_eu_hospitals_2009.pdf. Accessed 3 Oct 2016.
29. Federation of Infection Society, Glasgow, 2015. In: Federation of Infection Society annual conference 2015. 2015
30. BASHH Spring Conference 2015 Abstract Presentations 1–3 June 2015 Royal Concert Halls, Glasgow, Scotland. In: Sexually Transmitted Infections (STI). Vol 91, 2015; A1–104. Available at: https://www.bashh.org/documents/Final%20BASHH%202015%20Abstract%20book.pdf/. Accessed 3 Oct 2016.
31. British Orthopaedic Association Annual Congress 2015, 15–18 September - ACC Liverpool. In: British Orthopaedic Association. Liverpool, 2015
32. Winter Scientific Meeting 25–17 November 2015, The Vox Conference Centre, Resorts World Birmingham. In: British Association of Plastic Reconstructive and Aesthetic Surgeons. Birmingham, 2015
33. ABN Annual Meeting 2015 19–22 May 2015 - Harrogate International Centre, Harrogate. Assoc Br Neurol 2015. Available at: http://www.theabn.org/events/abn-events/harrogate.html. Accessed 3 Oct 2016.
34. Abstracts from UK EM 2015. Emerg Med J 2015; 32. Available at: http://emj.bmj.com/lookup/doi/10.1136/emermed-2015-205511. Accessed 3 Oct 2016.
35. The Royal College of Psychiatrists' International Congress 29 June - 2 July 2015 Birmingham, 2015. Available at: http://www.rcpsych.ac.uk/pdf/Full%20Programme%20web%20v56.pdf.
36. British Geriatrics Society. Abstracts of work presented at the 2015 BGS Autumn Meeting: Promoting better health in old age, Brighton, 2015. Available at: http://www.bgs.org.uk/pdf_cms/admin_archive/2015_autumn_abstracts.pdf.
37. Endocrine Abstracts. In: Society for Endocrinology BES 2015. Vol 38., 2015
38. Expanding horizons of care. In: Annual Primary Care Conference 2015., 2015
39. Ashiru-oredope D, Sharland M, Charani E, McNulty C, Cooke J. Improving the quality of antibiotic prescribing in the nhs by developing a new antimicrobial stewardship programme: Start smart-then focus. J Antimicrob Chemother. 2012;67:i51–63.
40. O'Neill J. Tackling Drug-Resistant Infections Globally: Final Report and Recommendations the Review on. 2016. Available at: https://amr-review.org/sites/default/files/160525_Final%20paper_with%20cover.pdf.
41. Kok G, Gottlieb NH, Peters G-JY, et al. Tables and Figure for: A Taxonomy of Behavior Change Methods; an Intervention Mapping Approach. Health Psychol Rev. 2015;31:1–32. Available at: http://dx.doi.org/10.1080/17437199.2015.1077155.
42. Kwasnicka D, Dombrowski SU, White M, Sniehotta F. Theoretical explanations for maintenance of behaviour change: a systematic review of behaviour theories. Health Psychol Rev. 2016;7199:1–39.
43. 53rd ERA-EDTA Congress Abstracts2View™. Eur Ren Assoc Conf 2015. Available at: http://www.abstracts2view.com/era/. Accessed 3 Oct 2016.
44. Abstracts of the AAGBI Annual Congress, 23–25 September 2015, Edinburgh, UK. Anaesthesia. 2015;70(4 Suppl):1–91. doi:10.1111/anae.13223.
45. ABS Conference Annual Meeting - 2015. In: Association of Breast Surgery., 2015. Available at: http://www.associationofbreastsurgery.org.uk/abs-events/past-meetings/abs-conference-agm-2015/. Accessed 3 Oct 2016.
46. BCS annual conference, 'Hearts and Genes' June 8–10, Manchester, UK, 2015. Heart 2015; 101. Available at: http://heart.bmj.com/content/101/Suppl_4.toc#Clinical. Accessed 3 Oct 2016.
47. British Association of Dermatologists Annual Meeting, 2015, Manchester. Br J Dermatol 2015; 173: 1–2. Available at: http://doi.wiley.com/10.1111/bjd.13800. Accessed 3 Oct 2016
48. 2nd Digestive Disorders Federation Conference 22–25 June 2015 Abstracts. Gut 2015. Available at: http://gut.bmj.com/content/64/Suppl_1.toc. Accessed 3 Oct 2016.
49. ASGBI abstracts. Br J Surg 2015; 102: 88–177. Available at: http://doi.wiley.com/10.1002/bjs.9941. Accessed 3 Oct 2016.
50. The Association of Surgeons in Training Conference: #ASiT2015 Glasgow. Int J Surg 2015; 23: S1–4. Available at: http://linkinghub.elsevier.com/retrieve/pii/S1743919115012935.
51. Abstracts of the 55th Annual Scientific Meeting of the British Society for Haematology, 20–22 April 2015, Edinburgh, UK. In: British Journal of Haematology. Vol 169., 2015; 1–104. Available at: http://doi.wiley.com/10.1111/bjh.13350. Accessed 3 Oct 2016.
52. State of the Art Scientific Abstracts. J Intensive Care Soc 2015; 16. Available at: http://inc.sagepub.com/lookup/doi/10.1177/1751143715615276. Accessed 3 Oct 2016
53. Proceedings of the Society of British Neurological Surgeons: 58th Meeting. In: Journal of Neurology, Neurosurgery & Psychiatry. 2015. Available at: http://jnnp.bmj.com/cgi/doi/10.1136/jnnp.22.1.77 . Accessed 3 Oct 2016.
54. Abstracts of the RCOG World Congress 2015, 12–15 April, Brisbane, Queensland, Australia. In: Royal College of Obstetrics & Gynaecology. Vol 122., 2015; 1–414. Available at: http://onlinelibrary.wiley.com/doi/10.1111/1471-0528.13365/abstract. Accessed 3 Oct 2016.
55. Annual Congress 2015, 19–21 May 2015 - The ACC Liverpool. In: The Royal College of Ophthalmologists. 2015
56. BAPS Papers. In: Journal of Pediatric Surgery. Vol 51., 2016. Available at: http://www.sciencedirect.com/science/journal/00223468/51/2. Accessed 4 Oct 2016.
57. Royal College of Paediatrics and Child Health, Abstracts of the Annual Conference, 28–30 April 2015, The ICC, Birmingham. 2015. Available at: http://adc.bmj.com/content/100/Suppl_3.toc. Accessed 3 Oct 2016.
58. British Thoracic Society Winter Meeting, The Queen Elizabeth II Centre Broad Sanctuary Westminster London SW1P 3EE 2 to 4 December 2015 Programme and Abstracts. In: Thorax., 2015; Vol 70; Suppl 3. Available at: http://thorax.bmj.com/content/70/Suppl_3.toc.
59. Rheumatology 2015 Abstracts. In: Rhematology., 2015; Volume 54 suppl 1. Available at: http://rheumatology.oxfordjournals.org/content/54/suppl_1.toc. Accessed 3 Oct 2016.
60. British Transplantation Society and Nederlandse Transplantatie Vereniging Joint Congress 2015. In: British Transplantation Society. Bournemouth, 2015. Available at: http://www.btscongress.com/abstracts.html.
61. BAUS 2015 Annual Scientific Meeting. Br Assoc Urol Surg 2015. Available at: http://baus.multilearning.com/baus/#!*menu = 6*browseby = 7*sortby = 1*media = 3*ce_id = 822.
62. Special Issue: VSGBI abstracts from The Vascular Societies' Annual Scientific Meeting, 11–13 November 2015. Br J Surg 2016; 103: 1–30. Available at: http://doi.wiley.com/10.1002/bjs.10271.

The knowledge, attitudes and practices of doctors regarding antibiotic resistance at a tertiary care institution in the Caribbean

Alison Nicholson[1*], Ingrid Tennant[2], Livingston White[3], Camille-Ann Thoms-Rodriguez[1], Loraine Cook[4], Stephen Johnson[5], Tamara Thompson[6], Jasper Barnett[7] and Lundie Richards[7]

Abstract

Background: Antibiotic resistance (ABR) is a serious threat that requires coordinated global intervention to prevent its spread. There is limited data from the English-speaking Caribbean.

Methods: As part of a national programme to address antibiotic resistance in Jamaica, a survey of the knowledge, attitudes and antibiotic prescribing practices of Jamaican physicians was conducted using a 32-item self-administered questionnaire.

Results: Of the eight hundred physicians targeted, 87% responded. The majority thought the problem of resistance very important globally (82%), less nationally (73%) and even less (53%) in personal practices. Hospital physicians were more likely to consider antibiotic resistance important in their practice compared to those in outpatient practice or both ($p < 0.001$). Composite knowledge scores were generated and considered good if scored > 80%, average if 60–79% and poor if < 60%. Most had good knowledge of factors preventing resistance (83%) and resistance inducing potential of specific antibiotics (59%), but only average knowledge of factors contributing to resistance (57%). Knowledge of preventative factors was highest in females ($p = 0.004$), those with postgraduate training ($p = 0.001$) and those > four years post graduation ($p = 0.03$). Empiric therapy was often directed by international guidelines and cultures were not routinely done. Limited laboratory and human resources were identified as challenges.

Conclusion: Physicians in this study were aware of the problem of ABR, but downplayed its significance nationally and personally. These results will guide a national antibiotic stewardship programme.

Keywords: Antibiotic, Prescribing, Practices, Resistance, Knowledge, Attitudes

Background

Antibiotic resistance (ABR) has emerged as a significant threat to the quality of health care in the twenty-first century [1]. This, combined with decreased production of new antimicrobial agents, has precipitated a global crisis with the emergence of bacteria resistant to most antibiotics [2–5].

The inability of previously effective antibiotics to treat common bacterial infections has far reaching consequences [1]. The success of many modern advancements in medicine is predicated on the availability and efficacy of antibiotics. These include surgery using prostheses, organ transplantation and chemotherapy [4]. The effects of ABR extend beyond increased mortality (63,000/year in the US and 25,000/year in the EU) [6] and morbidity to include increased hospital stay and costs. In the USA, ABR has been estimated to cost over 55 billion dollars per annum [7]. In Europe, estimated costs are at least €1.5 billion per year [6]. However, the real costs are higher when the impact of ABR on the entire health care system and national productivity is taken into account.

Of the over 20 countries in the English speaking Caribbean, data on antibiotic resistance are limited largely to reports from Jamaica, Trinidad and Tobago and Barbados [8–13]. This is concerning, as the Caribbean is a popular destination especially for North

* Correspondence: alison.nicholson@uwimona.edu.jm
[1]Department of Microbiology, The University of the West Indies (UWI), Kingston, Jamaica
Full list of author information is available at the end of the article

Americans and Europeans and this would have implications for the types of multiple drug resistant organisms (MDROs) present. A multiple drug resistant organism is defined as one that is resistant to one or more drugs in three or more drug classes [14]. In Jamaica, globally recognized "problem organisms" that have been identified include Methicillin resistant *Staphylococcus aureus* (MRSA), extended spectrum betalactamases (ESBL) *Klebsiella pneumoniae, Escherichia coli* and *Enterobacter sp.*, New Delhi metallo-beta-lactamase (NDM-1) *Klebsiella pneumoniae,* carbapenem resistant *Pseudomonas aeruginosa* and *Acinetobacter spp.* as well as Vancomycin resistant Enterococcus (VRE) [13, 15–17]. A 2009 study in a university-affiliated hospital in Kingston, Jamaica showed that resistance among Gram-positive organisms was much lower than among Gram-negative organisms [16].

Antimicrobial abuse is an important cause of ABR and is a compelling target for attention. "Antimicrobial abuse" is an umbrella term for a wide range of breaches including overuse, inappropriate choice, incorrect dosage, incorrect duration of therapy, incorrect dosing interval and suboptimal route of delivery [4, 18].

A single-centre study from Jamaica showed that although physicians were aware of ABR and contributing factors, this did not influence their prescribing practices [19]. With a desire to slow the emergence of antimicrobial resistance by determining the strategies necessary to improve prescribing practices among Jamaican physicians, a much larger all island multicentre study was carried out.

Methods

Aim and study design

A cross-sectional study was performed to identify the knowledge, attitudes and practices of Jamaican physicians towards antibiotic resistance and antibiotic prescribing practices. This information will help in the development of national antibiotic guidelines and workshops for healthcare workers. A problem with such strong global significance requires every country to define its challenges and make its voice heard.

Study sampling and study instrument

This study was conducted across Jamaica, the third largest Caribbean island, 11,424 km^2, with a population of approximately 2.8 million [20, 21]. Approximately 4000 public and private doctors were identified as currently providing medical care from national registration records (Jamaican Medical Council). We targeted 20% or 800 doctors. With this sample size, we calculated that we would have a margin of error of 4% and a 99% confidence level, assuming a conservative response distribution of 50%. We recruited through medical conferences, hospital meetings and visits to private practices across the four Jamaican health regions- South, Southeast, Northeast and West. Physician registration with the local medical council requires regular attendance at conferences or meetings to obtain continuing medical education credits (CMEs). In addition, we did not target microbiological conferences or those on antibiotics or resistance, but included a wide cross-section of meetings. Therefore, we do not believe that our sample was biased towards physicians with better knowledge of ABR. Data collection was done between October 2014 and September 2015.

The instrument used was a 32-item self-administered questionnaire comprising questions related to demographics (eight questions), knowledge (six questions), attitudes (five questions) and practices associated with antibiotic use (13 questions). Ethical approval was obtained from the Faculty of Medical Sciences, UWI (ECP 183 13/14) and Ministry of Health (MOH) Ethics Committees (2014/26) and informed consent was obtained from each participant.

Data analysis

Data were analysed using Statistical Analysis in the Social Sciences (SPSS) version 19 and correlations assessed using the Chi-square test. A p-value of less than 0.05 was considered statistically significant.

Physicians' knowledge of factors contributing to development of ABR and factors useful in containing resistance were examined. Each factor was analyzed on a scale of 0 to 3 (0 = don't know, 1 = minimally important, 2 = moderately important and 3 = very important) and showed how the respondents ranked their importance. Knowledge of antibiotics more prone to inducing resistance was also assessed, and each was scored between 0 and 2 (0 = don't know, 1 = less likely, 2 = more likely).

Composite knowledge scores were also calculated. The first score *"Factors contributing to development of ABR"*, represents a computation of 9 variables, each with 4 categories scored from 0 to 3 as follows: 0 = Don't Know, 1 = Minimally Important, 2 = Moderately Important, 3 = Very Important. To ensure the variables were compatible with parametric analysis, the scale variable was converted to an ordinal variable; created by recoding into the following categories (9 to15 = Poor knowledge; 16 to 21 = Average knowledge, 22 to 27 = Good knowledge). This score was then cross-tabulated against physician variables to determine significant predictors.

The second score *"Factors useful in containing resistance"* was created from 8 variables, each with four categories (0 = Don't Know, 1 = Not Useful, 2 = May be useful, 3 = Useful). This scale was recoded into three categories (Poor knowledge = 8–12; Average knowledge = 13–16; Good knowledge = 17–24).

The third score *"Antibiotics more prone to inducing resistance"* (which refers to the potential of an antibiotic to cause the emergence of resistance over time [22]) was created from 7 variables, each with three categories (0 = Don't Know, 1 = Less likely, 2 = More likely). The overall score was calculated based on the number of correct responses, with a maximum of 14 points. This scale was recoded into three categories; (Poor knowledge = 0–4; Average knowledge = 5–9; Good knowledge = 10–14).

Reliability analyses using Cronbach alpha were done to determine the level of internal consistency among the items comprising the individual scales. Results indicated high Cronbach's alpha scores of 0.749 to 0.859 for most of the scales. Only *"Factors contributing to development of ABR"* had a lower Cronbach's alpha of 0.631, which is still acceptable [23].

Results

Respondent demographics

A total of 695 physicians completed the questionnaire, a response rate of 87%, with 51% female. The majority stated that their practice was mainly hospital based (60%) and 51% had postgraduate training. About a third (32%) were less than four years post registration and 33% were residents. (Table 1) The Southeast region accounted for 62% of the respondents, the Western region 22%, the Northeast region 5% and the Southern region 11%. This corresponded fairly well with data from the Ministry of Health, which indicated the following distribution of physicians: Southeast region 55%, Western region 20%, Northeast 15% and South 10% (J Barnett, pers. comm.).

Opinion on the magnitude of the problem

Most of the respondents (82%) felt the global problem of ABR was very important, but less considered the national problem very important (73%). In their personal practice, however, only 53% assessed resistance as being very important; and 15% did not think it was important at all. Hospital physicians were more likely to consider ABR very important in their practice than outpatient-based, or physicians who practiced in both areas (65% vs. 39% and 35% respectively, $p < 0.001$).

Knowledge

Factors contributing to resistance

Widespread use of antibiotics was thought to be most important, with a mean score of 2.79 ± 0.48 followed by overuse of broad-spectrum antibiotics (2.74 ± 0.55) and inappropriate use of antibiotics (2.61 ± 0.60). Inadequate hand washing (1.47 ± 0.95) and use of antibiotics in the livestock industry (1.41 ± 1.03) were considered least important. (Table 2).

Table 1 Physician Demographics

	Category	Frequency	Percent
Gender	Male	338	49%
	Female	348	51%
Current Practice	Mainly hospital based	387	60%
	Mainly outpatient or clinic based	158	25%
	An equal proportion of both	97	15%
	Total	642	100%
Position	Intern/SHO	118	17%
	Intern/resident	186	27%
	Senior/chief resident	43	6%
	Consultant	156	22%
	Private GP	120	17%
	Specialist private practice	38	5%
	Government clinic medical officer	34	5%
	Total	695	100%
Postgraduate Training	Yes	338	51%
	No	328	49%
	Total	666	100%
Specialty	Anaesthesia/intensive care	56	17
	Internal medicine	64	19
	Surgical specialty	102	31
	Paediatrics	27	8
	Obstetrics and gynaecology	24	7
	Accident and emergency	13	4
	Family medicine	42	13
	Clinical microbiologist	6	2
	Total	334	100%
Years Post Registration	0–4 years	218	32%
	5–9 years	130	19%
	10–14 years	87	13%
	15–19 years	61	9%
	>_ 20 years	176	26%
	Total	672	100%

N.B. Total sample size for this study is 695. Differences in totals for each subsection occur because of missing values

Based on their overall score, the majority (57.4%) had average knowledge, 29.2% had good knowledge and 13.5% had poor knowledge of factors contributing to ABR. Higher knowledge of these factors was positively

Table 2 Knowledge of Factors Contributing to Antibiotic Resistance

	Mean	SD
Widespread use of antibiotics	2.79	.48
Overuse of broad spectrum antibiotics	2.74	.55
Inappropriate use of antibiotic therapy	2.61	.60
Inappropriate initial choice of antibiotics	2.58	.62
Lack of guidelines on antibiotic usage	2.17	.81
Patients' demand for antibiotics	1.90	.80
Role of pharmaceutical companies in promoting the use of antibiotics	1.75	.79
Inadequate hand washing	1.47	.95
Use of antibiotics in the livestock industry	1.41	1.03

correlated to female sex ($p = 0.004$), having postgraduate training ($p = 0.001$) and > four years post graduation ($p = 0.03$).

Knowledge of preventing or containing antibiotic resistance

Physician education programmes (2.67 ± 0.66) and access to timely laboratory reports (2.67 ± 0.67) were both considered most important and antibiotic restriction (2.04 ± 0.80) and cycling (1.97 ± 0.92) least important (Table 3).

The overall score for knowledge of factors to contain resistance showed the majority of respondents had good knowledge (83%), 9.5% had average knowledge and 7.5% poor. A good score was positively correlated to type of current practice ($p = 0.04$), with the highest scores in physicians whose practice was mainly hospital based.

Antibiotics more prone to inducing resistance

Respondents incorrectly thought that amoxicillin-clavulanic acid had the greatest potential to induce resistance (1.51 ± 0.7), but correctly identified ceftriaxone (1.31 ± 0.75) and ciprofloxacin (1.23 ± 0.78) as inducers of resistance. Antibiotics thought to have the least potential to induce resistance were amikacin (0.94 ± 0.7) and the carbapenems (0.98 ± 0.7). (Table 4).

Most (58.7%) had good knowledge, 25% had average knowledge and the remainder's knowledge was poor (16%). This score was correlated to type of practice ($p = 0.005$); years post graduation ($p = 0.018$) and postgraduate training ($p = 0.013$). Physicians who were primarily hospital-based, who had been in practice between 10 and 14 years or had postgraduate training had the highest scores.

Optimal duration of therapy

Most physicians would treat an uncomplicated urinary tract infection for 7–10 days (43%), 30% would treat for five days and 24% for less than five days. For a group A streptococcus pharyngitis, 64% would treat for seven to ten days, 19% for five days and 12% for 14 days. A community-acquired pneumonia would be treated for 7–10 days by the majority (75%), and five days (13%) and 14 days (8%) by the remainder. A *Staphylococcus aureus* bacteremia would be prescribed 14 days of antibiotics by 48% of respondents, seven to ten days by 36% and > 14 days by 12%.

Complications related to antibiotic resistance

Respondents felt that increased costs related to care (73%) and prolonged hospital stay (66%) were the most frequent complications of ABR. Death and organ failure (33% respectively) were thought to be less common.

Attitude

Opinion on restriction of antibiotics

The antibiotics considered suitable for a hospital-restricted list (multiple antibiotics could be chosen) included vancomycin (81%), carbapenems (79%) and piperacillin/tazobactam (65%). Most did not think that ciprofloxacin (27%), ceftazidime (28%) or ceftriaxone (14%) should be restricted. 36% of respondents felt the current level of restriction should be increased, 25% felt they should be maintained and 4% advocated a decrease.

Table 3 Knowledge of Preventing or Containing Antibiotic Resistance

	Mean	SD
Ongoing physician educational programmes	2.67	.659
Access to timely lab reports	2.67	.674
Development of national antibiotic guidelines	2.63	.684
Access to microbiology consultations	2.58	.694
Development of better diagnostic tests to differentiate bacterial from viral infection	2.53	.745
Public educational programmes	2.44	.753
Antibiotic restriction: requiring a countersignature by a consultant or microbiologist	2.04	.800
Antibiotic cycling: switching routine use from one class to another at a regular intervals	1.97	.920

Table 4 Knowledge of Inducing Antibiotic Resistance

	Mean	SD
Amoxicillin-clavulanic acid	1.51	.70
Ceftriaxone	1.31	.75
Ciprofloxacin	1.23	.78
Ceftazidime	1.13	.74
Piperacillin-tazobactam	1.01	.70
Meropenem/Imipenem	.98	.70
Amikacin	.94	.65

(0 = don't know, 1 = less likely, 2 = more likely)

Practice

Personal experience with MDROs

Physicians identified MRSA (65% of respondents), multi-resistant *Pseudomonas aeruginosa* and ESBL *Eschericha coli* (35% each), ESBL *Klebsiella pneumoniae* (28%), penicillin resistant *Streptococcus pneumoniae* (PRSP, 27%) and Vancomycin Resistant Enterococcus (VRE) (19%) within their personal practices. Hospital physicians and those with both a hospital and outpatient-based practice consistently reported higher personal experience with MDROs, except for PRSP. Hospital physicians reported less experience with PRSP (22%) than outpatient-based (30%) and those with a combined practice (34%, $p = 0.03$). 75% hospital-based, 72% of both and 41% outpatient-based physicians had experience with MRSA ($p < 0.001$).

Choice of antibiotics

The factors that commonly affected antibiotic choice included severity (91%) and site (90%) of infection; patient factors such as renal disease, immunocompromise and allergy (84%); availability of antibiotics (84%) and cost (58%). Knowledge of patterns of ABR was important for 54%. Only 5% of respondents admitted to being influenced by requests from the patient or their family and 2% to pressure from pharmaceutical companies.

For a community-acquired pneumonia, the most common initial empiric choices were amoxicillin-clavulanic acid (77%) and erythromycin (38%). For a hospital acquired pneumonia, ceftriaxone (38%), ceftazidime (33%) and piperacillin/tazobactam (31%) were the most popular choices. Trimethoprim-sulfamethoxazole (52%), amoxicillin-clavulanic acid (44%) and ciprofloxacin (41%) were commonly used for uncomplicated urinary tract infections. (Table 5) Physicians were allowed to choose more than one antibiotic for each type of infection, and so totals are greater than 100%.

Forty-three percent (43%) of respondents frequently take cultures prior to starting a course of antibiotics, 47% occasionally and only 7% always take cultures. Frequently taking cultures was more common amongst hospital physicians (53%) than outpatient-based (24%) or those who had a combined practice (44%, $p < 0.001$). Most (53%) are able to get results within four to seven days, and 16% in less than three days. However, 27% complained that results would take over 1 week. 41% of respondents felt that their initial choice was correct based on laboratory reports "somewhat often" and 31% "sometimes" 5% had never checked.

Responses to culture reports

Physicians were asked what their response would be to a culture report indicating the organisms isolated were resistant to the empiric antibiotic/s in a patient responding clinically. The majority (54%) would change to antibiotics indicated by the report, 31% would continue the present antibiotics, and 16% would add one of the susceptible antibiotics indicated by the report. When asked what their response would be to a culture report showing an isolate sensitive to current antibiotics, but also to a narrower-spectrum antibiotic in a patient who is responding clinically, only 21% would de-escalate to the narrow-spectrum therapy.

Physicians' treatment decisions when antibiotics are not indicated

When asked about their practice if they thought antibiotics were not indicated, 92% would explain to their patients why they were not needed, 88% would guide them on seeking follow-up care if symptoms do not improve, 84% would provide medications for relief of symptoms and 71% would educate on the harm of taking unnecessary antibiotics. Only 6% admitted to prescribing antibiotics if the patient demanded it. However, when further asked if they had ever prescribed antibiotics only because of patients' insistence, 21% (12% hospital based, 31% outpatient based) admitted to doing that.

Additional training

Only 34% of respondents thought that their knowledge of antibiotics and ABR was good or very good; the majority (53%) felt it was average and this was the same for both hospital and outpatient-based physicians. The majority of respondents (86%) thought they needed a refresher course in ABR and prescription. Just over half of the respondents (52%) had further training in the use of antibiotics post graduation, either through a seminar (86%) or a formal course (14%).

The majority of physicians (74%) turned to the Internet when they needed further information on infection management. Other sources included consultation with local experts (54%), other colleagues (43%), national guidelines (41%) and textbooks (40%). Only 35% would consult institutional guidelines.

Table 5 Choices of Empiric Antibiotics

	Community acquired pneumonia	Hospital acquired pneumonia	Uncomplicated urinary tract infection	Overall
Amoxicillin-clavulanic acid	77%	21%	44%	53%
Erythromycin	38%	11%	3%	14%
Ceftriaxone	21%	38%	6%	22%
Cefuroxime	15%	16%	10%	14%
Ciprofloxacillin	7%	13%	41%	20%
Bactrim	7%	5%	52%	18%
Ceftazidime	7%	33%	3%	13%
Metronidazole	6%	8%	5%	13%
Piperacillin/tazobactam	6%	31%	3%	11%
Meropenem	4%	12%	2%	5%
Amikacin	3%	9%	4%	5%

Discussion

This is the first national survey of Jamaican doctors regarding their knowledge and opinions on antibiotic resistance and their prescribing practices. Physicians from all health regions were included from a wide range of disciplines and clinical experience.

Knowledge and attitudes

Eight out of 10 doctors (82%) recognized the magnitude of ABR globally, but less were convinced of this locally (73%) and even less so in their personal practice (53%). The danger of this finding is that physicians could become detached from the problem, making them less likely to try to contain it. ABR is more common in the hospital setting and this was reflected in the responses of the hospital doctors. The authors have observed that the prohibitive cost and delay in retrieving microbiology reports in some areas have adversely affected the Jamaican physicians' perceptions of the value of obtaining routine cultures. This could explain why only 7% of physicians always take cultures for a suspected infection. Hence, there is little reminder of prevailing resistance patterns.

Most physicians appreciated the influence of widespread use, inappropriate choices and overuse of broad-spectrum antibiotics as drivers of ABR [4, 18]. However a significant number failed to recognize important drivers of resistance such as inadequate hand hygiene and antibiotic usage in the livestock industry [4, 5]. When the objective assessment of their overall knowledge of ABR was compared to their own personal assessment, there was good correlation with 57% receiving an average score objectively, and 54% perceiving their knowledge as average.

Ongoing educational programmes, the development of national antibiotic guidelines, access to microbiology consultation, as well as improved laboratory services were thought to be most useful in containing ABR. There are only two medical microbiologists and one infectious disease specialist for the public health sector across the entire island. This needs to be urgently addressed as part of a national programme. Access to timely laboratory reports continues to be a challenge in this resource limited setting, where there are only few laboratories with limited diagnostic capacity, often using manual systems. Although this problem would appear to be a local one, its potential impact could be global because of Jamaica's position as a popular destination. The role of inadequate rapid point of care (POC) tests to differentiate between viral and bacterial infections was also clearly appreciated by the respondents as being an important factor to contain resistance. POC tests are those that are performed at the bedside and generate convenient and rapid results [24]. These would quickly differentiate between viral and bacterial infections such as Group A Streptococcus and urinary Streptococcus pneumoniae. Unfortunately there are only a few rapid POC tests and this is a problem internationally [25]. This is particularly highlighted by upper respiratory tract infections which are common worldwide and are often overtreated by antibiotics in the absence of rapid POCs [26]. Factors such as antibiotic cycling and restriction, that would confine the physicians' prescribing practice, were not perceived to be as important. This was confirmed by the fact that only just over one third (36%) thought that current antibiotic restriction policies should be increased.

Just over half of the physicians (59%) surveyed understood that some antibiotics are more prone to inducing resistance than others. As expected, physicians in the hospital setting had better knowledge, but there is room for more education across the board, such as seminars, workshops, conferences, newsletters and official antibiotic guidelines. Although the third generation cephalosporins and fluoroquinolones have a high propensity towards resistance induction [27] they remain some of the more prescribed antibiotics. Ceftriaxone was the second most commonly chosen empiric antibiotic overall followed by ciprofloxacin. The response to optimal duration of antibiotic therapy varied widely and highlights the need for national and institutional guidelines.

Practice

Although 65% of the respondents identified MRSA as the most common resistant organism seen in their practice, it should be noted that at the major referral hospital in the island, MRSA prevalence rate for the past three years has been less than 4% [16]. This information has been widely communicated to local physicians through conferences and workshops. Typing of the MRSA isolates retrieved from this hospital showed that only 29% were scc mec IV type (E. Finlayson, unpub. Data [28]. It should also be noted that 30% and 24% of the MRSA isolates retrieved in 2008 were resistant to low level and high level mupirocin respectively [29] highlighting again the need for constant surveillance.

Similarly, the prevalence rates for VRE have been less than 1% for the past four years in the same hospital (A Nicholson, unpub. data), even though 19% of physicians reported having seen this organism in their practice. As to be expected, hospital physicians reported a higher incidence of MDROs, and PRSPs were more commonly seen in the community.

Although factors influencing choice were appropriate, knowledge of local antibiograms was not always included. Again, this could be related to limited laboratory resources that reduce the availability of culture results and objective data. In the absence of national guidelines, the tendency is for the physicians to use international guidelines, as evidenced by the empiric choices for community and hospital acquired pneumonia and urinary tract infections. This finding also corresponds with the physicians' high use of the Internet for information (74%), far more than consulting local experts (54%). From the limited susceptibility data available, it is clear that local susceptibility patterns, eg *Staphylococcus aureus* (3.2% MRSA) and *Enterococcus,* (< 1% VRE) (are different from those reported in developed countries, and hence empiric choices should not be solely based on international guidelines. *Streptococcus pneumoniae* is recognized as the commonest cause of community acquired pneumonia and recent data showed a 8% resistance to penicillin (IV) for all isolates nationally (A. Foster, 2015 unpub. data), which is far less than the 24% resistance seen in North America [30]. Where penicillin resistance is low, the use of penicillin/amoxicillin-clavulanic acid for first line therapy is appropriate.

Physicians were more inclined to change to broad-spectrum antibiotics and reluctant to de-escalate, even in the face of laboratory data [31]. This type of practice is expensive, and ultimately drives resistance [32]. In this era of ABR it is important for physicians to achieve optimal outcomes by combining laboratory and clinical data. This study found that only 21% of physicians would de-escalate therapy, while a 2010 single-centre Jamaican study showed that only 7.7% actually practiced de-escalation [33]. There has been some improvement through education of physicians as to the importance of the practice, and attention had been drawn to the results of the 2010 study in conferences, workshops and small group sessions by local microbiologists. Encouragement to de-escalate should continue to be a target in future programmes.

It is encouraging to see that the physicians were paying attention to the need for patient education ranging from explanations of the dangers of unnecessary antibiotics to guiding them to seek follow-up care if necessary. Although 6% admitted to prescribing antibiotics on demand, a further 15% admitted to having done so in the past. This may be the result of increased of continuing education via conferences and workshops, some of which are mandatory. We would have expected more response to patient pressure, especially in the private setting. This is a positive finding, but more work is needed to further reduce this figure.

The majority of physicians were interested in further educational courses on antibiotic resistance. The results of this survey will guide the development of these courses, which could be in the form of hospital based workshops, orientation of new staff and medical conferences.

The major limitation of this study is that it relied on self-reporting by physicians as well as recall of past practices. This could have led to either under or over reporting and recall bias, which may have affected results. Further qualitative research using focus groups, for example, could highlight reasons for some of the practices seen, such as the reluctance to de-escalate therapy, and this could guide interventions.

Conclusions

Physicians in this study were aware of the problem of ABR, but downplayed its significance nationally and personally. Most had only average knowledge of factors driving resistance, but good knowledge of factors to control resistance. They tended to use international guidelines when making empiric choices, to choose high-powered antibiotics even when patients were improving and to resist de-escalation when appropriate. These are all important targets for a national campaign. Strengthening laboratory medicine in resource limited countries such as Jamaica and most of the English speaking Caribbean countries would play a major role in restricting the emergence of antibiotic resistance. This would also involve training more clinical microbiologists, infectious disease physicians, pharmacists and other experts. This would help to determine prevalent organisms and their antibiograms resulting in more accurate and cost effective therapy. The savings from this could then be invested in an antimicrobial stewardship programme. Policy changes are also needed from local Ministries of Health and national medical associations to provide guidance and monitoring.

Abbreviations

ABR: Antibiotic resistance; ESBL: Extended spectrum betalactamase; MDROs: Multidrug resistant organisms; MOH: Ministry of Health; MRSA: Methicillin resistant *Staphylococcus aureus*; PRSPs: Penicillin resistant *Streptococcus pneumoniae*; SPSS: Statistical Analysis in the Social Sciences; VRE: Vancomycin resistant Enterococcus

Acknowledgments

This project was supported by the National Health Fund, Jamaica.

Disclaimers

The opinions expressed by authors contributing to this journal do not necessarily reflect the opinions of the National Health Fund, Jamaica or the institutions with which the authors are affiliated.

Funding

Funding for this project was obtained through a grant received from the National Health Fund. The funds received were used for data collection and analysis.

Authors' contributions

AN being the primary author of this paper participated in every aspect of this research project from its conceptualization to its execution and write up. IT, LW, LC, SJ, JB and LR also helped to design the study. CT-R helped with data collection. All authors helped to analyse the data and write the paper. All authors have read and approved the final manuscript.

Authors' information

Dr. Alison Nicholson is a Consultant Medical Microbiologist in the Department of Microbiology at the University of the West Indies, Mona, where she is currently the Head of Department. Dr. Nicholson has an interest in antibiotic resistance and infection control.

Consent for publication

N/A

NB Study participants gave consent to participate in the study, however there is nothing in the paper that can be used to uniquely identify them.

Competing interests

The authors declare they have no competing interests.

Author details

[1]Department of Microbiology, The University of the West Indies (UWI), Kingston, Jamaica. [2]Department of Surgery, Radiology, Anaesthesia and Intensive Care, UWI, Kingston, Jamaica. [3]UWI CARIMAC, Kingston, Jamaica. [4]School of Education, UWI, Kingston, Jamaica. [5]Department of Government, UWI, Kingston, Jamaica. [6]Department of Medicine, UWI, Kingston, Jamaica. [7]Ministry of Health, Kingston, Jamaica.

References

1. Levy SB, O'Brien TF. Global Antimicrobial Resistance Alerts and Implications. CID. 2005;41:219–20. (Suppl 4)
2. Livermore D. Current epidemiology and growing resistance of gram-negative pathogens. Korean J Intern Med. 2012;27:28–142.
3. Laxminarayan R, Duse A, Wattal C, Zaidi A, Wertheim H, Sump N, et al. Antibiotic resistance—the need for global solutions. Lancet Infect Dis. 2013; 13(12):1057–98.
4. Ventola C. The antibiotic resistance crisis. Pharm Ther. 2015;40(4):277–83.
5. The World Health Organization. Antimicrobial Resistance. The World Health Organization Media Centre. Fact sheet N°194. 2015. https://warwick.ac.uk/fac/sci/lifesci/outreach/headstart_2016/who__antimicrobial_resistance.pdf. Accessed 1 Sept 2016.
6. Aminov R. A brief history of the antibiotic era: lessons learned and challenges for the future. Front Microbiol. 2010;1:134.
7. Smith R, Coast J. The true cost of antimicrobial resistance. BMJ. 2013;346:1–5.
8. Akpaka PE, Swanston WH. Phenotypic detection and occurrence of extended-spectrum beta-lactamases in clinical isolates of *Klebsiella pneumoniae* and *Escherichia coli* at a tertiary Hospital in Trinidad & Tobago. Braz J Infect Dis. 2016;12(6):516–20.
9. Akpaka PE, Kissoon S, Jayaratne P. Molecular Analysis of Vancomycin-Resistant Enterococci Isolated from Regional Hospitals in Trinidad and Tobago. Adv Med. 2016; https://www.hindawi.com/journals/amed/2016/8762691/. Accessed 01 Sep 2016.
10. Akpaka PE, Roberts R, Monecke S. Molecular characterization of antimicrobial resistance genes against Staphylococcus aureus isolates from Trinidad and Tobago. J Infect Public Health. 2016; http://www.ncbi.nlm.nih.gov/pubmed/27328777. Accessed 01 Sep 2016
11. Hariharan S, Nanduri SB, Moseley HS, Areti KY, Jonnalagadda R. Spectrum of microbes and antimicrobial resistance in a surgical intensive care unit. Am J Infect Control. 2003;31(5):280–7.
12. Levett PN, Holt HA, McGowan AP. Resistance to third-generation cephalosporins in Barbados. West Indian Med J. 1993;42(2):69–71.
13. Thoms-Rodriguez CA, Mazzulli T, Christian N, Willey B, Boyd DA, Mataseje LF, et al. New Delhi metallo-β-lactamase in Jamaica. J Infect Dev Ctries. 2016;10(2):183–7.
14. Souli M, Galani I, Giamarellou H. Emergence Of extensively drug-resistant and pandrug-resistant gram-negative bacilli in Europe. Euro Surveill. 2008; 47(13):1–11.
15. Christian N, Roye-Green K, Smikle M. Molecular epidemiology of multidrug resistant extended spectrum beta-lactamase producing Klebsiella pneumoniae at a Jamaican hospital, 2000–2004. BMC Microbiol:2010. http://bmcmicrobiol.biomedcentral.com/articles/10.1186/1471-2180-10-27. Accessed 01 Sep 2016.
16. Nicholson AM, Ledgister S, Williams T, Robinson S, Gayle P, Lindo T, et al. Distribution of nosocomial organisms and their resistance patterns in the intensive care unit of the University Hospital of the West Indies, Kingston. Jam W Indian Med J. 2009;58(2):142–8. (ISSN 0043-3144)
17. Thoms-Rodriguez C, Mazzulli T, Christian N, Willey B, Nicholson AM. Meropenem Efflux in *Pseudomonas aeruginosa* at a Tertiary Care Hospital in Jamaica. W Indian Med J. 2016; https://www.mona.uwi.edu/fms/wimj/article/2678. Accessed 01 Sep 2016
18. Hamilton-Miller JMT. Use and abuse of antibiotics. Br J Clin Pharm. 1984;18:469–74.
19. Tennant I, Nicholson A, Gordon-Strachan GM, Thoms C, Chin V, Didier MA. A survey of physicians' knowledge and attitudes regarding antimicrobial resistance and antibiotic prescribing practices at the university hospital of the west indies. W Indian Med J. 2010;59(2):165–70.
20. Johnson K and Bartlett K. The role of tourism in national human resource development: a Jamaican perspective. Human Resource Development International. 2013. http://www.tandfonline.com/doi/abs/10.1080/13678868.2013.771867. Accessed 01 Sep 2016.
21. The Statistical Institute of Jamaica. The Statistical Institute of Jamaica Website. 2014. http://statinja.gov.jm/demo_socialstats/population.aspx. Accessed 01 Sep 2016.
22. The World Health Organization. Second Meeting of the Subcommittee of the Expert Committee on the Selection and Use of Essential Medicines. Use of Ceftazidime in Children and Options for Treating Pseudomonas Infections. Geneva : s.n., 2008.
23. Pedhazur EJ, Pedhazur-Schmelkin LP. Measurement, design and analysis: an integrated approach. New York: Psychology Press; 1991. p. 109.
24. Peeling RW, Mabey D. Point-of-care tests for diagnosing infections in the

developing world. Clin Microbiol Infect. 2010;18(16):1062–9.

25. Society for Healthcare Epidemiology of America and Infectious Diseases Society of America. Policy statement on antimicrobial stewardship by the Society for Healthcare Epidemiology of America (SHEA), the Infectious Diseases Society of America (IDSA), and the Pediatric Infectious Diseases Society (PIDS). Infect Control Hosp Epidemiol. 2012; 33(4):322–3.
26. Leichman AK. New diagnostic test distinguishes bacterial from viral infections. Israel 21C. https://www.israel21c.org/new-diagnostic-test-distinguishes-bacterial-from-viral-infections/. Accessed 16 Jan 2018.
27. Ruiza J, Jurado A, Garcia-Méndez E, Marco F, Aguilar L, Jiménez de Anta T, et al. Frequency of selection of fluoroquinolone-resistant mutants of *Neisseria gonorrhoeae* exposed to gemifloxacin and four other quinolones. J Antimicrob Chemother. 2001;48(4):545–8.
28. Brown P. Multiple-locus VNTR analyses of methicillin-resistant *Staphylococcus aureus* from Jamaica. Infect Dis (Auckl). 2015;8:31–8.
29. Nicholson AM, Thoms C, Wint H, Didier M, Willis R, McMorris N, et al. The detection of mupirocin resistance and the distribution of methicillin-resistant *Staphylococcus aureus* at the University Hospital of the West Indies, Jamaica. West Indian Med J. 2010;59(5):509–13.
30. Whitney C, Farley M, Hadler J, Harrison L, Lexau C, Reingold A, et al. Increasing prevalence of multidrug-resistant *Streptococcus pneumoniae* in the United States. N Engl J Med. 2000;343:1917–192.
31. Masterton R. Antibiotic De-Escalation. Crit Care Clin. 2011;27:149–62.
32. Hayashi Y, Paterson D. Strategies for reduction in duration of antibiotic use in hospitalized patients. CID. 2011;52:1232–40.
33. Chin V, Harding HE, Tennant I, Soogrim D, Gordon-Strachan GM, Frankson MA. Dynamics of antibiotic usage in the intensive care unit at the University Hospital of the West Indies. West Indian Med J. 2010; 59(2):159–64.

8

Frequency of antiseptic resistance genes in clinical staphycocci and enterococci isolates in Turkey

Seyda Ignak[1*], Yasar Nakipoglu[2] and Bulent Gurler[2]

Abstract

Background: Disinfectants and antiseptics are biocides widely used in hospitals to prevent spread of pathogens. It has been reported that antiseptic resistance genes, *qac*'s, caused tolerance to a variety of biocidal agents, such as benzalkonium chloride (BAC) and chlorhexidine digluconate (CHDG) in *Staphylococcus spp.* isolates. We aimed to search the frequency of antiseptic resistance genes in clinical *Staphylococcus spp.* and *Enterococcus spp.* isolates to investigate the possible association with antiseptic tolerance and antibiotic resistance.

Methods: Antiseptic resistance genes (*qacA/B*, *smr*, *qacG*, *qacH*, and *qacJ)* isolated from Gram-positive cocci (69 *Staphylococcus spp.* and 69 *Enterococcus spp.*) were analyzed by PCR method. The minimum inhibitory concentrations (MICs) of BAC and CHDG were determined by agar dilution method, whereas antibiotic susceptibility was analyzed by disk diffusion method according to Clinical and Laboratory Standards Institute (CLSI) criteria.

Results: The frequency of antiseptic resistance genes was found to be high (49/69; 71.0%) in our clinical staphylococci isolates but absent (0/69; 0%) in enterococci isolates. The frequency of *qacA/B* and *smr* genes was higher (25/40; 62.5% and 7/40; 17.5%, respectively) in coagulase negative staphylococci (CNS) when compared to *Staphylococcus aureus* strains (3/29; 10.3%, and 4/29; 13.8%, respectively). In contrast, the frequency of *qacG* and *qacJ* genes was higher (11/29; 37.9% and 8/29; 27.5%, respectively) in *S. aureus* than those of CNS (5/40; 12.5%, 10/40; 25.0%) strains. *qacH* was not identified in none of the strains. We found an association between presence of antiseptic resistance genes and increased MIC values of BAC (>4 μg/mL) in staphylococci and it was found to be statistically statistically significant ($p < 0.01$). We also showed that MICs of BAC and CHDG of vancomycin-resistant enterococci (VRE) isolates were significantly higher than those of vancomycin-susceptible enterococci (VSE) isolates ($p < 0.01$).

Conclusions: For our knowledge, our study is the first to investigate antiseptic resistance genes in enterococci and also *qacG*, *qacH*, and *qacJ* genes in staphylococci isolates in Turkey. Further studies are needed to revise the biocide policy and to support infection control programs to avoid the development of new resistance mechanisms.

Keywords: *Staphylococcus spp.*, *Enterococcus spp.*, *qac* genes, Antiseptic, Biocide, Resistance

* Correspondence: seyda_ignak@hotmail.com
[1]Department of Medical Biology, Bahcesehir University School of Medicine, Sahrayıcedid Mah. Batman Sok. No:66-68, Yenisahra-Göztepe, Istanbul, Turkey
Full list of author information is available at the end of the article

Background

Staphylococcus aureus causes a wide range of clinical infections such as skin and soft tissue infections, surgical site infections, endocarditis, and bacteremia. Traditionally, coagulase-negative staphylococci (CNS) isolates were considered a as non-pathogenic commensals but in recent years the clinical importance of CNS has been increased significantly due to its role in some diseases like catheter related bloodstream infections. *Enterococcus spp.* found in the gastrointestinal tract of humans is a commensal bacteria and considered to be harmless for many years. Nowadays, it is considered to be one of the most common nosocomial pathogen especially due to strains of vancomycin resistant enterococci, VRE [1, 2]. There has been a significant increase in the incidence of nosocomial infections caused by *Staphylococcus spp.* and *Enterococcus spp.* which are multiresistant to various antibiotics in recent years [3].

Some antiseptic and disinfectant agents in the hospital setting such as quaternary ammonium compounds like benzalkonium chloride (BAC) and divalent cations like chlorhexidine digluconate (CHDG) are used to prevent infections within healthcare facilities. It has been reported in many studies that extensive use of biocidal agents reduce susceptibility to antiseptics in *Staphylococcus spp.* [4–6].

Antiseptic resistance genes (*qacAB, smr, qacG, qacH, qacJ*), encoding multidrug efflux pumps which are carried by plasmids, were identified in *Staphylococcus* genus for the first time [7–10]. Antiseptic resistance gene studies of *qacA/B* and *smr* mostly focused on *S. aureus* [10–12] but there are a limited number of studies in CNS strains [13, 14]. Moreover, the studies concerning the prevalance of *qacG, qacH,* and *qacJ* genes mostly focused on CNS obtained from animal and food sources [15, 16].

Despite the rising significance of *Enterococcus spp.* as nosocomial pathogen there are insufficient number of studies on *qac* genes in clinical isolates. Bischoff et al. [17] detected the first *qacA/B* gene-positive *Enterococcus faecalis* isolate in clinical blood samples. Thus far, there are no *qac* genes reported in enterococci other than *qacC, qacEΔ1, qacZ* and *qacA/B*. Increase in minimum inhibitory concentration (MIC) values to biocides does not mean "resistance" because these agents can be used at high concentrations without encountering toxicity [18]. Thus the terms "reduced susceptibility" or "increased tolerance" are more suitable for pathogens exhibiting an elevated MIC to a biocides [19].

In this study, we aimed; 1. To investigate *qacAB, smr, qacG, qacH, qacJ* genes in *Staphylococcus spp.* and *Enterococcus spp.* isolates, 2. To determine the susceptibility of the strains to antibiotics and two antiseptic agents, including BAC and CHDG, 3. To show relationship between MIC values of antiseptic agents/resistance to antibiotics and presence of antiseptic resistance genes. For our knowledge, this is the first study in Turkey that investigated antiseptic resistance genes in enterococci isolates and also first in terms of showing the presence of *qacH, qacG,* and *qacJ* genes in staphylococci isolates.

Methods

Bacterial isolates

In our study, 69 *Staphylococcus spp.* (10 methicillin-resistant *S.aureus* (MRSA), 19 methicillin-susceptible *S.aureus* (MSSA), 27 MRCNS, 13 of methicillin-susceptible CNS (MSCNS)) and 69 of *Enterococcus spp.* were collected from different clinical samples such as blood, cerebrospinal fluid, urine, abscess, catheter tips, nasal secretions and endotracheal aspiration fluid between January 2010–March 2011 in a university hospital with more than 1500 beds. This study was conducted in accordance with revised Helsinki Declaration and approved by the institutional clinical research ethic commitee.

All samples were cultured on suitable bacteriological media and identified by the conventional method. *Staphylococcus spp.* isolates were identified by API-Staph commercial identification kit (API Staph System, bioMèrieux, France).

Minimum inhibitory concentration of antiseptics

MICs of BAC and CHDG were detected by a modified agar dilution method according to the recommendations of Clinical and Laboratory Standards Institute (CLSI) [20]. The MICs of the BAC and CHDG in negative control strain (*S.aureus ATCC 6538*) which is negative for antiseptic resistance genes were considered as baseline and any MICs above these values were accepted as "tolerance concentration".

Antibiotic susceptibility test

In this study, antibiotic sensitivity testing was performed via disc diffusion method by using following antibiotics; tetracycline, ciprofloxacin, tobramycin, trimethoprim-sulfamethoxazole, rifampin, and chloramphenicol. Methicillin and iMLSB (inducible macrolide-lincosamide-streptogramin B) resistance tests were implemented to *Staphylocccus spp.* isolates, while vancomycin resistance test to *Enterococcus spp.* isolates. All tests were performed according to CLSI [21] criteria.

The antibiotic susceptibility discs were purchased from OXOID (Hemakim, Istanbul, Turkey).

Detection of antiseptic resistant genes by multiplex PCR

Total genomic DNA of the strains were extracted using High Pure PCR Template Preparation Kit (Roche, Germany). All DNA extracts were stored at +4 °C prior to PCR.

A single primer pair was used for amplifying both *qacA* and *qacB* due to seven base difference between *qacA* and *qacB* genes. We made two multiplex PCR sets; one included primers of *A/B* and *smr* and second one contained primers of *qacG, qacH,* and *qacJ* genes as previously published [15, 22]. All primer sequences are shown in Table 1.

PCR Master Mix 2X (Fermentas, Canada) was used for PCR assays. According to recommendation of manufacturer, the final volume of each reaction in the PCR was 25 μL. Each reaction contained 12,5 μL master mix, for each primer; 1 μL (10 pmol) of forward primer, 1 μL (10 pmol) of reverse primer, 2 μL of DNA extract and final volume was 25 μL by adding sterile H_2O. PCR of *qacA/B* and *smr* genes were performed using an initial denaturation step 96 °C for 3 min, followed by 25 cycles of 95 °C for 20 s, 53 °C for 20 s, 72 °C for 20 s, and a final extension step at 72 °C for 5 min [22]. Whereas the cycling conditions for *qacG, qacH and qacJ* genes were as follows: DNA denaturation at 94 °C for 10 min, 25 cycles of 95 °C for 60 s, 48 °C for 45 s, 72 °C for 60 s, and a final extension step at 72 °C for 10 min [15]. Multiplex PCR products were run in 1% gel containing ethidium bromide and photographed under ultraviolet.

Positive control strains (*qacA/B, smr, qacG, qacH, qacJ*) were provided kindly by Jostein Bjorland from Norwegian School of Veterinary Science. *S.aureus ATCC 6538* was used as negative control strain.

Statistical analysis

The data analysis was conducted with the statistical package, IBM SPSS Statistics 22 (IBM.

SPSS, Turkey). The normal distribution of variables were checked by the Shapiro–Wilk test. Comparison of quantitive data between two groups were performed by Mann Whitney U test, while Continuity Correction and Fisher's Exact tests were used for comparison of qualitative data between two groups. *P* value less than 0.05 was considered statistically significant.

Results

We found that 15/29 (51.7%) *Staphylococcus aureus* and 34/40 (85.0%) CNS isolates, for a total of 49/69 (70.0%) *Staphylococcus spp.* isolates harbored at least one antiseptic resistance genes. Among the 49 strains positive for an antiseptic resistance gene; *qacA/B* genes were the most dominant (28/49; 57.1%) followed by *qacJ* (18/49; 36.7%), *qacG* (16/49; 32.6%), and *smr* (11/49; 22.4%) genes. We also found that 30/49 (61.2%) gene positive *Staphylococcus spp.* isolates had only one gene type, whereas the rest of the isolates (19/49; 38.7%) carried more than one gene type. None of the *Staphylococcus spp.* isolates carried the *qacH* gene. In addition, all *Enterococcus spp.* isolates were negative for any resistance genes (Table 2).

The MICs of BAC ranged from 1 to 16 μg/mL, and the MICs of CHDG ranged from 0.75 to 12 μg/mL in *Staphylococcus spp.* Baseline MIC concentrations of BAC and CHDG in the negative control strain (*S.aureus ATCC 6538*) were 4 and 1.5 μg/mL, respectively. Based on these measurements, we found a significant difference in MIC >4 μg/mL BAC between *Staphylococcus spp.* isolates positive and negative for an antiseptic resistance gene (p: 0.002; $p < 0.01$) but this relationship was not statistically significant for MICs of CHDG (>1.5 μg/mL; p: 0.925; $p > 0.01$) (Table 3).

All *Enterococcus spp.* isolates in this study were negative for antiseptic resistance genes. MIC levels of BAC and CHDG were 8–16 μg/ml and 6–12 μg/mL, respectively. We found that MICs of BAC and CHDG of VRE isolates were significantly higher than those of vancomycin-susceptible enterococci (VSE) isolates ($p < 0.01$) (Table 4).

A comparison of antibiotic resistance and the presence of antiseptic resistance genes in *Staphylococcus spp.* are shown in Table 5.

Table 1 Sequences of PCR primers

Primer	Gene	Primer Sequence (5′-3′)	Product Size	Reference
qacA/B F	*qacA/B*	GCA GAA AGT GCA GAG TTC G	361 bp	Noguchi et al. [22]
qacA/B R	*qacA/B*	CCA GTC CAA TCA TGC CTG		
smr F	*smr*	GCC ATA AGT ACT GAA GTT ATT GGA	195 bp	Noguchi et al. [22]
smr R	*smr*	GAC TAC GGT TGT TAA GAC TAA ACC T		
qacG F	*qacG*	CAA CAG AAA TAA TCG GAA CT	275 bp	Bjorland et al. [15]
qacG R	*qacG*	TAC ATT TAA GAG CAC TAC A		
qacH F	*qacH*	ATA GTC AGT GAA GTA ATA G	295 bp	Bjorland et al. [15]
qacH R	*qacH*	AGT GTG ATG ATC CGA ATG T		
qacJ F	*qacJ*	CTT ATA TTT AGT AAT AGC G	301 bp	Bjorland et al. [15]
qacJ R	*qacJ*	GAT CCA AAA ACG TTA AGA		

Table 2 The presence of antiseptic resistance genes in *Staphyloccus spp.*

RESISTANCE GENES (n:49)	MRSA (n: 10)	MSSA (n:19)	MRCNS (n:27)	MSCNS (n:13)
One gene (n: 30)				
qacA/B (n:18)	-	-	14	4
smr (n:6)	-	2	2	2
qacG (n:3)	2	1	-	-
qacH (n:0)	-	-	-	-
qacJ (n:3)	-	1	1	1
Two genes (n: 14)				
qacA/B, smr (n:3)	-	1	2	-
qacA/B, qacG (n:1)	1	-	-	-
qacA/B, qacJ (n:3)	-	-	1	2
qacG,qacJ (n:7)	3	2	2	-
Three genes (n: 5)				
qacA/B, qacG, qacJ (n:3)	-	1	-	2
smr, qacG, qacJ (n:2)	1	-	-	1

MRSA Methicillin-resistant *Staphylococcus aureus*; *MSSA* Methicillin-susceptible *Staphylococcus aureus*; *MRCNS* Methicillin-resistant coagulase-negative staphylococci; *MSCNS* Methicillin-susceptible coagulase-negative staphylococci

Discussion

MRSA, MRCNS, and VRE strains are opportunistic pathogens transmitted by the hands of health care workers. BAC and CHDG are handwashing and skin antiseptics used extensively to the control and prevent hospital infections. Many studies have shown both the presence of plasmid-mediated antiseptic resistance genes such as *qacA/B*, *smr*, *qacG*, *qacH*, and *qacJ* and reduced susceptibility to antiseptic agents. Other researchers have reported that plasmids carry antiseptic resistance genes together with antibiotic resistance genes and contribute to the development of resistance in pathogens [23–25]. In this study, we tried to find a possible association between the presence of antiseptic resistance genes and reduced susceptibility to antiseptics or resistance to various antibiotics in clinical isolates of *Staphylococcus spp.* and *Enterococcus spp.*. We observed that 15 (51.7%) of 29 *S.aureus* and 34 (85.0%) of 40 CNS isolates, for a total of 49 (71%) out of 69 staphylococci isolates harbored at least one antiseptic resistance gene. We also determined that among the 49 *Staphylococcus spp.* isolates positive for a gene, *qacA/B* genes were the most dominant (57.1%) followed by *qacJ* (36.7%), *qacG* (32.6%), and *smr* (22.4%) genes. The *qacH* gene was not found in any tested isolates. Our *Enterococcus spp.* isolates were free from any antiseptic resistance genes.

To date, two studies [26, 27] have been published on the antiseptic resistance genes of staphylococci in Turkey in addition to our previous study in 2012 [25]. Duran et al. [26] reported that the frequency of *qacA/B* and *smr* genes among amikacin-resistant *S.aureus* was 47.4% and 28.9% in Turkey, respectively, and this finding was statistically significant ($p < 0.05$). In the same study, the frequency of *qacA/B* and *smr* in CNS was 37.9% and 20.7%, respectively ($p < 0.05$). In another study conducted in Turkey, Aykan et al. [27] reported that 11.6% of MRSA isolates harbored *qacA/B* resistance genes. In this study, we found that 10% of our MRSA strains harbored the *qacA/B* gene, and our results were compatible with the results of Aykan et al. [27]. In our previous study, (25) we found that *smr* genes were more prevalent (36.0%) in MRSA whereas *qacA/B* genes more prevalent (4.0%) in MSSA strains. In addition, the presence of the iMLSB resistance phenotype in 8/18 (44.5%) *smr*-positive strains compared to 2/32 (6.25%) *smr*-negative strains was statistically significant ($p < 0.001$) [25]. However, unlike our previous work, *smr* and *qacA/B* genes existed in equal frequency (10.0%) in MRSA strains in this study. In addition, *smr* genes were more prevalent (15.7%) than *qacA/B* (10.5%) in MSSA strains. Moreover, we could not find any significant relationship between the presence of antiseptic resistance genes and antibiotic resistance.

Mayer et al. [7] reported results of the SENTRY European study group on the distribution of *qacA/B* and *smr* in 297 MRSA and 200 MSSA strains isolated between 1997 and 1999 in 24 different European university hospitals in 14 countries. They found that 42.0% of *S.aureus* (63.0% of MRSA and 12.0% of MSSA) harbored *qacA/B* genes, and *qacA/B* genes were more prevalent than the *smr* gene, which was detected in 5.8% of *S. aureus* (6.4% of MRSA and 5.0% of MSSA). They emphasized that the

Table 3 Comparison between MICs of BAC and CHDG, and presence of antiseptic resistance genes in staphylocci isolates

Antiseptic	MIC	Gene (+) Bacteria (*n* = 49) *n* (%)	Gene (–) Bacteria (*n* = 20) *n* (%)	Z	*p*
BAC	≤4 μg/mL	23 (46.9%)	18 (90%)	9.209	0.002**
	>4 μg/mL	26 (53.1%)	2 (10%)		
CHDG	≤1.5 μg/mL	32 (65.3%)	14 (70%)	0.009	0.925
	>1.5 μg/mL	17 (34.7%)	6 (30%)		

Continuity Correction
$^{**}p < 0.01$

Table 4 Comparison between MIC (μg/mL) of BAC and CHDG in VSE and VRE isolates

MIC (μg/ml)	VSE (n = 56) Mean ± SD (Median)	VRE (n = 13) Mean ± SD (Median)	Z	p
BAC (8–16 μg/mL)	8.00 ± 0.00 (8)	11.69 ± 4.15 (8)	-5.282	0.001**
CHDG (6–12 μg/mL)	11.78 ± 1.12 (12)	10.15 ± 2.88 (12)	−3.112	0.002**

Mann Whitney U Test
***p < 0.01*

prevalence of antiseptic resistance genes is a widespread problem in European hospitals. Our study demonstrated that the presence of *qacA/B* genes in clinical *S.aureus* strains was lower (10.3%) than *smr* genes, which were more prevalent (13.8%) than European strains. Vali et al. [10] reported that in the UK, *smr* (44.2%) genes were most prevalent, followed by *qacA/B* (8.3%) and *qacH* (3.3%), and that *qacA/B* and *smr* were detected concomitantly in 4.2% of isolates; however they did not find *qacG* in 120 clinical MRSA strains. In contrast to Vali et al. we found a high frequency of *qacG* (7/10; 70.0%) in MRSA strains; but the *qacH* gene was not seen. We also detected *qacA/B* genes concomitantly with *smr* in 5.2% (1/19) of MSSA and 7.4% (2/27) of MRCNS, with *qacG* in 50.0% (5/10) of MRSA, and *qacJ* in 11.2% (3/27) of MRCNS and 38.4% (5/13) of MSCNS.

Longtin et al. [28] reported that *smr* genes were more frequent (7.0%) than *qacA/B* genes (2%) in 334 MRSA isolates collected from two Canadian intensive care units between 2005 and 2009, and no strain contained both genes. Noguchi et al. [22] detected *qacA/B* genes in 14.0% and *smr* genes in 28.0% of 71 clinical MRSA isolates in Japan. Alam et al. [29] reported that in 522 clinical *S. aureus* isolates from a hospital in Japan, *qacA/B* was more prevalent in MRSA (32.6%) and more prevalent in MSSA (7.5%) than *smr* genes, which had a frequency of 3.3% in MRSA and 5.9% in MSSA.

Table 5 Comparison between the antibiotic resistances and presence of antiseptic resistance genes in staphylococci isolates

Antibiotic	Gene (+) Bacteria (n = 49) n (%)	Gene (–) Bacteria (n = 20) n (%)	χ^2	p
iMLSB	22 (44.9%)	10 (50%)	0.014	0.905
Tetracycline	21 (42.9%)	8 (40%)	0.001	1.000
Ciprofloxacin	16 (32.7%)	5 (25%)	0.115	0.735
Tobramycin	14 (28.6%)	5 (25%)	0.001	1.000
SXT	12 (24.5%)	2 (10%)	-	0.322
Rifampin	11 (22.4%)	7 (35%)	0.601	0.438
Chloramphenicol	6 (12.2%)	0 (0%)	-	0.171

Continuity Correction and Fisher's Exact Test
iMLSB Inducible macrolide-lincosamide-streptogramin B;
SXT Trimethoprim-sulfamethoxazole

Zhang et al. [30] reported that 50.0% of MRSA and 16% of MSSA strains were positive for *qacA/B* gene, and this difference was statistically significant (p: 0.003). In our study, *smr* and *qacA/B* genes existed in equal frequency (10.0%) in MRSA strains, and *smr* genes were more prevalent (15.7%) than *qacA/B* (10.5%) in MSSA strains.

Zhang et al. [30] reported that CNS carried more *qacA/B genes* (56.7%) and *smr* genes (18.1%) than *S. aureus* (41.2% and 11.8%, respectively) in strains isolated from nares of nurses in a hospital in Hong Kong. In the same study, they detected a significant difference in the frequency of *qacA/B* between MRCNS (66.9%) and MSCNS (35.1%) strains ($p < 0.001$). They observed similar findings for *smr* (p: 0.001). In our study, the frequency of *qacA/B* and *smr* genes in MRCNS (63% and 14.8%, respectively) was very close to that of MSCNS (61.5% and 23.0%, respectively).

Ye et al. [16] examined the frequency of *qacG, qacH* and *qacJ* in 237 *S. aureus* (including 12 MRSA) and 604 CNS isolates (139 of which were methicillin resistant). They found that *S. aureus* isolates from a nurse (1.9%) harbored *qacJ*. Of the *qacG*-positive isolates, one of them harbored *qacA/B* and another harbored *smr*. In the same study, they detected that MICs of gene-positive strains were 2-fold higher than those of negative controls, and the presence of a second *qac* gene further elevated the MICs. The frequency of resistance to gentamicin, fusidic acid, clindamycin, and tetracycline increased in gene-positive isolates, but the MRSA isolates did not harbor these genes.

Liu et al. [11] found that 94.6% (53/56) of QAC-tolerant *S.aureus* isolates was positive for the *qacA/B* gene. The frequencies of *smr* and *qacH* were 3.6% and 7.1%, respectively. *QacG* was not detected in any isolates. The researches concluded that *S. aureus* isolates of China could survive at proper in-use concentrations of some biocides.

Zhang et al. [30] found an association between the presence of antiseptic resistance genes, and resistance to some anibiotics (cefoxitin, penicillin, ciprofloxacin, SXT, tetracycline, clindamycin) and reduced susceptibility to antiseptics (BAC: MIC ≥4 μg/mL, and CHDG: MIC ≥2–4 μg/mL). We also found a significant difference ($p < 0.01$) between the presence of antiseptic resistance genes and the BAC value (MIC > 4 μg/mL) but not antibiotic resistance ($p > 0.05$) in staphylococci isolates.

A limited number of antiseptic resistance gene studies have involved clinical *Enterococcus spp.* isolates. Bischoff et al. [17] found that 1 out of 42 (2.38%) *E. faecalis* isolates from blood samples carried *qacA/B*; 1 out of 109 (0.92%) *E. faecalis* isolates from stool samples harbored *smr*; and no *Enterococcus spp.* isolates were positive for *qacG*, *qacH*, or *qacJ* genes. In contrast to Bischoff et al. [17] we could not find any *qacA/B* and *smr* genes in *Enterococcus spp.* Thus far, no *qac* genes have been reported in enterococci other than *qacC*, *qacEΔ1*, *qacZ* and *qacA/B*. We also did not find *qacG*, *qacH*, or *qacJ* genes in enterococci isolates.

Bhardaj et al. [31] reported that MIC values of *E. faecium* and *E. faecalis* to CHDG ranged from 0.5 to 16 μg/mL. They also found that VanA-type resistance genes (VRE) are induced by sub-bactericidal levels of CHDG. It is a major concern whether exposure to sub-MIC CHDG results in cross-resistance to antibiotics in clinical use. MICs of BAC and CHDG in our *Enterococci spp.* isolates ranged from 8 to 16 μg/mL and 6 to 12 μg/mL, respectively. However there was a statistically significant difference ($p < 0.01$) of MICs in BAC and CHDG between VRE and VSE strains.

Our study has some limitations. This study focused on antiseptic resistance genes such as *qacA/B*, *smr*, *qacG*, *qacH*, and *qac J*, which are mostly isolated in Gram-positive bacteria, but other genes, such as *qacEΔ*, *qac F*, and *qacZ*, should be investigated in the future. In addition, the small sample size might have affected the possible relationship between antiseptic resistance genes and the resistance pattern of antibiotics and antiseptic agents.

Conclusion

The frequency of antiseptic resistance genes was high (71.0%) in our *Staphylococcus spp.* and absent (0%) in *Enterococcus spp.* isolates. The frequency of *qacA/B* and *smr* genes was higher (62.5% and 17.5%, respectively) in CNS isolates compared to *S. aureus* strains (10.3% and 13.8%, respectively). In contrast, the frequency of *qacG* and *qacJ* genes was higher (37.9% and 27.5%, respectively) in *S. aureus* strains compared to CNS strains (12.5% and 25.0%, respectively). We found statistically significant ($p < 0.01$) association between the presence of antiseptic resistance genes and the MIC of BAC (>4 μg/mL) in staphylococci. They may be a marked difference in the frequency and type of antiseptic resistance genes between countries or even between different hospitals in the same country, and therefore each hospital should review its antimicrobial policy and support continuing education to avoid developing new antimicrobial resistance mechanisms.

Abbreviations

BAC: Benzalkonium chloride; CHDG: Chlorhexidine digluconate; CLSI: Clinical and Laboratory Standards Institute; iMLSB: Inducible macrolide-lincosamide-streptogramin B; MIC: The minimum inhibitory concentration; MRCNS: Methicillin-resistant coagulase-negative staphylococci; MRSA: Methicillin-resistant *Staphylococcus aureus*; MSCNS: Methicillin-susceptible coagulase-negative staphylococci; MSSA: Methicillin-susceptible *Staphylococcus aureus*; SXT: Trimethoprim-sulfamethoxazole; VRE: Vancomycin resistant enterococci; VSE: vancomycin susceptible enterococci

Acknowledgements

We thank Dr. Jostein Bjorland from Norwegian School of Veterinary Science for providing *qac* genes positive control strains.

Funding

The present work was supported by the Research Fund of Istanbul University with Project No. 7214.

Author's contributions

All authors participated in the design of the work. SI performed the test and data collection. SI and YN wrote the manuscript. All authors read and approved the final manuscript.

Consent for publication

Not applicable.

Competing interests

The authors declare that they have no competing interests.

Author details

[1]Department of Medical Biology, Bahcesehir University School of Medicine, Sahrayıcedid Mah. Batman Sok. No:66-68, Yenisahra-Göztepe, Istanbul, Turkey. [2]Istanbul Faculty of Medicine, Department of Medical Microbiology, Istanbul University, Istanbul, Turkey.

References

1. Casey AL, Lambert PA, Elliott TS. Staphylococci. Int J Antimicrob Agents. 2007;29:23–32.
2. Fisher K, Phillips C. The ecology, epidemiology and virulence of enterococcus. Microbiology. 2009;155:1749–57.
3. Alanis AJ. Resistance to antibiotics: are we in the post-antibiotic era? Arch Med Res. 2005;36:697–705.
4. McBain AJ, Rickard AH, Gilbert P. Possible implications of biocide accumulation in the environment on the prevalence of bacterial antibiotic resistance. J Ind Microbiol Biotechnol. 2002;29:326–30.
5. Gilbert P, Mcbain AJ. Potential impact of increased use of biocides in consumer products on prevalence of antibiotic resistance. Clin Microbiol Rev. 2003;16:189–208.
6. Maillard JY. Antimicrobial biocides in the healthcare environment: efficacy, usage, policies and perceived problems. Ther Clin Risk Manag. 2005;1:307–20.
7. Mayer S, Boos M, Beyer A, Fluit AC, Schmitz FJ. Distribution of the antiseptic resistance genes qacA, qacB and qacC in 497 methicillin-resistant and susceptible European isolates of Staphylococcus Aureus. J Antimicrob Chemother. 2001;47:896–7.
8. Noguchi N, Suwa J, Narui K, Sasatsu M, Ito T, Hiramatsu K, Song JH. Susceptibilities to antiseptic agents and distribution of antiseptic-resistance genes qacA/B and smr of methicillin-resistant Staphylococcus Aureus isolated in Asia during 1998 and 1999. J Med Microbiol. 2005;54:557–65.
9. Bjorland J, Steinum T, Sunde M, Waage S, Heir E. Novel plasmid-borne gene qacJ mediates resistance to quaternary ammonium compounds in equine Staphylococcus Aureus, Staphylococcus Simulans and Staphylococcus Intermedius. Antimicrob Agents Chemother. 2003;47:3046–52.

10. Vali L, Davies SE, Lai LLG, Dave J, Amyes SGB. Frequency of biocide resistance genes, antibiotic resistance and the effect of clorhexidine exposure on clinical methicillin resistant Staphylococcus Aureus isolates. J Antimicrob Chemother. 2008;61:524–32.
11. Liu Q, Liu M, Wu Q, Li C, Zhou T, Ni Y. Sensitivities to biocides and distribution of biocide resistance genes in quaternary ammonium compound tolerant Staphylococcus Aureus isolated in a teaching hospital. Scand J Infect Dis. 2009;41:403–9.
12. Miyazaki NH, Abreu AO, Marin VA, Rezende CA, Moraes MT, Villas Bôas MH. The presence of qacA/B gene in Brazilian methicillin-resistant Staphylococcus Aureus. Mem Inst Oswaldo Cruz. 2007;102:539–40.
13. Teixeira CF, Pereira TB, Miyazaki NH, Villas Boas MH. Widespread distribution of qacA/B gene among coagulase-negative staphylococcus spp. in Rio de Janeiro, Brazil. J Hosp Infect. 2010;75:333–44.
14. Leelaporn A, Paulsen IT, Tennent JM, Littlejohn TG, Skurray RA. Multidrug resistance to antiseptics and disinfectants in coagulase-negative staphylococci. J Med Microbiol. 1994;40:214–20.
15. Bjorland J, Steinum T, Kvitle B, Waage S, Sunde M, Heir E. Widespread distribution of disinfectant resistance genes among staphylococci of bovine and caprine origin in Norway. J Clin Microbiol. 2005;43:4363–8.
16. Ye HF, Zhang M, O'Donoghue M, Boost M. Are qacG, qacH and qacJ genes transferring from food isolates to carriage isolates of staphylococci? J Hosp Infect. 2012;80:95–6.
17. Bischoff M, Bauer J, Preikschat P, Schwaiger K, Mölle G, Hölzel C. First detection of the antiseptic resistance gene *qacA/B* in Enterococcus Faecalis. Microb Drug Resist. 2012;18:7–12.
18. Meyer B, Cookson B. Does microbial resistance or adaptation to biocides create a hazard in infection prevention and control? J Hosp Infect. 2010;76: 200–5.
19. Weber DJ, Rutala WA. Use of germicides in the home and the healthcare settings: is there a relationship between germicide use and antibiotic resistance? Infect Control Hosp Epidemiol. 2006;27:1107–19.
20. Clinical and Laboratory Standards Institute. Methods for dilution antimicrobial susceptibility tests for bacteria that grow aerobically. Approved Standard M7-A7. 7th ed. Wayne, PA: CLSI; 2006.
21. Clinical and Laboratory Standards Institute. Performance standards for antimicrobial susceptibility testing. Approved Standard M100-S17. Wayne, PA: CLSI; 2007.
22. Noguchi N, Hase M, Kitta M, Sasatsu M, Deguchi K, Kono M. Antiseptic susceptibility and distribution of antiseptic resistance genes in methicillin-resistant Staphylococcus Aureus. FEMS Microbiol Lett. 1999;172:247–53.
23. Wassenaar TM, Ussery D, Nielsen LN, Ingmer H. Review and phylogenetic analysis of qac genes that reduce susceptibility to quaternary ammonium compounds in Staphylococcus species. Eur J Microbiol Immunol (Bp). 2015;5:44–61.
24. Prag G, Falk-Brynhildsen K, Jacobsson S, Hellmark B, Unemo M, Söderquist B. Decreased susceptibility to chlorhexidine and prevalence of disinfectant resistance genes among clinical isolates of Staphylococcus Epidermidis. APMIS. 2014;122:961–7.
25. Nakipoğlu Y, Iğnak S, Gürler N, Gürler B. The prevalence of antiseptic resistance genes (qacA/B and smr) and antibiotic resistance in clinical Staphylococcus Aureus strains. Mikrobiyol Bul. 2012;46:180–9.
26. Duran N, Temiz M, Duran GG, Eryılmaz N, Jenedi K. Relationship between the resistance genes to quaternary ammonium compounds and antibiotic resistance in staphylococci isolated from surgical site infections. Med Sci Monit. 2014;20:544–50.
27. Aykan SB, Cağlar K, Engin ED, Sipahi AB, Sultan N, Yalınay ÇM. Investigation of the presence of disinfectant resistance genes qacA/B in nosocomial methicillin-resistant Staphylococcus Aureus isolates and evaluation of their in vitro disinfectant susceptibilities. Mikrobiyol Bul. 2013;47:1–10.
28. Longtin J, Seah C, Siebert K, McGeer A, Simor A, Longtin Y, Low DE, Melano RG. Distribution of antiseptic resistance genes qacA, qacB, and smr in methicillin-resistant Staphylococcus Aureus isolated in Toronto, Canada, from 2005 to 2009. Antimicrob Agents Chemother. 2011;55:2999–01.
29. Alam MM, Ishino M, Kobayashi N. Analysis of genomic diversity and evolution of the low-level antiseptic resistance gene smr in Staphylococcus Aureus. Microb Drug Resist. 2003;9:1–7.
30. Zhang M, O'Donoghue MM, Ito T, Hiramatsu K, Boost MV. Prevalence of antiseptic-resistance genes in Staphylococcus Aureus and coagulase-negative staphylococci colonising nurses and the general population in Hong Kong. J Hosp Infect. 2011;78:113–7.
31. Bhardwaj P, Ziegler E, Palmer KL. Chlorhexidine induces VanA-type vancomycin resistance genes in enterococci. Antimicrob Agents Chemother. 2016;60:2209–21.

Prevalence and antibiotic resistance of bacteria isolated from the cerebrospinal fluid of neurosurgical patients at Peking Union Medical College Hospital

Jian-bo Chang[1†], Hao Wu[1†], He Wang[2], Bai-tao Ma[1], Ren-zhi Wang[1] and Jun-ji Wei[1*]

Abstract

Background: Postoperative central nervous system infections (PCNSIs) represent a serious complication, and the timely use of antibiotics guided by the identification of the causative pathogens and their antibiotic sensitivities is essential for treatment. However, there are little data regarding the prevalence of PCNSI pathogens in China. The aim of this study is to investigate the features of pathogens in patients with PCNSIs, which could help clinicians to choose the appropriate empirical antibiotic therapy.

Methods: We retrospectively examined the positive CSF cultures in patients who underwent craniotomy between January 2010 and December 2015. We collected data, including demographic characteristics, type of neurosurgery, laboratory data, causative organisms and antimicrobial susceptibility testing results.

Results: A total of 62 patients with 90 isolates out of 818 patients with 2433 CSF culture samples were available for data analysis. The estimated incidence and culture-positive rate of PCNSIs were approximately 0.9 and 7.5%, respectively. The predominant organism was coagulase-negative staphylococci, of which most were methicillin-resistant coagulase-negative staphylococci (MRCoNS). All were susceptible to vancomycin, linezolid, rifampicin and amoxicillin-clavulanate. *Acinetobacter baumannii* was the most frequent causative Gram-negative agent and was resistant to 12 out of 18 antimicrobials tested. The sensitivity rates for tigecycline and minocycline were only 40 and 33%, respectively.

Conclusion: PCNSIs could lead to high mortality. Although the MRCoNS were the predominant organism, the management of *Acinetobacter baumannii* was a major clinical challenge with few effective antimicrobials in PCNSIs.

Keywords: Prevalence, Antibiotic resistance, Central nervous system infections, Neurosurgery

Background

Postoperative central nervous system infections (PCNSIs) are relatively rare but serious complication following neurosurgery, especially craniotomies, resulting in poor patient outcomes and increasing the total cost of illness. Craniotomies are used for the treatment of head injury, brain tumor or intracranial hemorrhage, external ventricular device placement, and entriculostomy [1]. The incidence of infections after cranial surgery, mostly meningitis, varies from 0.3 to 7.8% [2, 3]. The diagnosis of PCNSIs requires a high degree of clinical suspicion and lumbar puncture for cerebrospinal fluid (CSF) culture. Once diagnosed, selection of the empirical antibiotic should be guided by knowledge of the causative pathogens and their sensitivities.

The epidemiology of bacterial infections varies with time, geographical distribution, age, race, underlying medical and/or neurosurgical conditions, means of contraction, status of vaccination, and use of antibiotics in the community [4]. Although the primary pathogens in PCNSI are still Gram-positive bacteria, such as *Staphylococcus aureus*, there is a possible trend towards greater numbers of Gram-negative bacteria, especially *Acinetobacter* [5, 6]. Another obvious change is the increased rates of multi-antibiotic

* Correspondence: weijunji@pumch.cn
†Equal contributors
[1]Department of Neurosurgery, Peking Union Medical College Hospital, Peking Union Medical College, Chinese Academy of Medical Sciences, No.1 Shuaifuyuan, Dongcheng District, Beijing 100730, China
Full list of author information is available at the end of the article

resistant strains such as methicillin-resistant *S. aureus* (MRSA) and strains that produce extended-spectrum β-lactamases (ESBL) in recent years [7]. The potential underlying cause is the widespread use of empirical vancomycin and antipseudomonal β-lactam antibiotics [8].

Both the species and the antibiotic resistance profile of bacteria, as well as the blood-brain barrier, are crucial components to consider when selecting the appropriate antibiotics. There have been many recent studies reporting the risk factors for PCNSIs [9–12] in China. Unfortunately, little data regarding prevalence and antibiotic resistance of bacteria have been published. Peking Union Medical College Hospital (PUMCH), founded by the Rockefeller Foundation in 1921, is a university general hospital and tertiary referral center in northern China, where the department of neurosurgery conducts approximately 1200 operations each year. As one of the largest pituitary centers in China, about half operations were endonasal trans-sphenoidal approach [13]. Recently, the average length of stay has been approximately 6 days. This research will report the features of pathogens and investigate the clinical characteristics of post-craniotomy PCNSIs in a single institution over the past 6 years.

Methods

This study was approved by the Ethics Committee of Peking Union Medical College Hospital (PUMCH). The results of CSF cultures isolated from inpatients were reviewed via a computerized log containing records from January 2010 to December 2015. The data of patients with positive culture isolates were collected from medical records using previously designed standardized evaluation forms (the details showed in Additional file 1) that included demographic characteristics, types of neurosurgery, laboratory data, causative organisms and antimicrobial susceptibility testing. The positive CSF culture result was the main inclusion criteria. The isolation of the same species from the same patient within 7 days was regarded as the same isolate and not counted multiple times. All the patients met clinical diagnostic criteria of nervous central infection [14]. Culture contamination was determined by specialists from the clinical laboratory and neurosurgery, which was based on the identity of the microorganism itself and its clinical features [14–16]. Previous cranial operation, including both elective and emergency procedures, was another inclusion criteria. Patients who underwent a spinal operation or simple wound revision without drilled holes were excluded from the study. Patients with evidence of concomitant chronic meningitis or encephalitis not due to microbial infection were also excluded.

All patients received 1.5 g of a second-generation cephalosporin as prophylactic therapy 1 h before incision and followed by a 24-h postoperative course. Strict precautions were taken throughout the operation, including the use of antibacterial film, to ensure that there was no perioperative breach in sterility [17]. We analyzed the results of antibiotic susceptibility based on the Clinical and Laboratory Standards Institution (CLSI) methods [15]. Pathogenic organisms were considered resistant if they were reported as intermediate or resistant to at least one of the agents, which included cephalosporins, fluoroquinolones, aminoglycosides, carbapenems, extended-spectrum penicillins, macrolides, and β-lactam/β-lactamase inhibitors.

Results

From 2010 to 2015, approximately 6500 in-hospital patients were treated with approximately 7500 operations in the department of neurosurgery. We obtained 2433 CSF culture samples from 818 patients. Of these, 78 patients with 108 positive isolates were identified, and their medical records were reviewed. Following review, 12 isolates were excluded due to contamination, and four patients were removed because they did not undergo surgery. Finally, 62 patients with 90 isolates met the inclusion criteria. Of them, two patients were failed to obtain the whole medical records and the sensitivity results of five isolates were not available. The incidence of PCNSIs was approximately 0.9% (62/6500) and the estimated culture-positive rate of infection was approximately 7.5% (62/818) and 16 patients with 44 isolates were infected with polymicrobial, in which six patients with more than two species.

Table 1 shows the characteristics of 60 patients with positive CSF cultures. The median days of hospitalization and the infection period postoperation were 46.5 (IQR = 38) days and 9 (IQR = 9) days, respectively. Half of the patients underwent surgery using the endonasal trans-sphenoidal approach, and most were diagnosed with a pituitary adenoma. Most patients treated with craniotomy were diagnosed with occupied lesions. CSF analysis indicated that the patients had low CSF glucose and high protein levels postoperatively. The mortality of culture-positive PCNSIs was 8%, which was approximately 16 times greater than the mortality of inpatients in general (0.49%, 32/6500).

As Table 2 shows, the distributions of Gram-positive, Gram-negative and Eumycetes were 56, 40 and 4%, respectively. The predominant Gram-positive isolate was coagulase-negative staphylococci (33%), followed by *Enterococcus faecalis* (8.9%) and *Staphylococcus aureus* (7.8%). *Acinetobacter spp.* was the predominant Gram-negative organism and was isolated in 16 (17.8%) isolates, followed by *Pseudomonas aeruginosa* in 6 (6.7%) and *Klebsiella pneumonia* in 5 (5.6%).

Table 3 shows the in vitro antibiotic sensitivities of the Gram-positive isolates; 24 coagulase-negative staphylococci isolates were sensitive to linezolid (95%), teicoplanin (100%), vancomycin (100%) and quinupristin-dalfopristin. The seven *Enterococcus faecalis* isolates were all sensitive

Table 1 Demographic and clinical characteristics of 62 patients with post-neurosurgical bacterial meningitis

Characteristic	Value
Demographic parameters	
Mean age (yr)	42.5
Sex, male:female	33:29
Interval between infection and the initial neurosurgery (median day)	9 (IQR[a] = 9)
Days in hospital (median)	46.5 (IQR = 38)
Death	5 (8%)
Operation types	
Endonasal trans-sphenoidal approach	28 (45.2%)
Craniotomy	21 (33.9%)
Shunt placement	9 (14.5%)
Decompressive craniectomy	4 (6.4%)
CSF data	
Leukocyte count (10^6/L)	median = 599.5 (IQR = 3573)
Glucose level (mmol/L)	median = 2.5 (IQR = 1.8)
Lactate level (mmol/L)	median = 119.5 (IQR = 7.5)
Protein level (g/L)	median = 1.3 (IQR = 2.8)

[a]*IQR* interquartile range

Table 2 Bacteria isolated from cerebrospinal fluid (*N* = 90)

Organism	*n* (%)
Gram-positive bacteria	51 (56)
Coagulase-negative staphylococci[a]	30 (33)
Enterococcus faecalis	8 (8.9)
Staphylococcus aureus	7 (7.8)
Others[c]	6 (6.7)
Gram-negative bacteria	36 (40)
Acinetobacter spp.[b]	16 (17.8)
Pseudomonas aeruginosa	6 (6.7)
Klebsiella pneumoniae	5 (5.6)
Enterobacter aerogenes	3 (4)
Enterobacter cloacae	2 (2.2)
Others[d]	4 (4.4)
Eumycetes	3 (4)
Candida albicans	2 (2.2)
Cryptococcus neoformans	1 (1.1)

[a]*Staphylococcus epidermidis* (*n* = 9), *Staphylococcus haemolyticus* (*n* = 5), *Staphylococcus capitis* (*n* = 4), *Staphylococcus warneri* (*n* = 3), *Staphylococcus hominis* (*n* = 3), *Staphylococcus sciuri* (*n* = 1), *Staphylococcus saprophyticus* (*n* = 1) and other unidentified coagulase-negative staphylococci (*n* = 4)
[b]*Acinetobacter baumannii* (*n* = 14). *Acinetobacter lwoffii* (*n* = 1), *Acinetobacter pittii* (*n* = 1)
[c]Gram-positive organisms: *Aerococcus* (*n* = 2), *Corynebacterium striatum* (*n* = 2), *Streptococcus pneumonia* (*n* = 2)
[d]Gram-negative organisms: *Brevundimonas diminuta* (*n* = 1), *Escherichia coli* (*n* = 1), *Bordetella Moreno-Lopez* (*n* = 1), *Serratia marcescens* (*n* = 1)

to chloramphenicol, cefoxitin, linezolid, nitrofurantoin and tigecycline, and the seven *Staphylococcus aureus* isolates were all sensitive to amoxicillin-clavulanate, linezolid, rifampicin, rifampicin, teicoplanin and vancomycin. Of the Gram-negative isolates, there were only five samples of the *Acinetobacter spp.* available for analysis, and they displayed low sensitivity to tigecycline (40%) and minocycline (33%), as Table 4 showed.

Discussion

PCNSIs are rare but severe complications with heavy disease burden following cranial operations. They are associated with increased costs, psychological and emotional trauma and a delay in postoperative adjuvant therapies [9, 12, 18]. The literature contains differing reports of the incidence of PCNSIs. All the PCNSI patients in this study were diagnosed by CSF culture, and the incidence was approximately 0.9% (62/6500), which was similar to some previous studies [3, 19, 20] ranging from 0.3 to 4.8%. However, other studies reported higher rates of PCNSIs, ranging from 6.5 to 7.4% [9, 12, 21]. One possible explanation may be the different inclusion criteria. In this research, only culture-positive post-operation patients were included, implying a lower false-positive rate. Different types of operations may be another reason for the discrepancy between studies. About half of the patients in this study underwent surgery using the endonasal trans-sphenoidal approach, which tends to have a low incidence of infection of approximately 1–10% [22].

The culture-positive rate of infection in previous studies, approximately 50% [9, 12, 21], which was also higher than the present study (7.5%). Possible reasons for the lower positive test rate may be the use of cefuroxime as a prophylactic antibiotic and the use of therapeutic antibiotics as soon as the infection was diagnosed [14]. Another cause could be that the same species of microorganisms cultured from different isolates within 7 days were counted as a single isolate.

The mortality rate of PCNSIs dropped drastically in past years, from 34% in 2005 [23] to 19% in 2011 [5], and a recent study reported that the mortality was 1.8% [9]. Compared to the research of Shi [9], the present study showed a higher mortality of PCNSIs (8%). A possible explanation for the higher fatality rate might be that the diagnosis of PCNSIs in this study depended on the isolation of a pathogen rather than clinical signs, which may mean that many infected patients without positive cultures were excluded. Underestimating the overall number of PCNSIs would lead to overestimating the mortality. Above all, the incidence, positive-culture rate and mortality of PCNSIs vary between studies and are hard to compare due to different inclusion criteria.

The predominant organism was Gram-positive bacteria, accounting for approximately 56% of the total isolates. Coagulase-negative staphylococci was the major organism,

Table 3 Gram-positive antibiotic sensitivity rates

Organism	AMC	AMP	CLI	CHL	CIP	ERY	FOX	GEN	LNZ	LVX	NIT	PEN	RIF	SXT	TCY	TEC	TGC	VAN	OXA	QDA
Coagulase-negative staphylococci [24]	33	–	33	–	46	23	40	61	95	57	–	15	86	52	85	100	–	100	25	100
Enterococcus faecalis [7]	–	67	–	100	75	0	100	67	100	–	100	67	–	–	20	83	100	83	–	–
Staphylococcus aureus [7]	100	–	33	–	83	28	83	43	100	–	–	0	100	50	83	100		100	83	100

AMC amoxicillin-clavulanate, *AMP* ampiclox, *CLI* clindamycin, *CHL* chloramphenicol, *CIP* ciprofloxacin, *ERY* erythromycin, *FOX* cefoxitin, *GEN* gentamycin, *LNZ* linezolid, *LVX* levofloxacin, *NIT* nitrofurantoin, *PEN* penicillin, *RIF* rifampicin, *SXT* sulfamethoxazole-trimethoprim, *TCY* tetracycline, *TEC* teicoplanin, *TGC* tigecycline, *VAN* vancomycin, *OXA* oxacillin, *QDA* quinupristin-dalfopristin

which included *Staphylococcus epidermidis*, *Staphylococcus haemolyticus*, and *Staphylococcus capitis*. *Acinetobacter baumannii* was the most frequent causative Gram-negative agent, accounting for 44% of the total isolates. The microbiological findings in this study were consistent with the majority of previous results, with the most common organisms grown in the culture being Gram-positive [10, 23, 24]. However, in most studies, the dominant Gram-positive organism is *Staphylococcus aureus* [23, 24]. Additionally, *Acinetobacter spp.* were the most commonly isolated Gram-negative bacteria in our study [11, 12, 25, 26], whereas Enterobacteriaceae were the most common in other studies [10, 20, 23, 24].

Of the coagulase-negative staphylococci, 18 (75%) were methicillin-resistant coagulase-negative staphylococci (MRCoNS), and all were susceptible to vancomycin, teicoplanin and quinupristin-dalfopristin. The results agreed with the results of previous studies [27, 28]. Approximately 25% (2 isolates) of *Staphylococcus aureus* isolates were methicillin-resistant *Staphylococcus aureus* (MRSA), and these isolates were susceptible to vancomycin, linezolid, rifampicin and amoxicillin-clavulanate. The incidence of MRSA in our study was higher than the 15.7% incidence Sipahi, O. R. reported [29] and lower than the 40% incidence reported by Rolston, K. V [18]. M.RSA was not a significant problem in our study, as only two samples were identified. However, it has been a major concern in recent years [30]. The results of both MRCoNS and MRSA in our study indicated that the three most effective antibiotics against the MRCoNS were vancomycin, teicoplanin, and linezolid. Vancomycin was the last resort and the drug of choice to treat infections caused by Gram-positive bacteria in CNS infection. Fortunately, all the MRCoNS and MRSA were sensitive to it. However, there were two vancomycin-resistant *Enterococcus faecalis* isolates, therefore, the emergence of resistance to vancomycin could be a serious concern for PCNSIs.

Of the Gram-negative isolates, only the susceptibility of *Acinetobacter baumannii* was analyzed; the others failed due to lack of isolates. There were 13 patients with 13 *Acinetobacter baumannii* isolates, and all 13 isolates were multidrug-resistant (MDR) bacteria with resistance to 12 out of 18 antimicrobials tested. Few studies have reported data on *Acinetobacter baumannii* isolates from CSF, but the SENTRY Antimicrobial Surveillance Program reported that the frequency of *Acinetobacter* spp. was approximately 7% [31]. However, the MDR rate was amazingly high, ranging from 50 to 70%, and the rate of carbapenem-resistant *Acinetobacter baumannii* (CRAB) has risen in recent years [32]. The emergence of MDR *Acinetobacter baumannii*, known as one of the ESKAPE pathogens [33], has become a serious medical problem worldwide [34, 35]. The data presented here could provide further evidence of the widespread distribution of multidrug-resistant *A. baumannii*. This increasing incidence is of great concern considering the lack of treatment options for dealing with MDR *Acinetobacter baumannii* infections. Similar to previous study [34], tigecycline and minocycline were the most effective antibiotic for *Acinetobacter baumannii*, however the sensitivity rates in our study were only 40 and 33%, respectively. More studies should investigate the treatment strategy in the future.

Early diagnosis and the timely use of antibiotics are essential for the treatment of PCNSIs [14]. Few studies from the Chinese mainland about the causative pathogens and their drug sensitivities were available. The present study not only showed the distribution of pathogens from a region, but reflected a similar trend to that observed worldwide, which could help clinicians choose the appropriate empirical antibiotic therapy for PCNSIs. There were a number of limitations to this study. First, the data did not yield highly specific information regarding clinical variables, such as the manifestation of CNS infection and the operative part of encephalic region, and we were not

Table 4 Gram-negative antibiotic sensitivity rates

Organism	AMK	CAZ	CIP	CRO	CSL	CTX	FEP	GEN	IPM	LVX	MEM	MNO	PIP	SAM	SXT	TCC	TGC	TZP
Acinetobacter spp.[b] [13]	8	0	0	0	17	0	0	0	18	0	20	33	0	0	0	0	40	0

AMK amikacin, *CAZ* ceftazidime, *CIP* ciprofloxacin, *CRO* ceftriaxone, *CSL* cefoperazone-sulbactam, *CTX* cefotaxime, *FEP* cefepime, *GEN* gentamycin, *IPM* imipenem, *LVX* levofloxacin, *MEM* meropenem, *MNO* minocycline, *PIP* piperacillin, *SAM* ampicillin-sulbactam, *SXT* sulfamethoxazole-trimethoprim, *TCC* piperacillin-clavulanate, *TGC* tigecycline, *TZP* piperacillin-tazobactam

able to provide insight with regards to these topics. Second, although the number of isolates in the present study was larger than some of previous [10, 11, 24, 34], there was still selection bias, and data from a single institution may not be representative of the entire population of China. Finally, the resistance feature of each isolate was not investigated at the molecular level.

Conclusion

Postoperative central nervous system infections (PCNSIs) are a serious complication and could lead to a higher mortality rate. MRCoNS was the predominant organism isolated and was totally susceptible to vancomycin, linezolid, rifampicin and amoxicillin-clavulanate. The management of *Acinetobacter baumannii* remains a major clinical challenge with few effective antimicrobials in PCNSIs.

Abbreviations

CLSI: Clinical and Laboratory Standards Institute; CSF: Cerebrospinal fluid; ESBL: Extended-spectrum β-lactamases; IQR: Interquartile range; MDR: Multidrug-resistant; MRCoNS: Methicillin-resistant coagulase-negative staphylococci; PCNSIs: Patients with postoperative central nervous system infections; PUMCH: Peking Union Medical College Hospital

Acknowledgements

Funding

The authors have no personal financial or institutional interest in any of the drugs, materials, or devices described in this article.

Authors' contributions

All the authors planned this study and contributed to the interpretation of the data, revisions, and inputs at all stages of the study. JC and HW contributed equally to this work. All authors read and approved the final manuscript.

Consent for publication

All the authors approve and agree the article to this publication.

Competing interests

The authors declare that they have no competing interests.

Author details

[1]Department of Neurosurgery, Peking Union Medical College Hospital, Peking Union Medical College, Chinese Academy of Medical Sciences, No.1 Shuaifuyuan, Dongcheng District, Beijing 100730, China. [2]Department of Laboratory Medicine, Peking Union Medical College Hospital, Peking Union Medical College, Chinese Academy of Medical Sciences, No.1 Shuaifuyuan, Dongcheng District, Beijing 100730, China.

References

1. Ottenhausen M, Bodhinayake I, Evins AI, Banu M, Boockvar JA, Bernardo A. Expanding the borders: the evolution of neurosurgical approaches. Neurosurg Focus. 2014;36(4):E11.
2. Leblebicioglu H, Erben N, Rosenthal VD, Sener A, Uzun C, Senol G, et al. Surgical site infection rates in 16 cities in Turkey: findings of the International Nosocomial Infection Control Consortium (INICC). Am J Infect Control. 2015;43(1):48–52.
3. Dashti SR, Baharvahdat H, Spetzler RF, Sauvageau E, Chang SW, Stiefel MF, et al. Operative intracranial infection following craniotomy. Neurosurg Focus. 2008;24(6):E10.
4. Chang CJ, Ye JJ, Yang CC, Huang PY, Chiang PC, Lee MH. Influence of third-generation cephalosporin resistance on adult in-hospital mortality from post-neurosurgical bacterial meningitis. J Microbiol Immunol Infect. 2010;43(4):301–9.
5. Tangden T, Enblad P, Ullberg M, Sjolin J. Neurosurgical gram-negative bacillary ventriculitis and meningitis: a retrospective study evaluating the efficacy of intraventricular gentamicin therapy in 31 consecutive cases. Clin Infect Dis. 2011;52(11):1310–6.
6. Rodriguez Guardado A, Blanco A, Asensi V, Perez F, Rial JC, Pintado V, et al. Multidrug-resistant Acinetobacter meningitis in neurosurgical patients with intraventricular catheters: assessment of different treatments. J Antimicrob Chemother. 2008;61(4):908–13.
7. van de Beek D, Cabellos C, Dzupova O, Esposito S, Klein M, Kloek AT, et al. ESCMID guideline: diagnosis and treatment of acute bacterial meningitis. Clin Microbiol Infect. 2016;22(Suppl 3):S37–62.
8. Kristich CJ, Rice LB, Arias CA. Enterococcal infection-treatment and antibiotic resistance. In: Gilmore MS, Clewell DB, Ike Y, Shankar N, editors. Enterococci: from commensals to leading causes of drug resistant infection. Boston: Massachusetts Eye and Ear Infirmary; 2014.
9. Shi ZH, Xu M, Wang YZ, Luo XY, Chen GQ, Wang X, et al. Post-craniotomy intracranial infection in patients with brain tumors: a retrospective analysis of 5723 consecutive patients. Br J Neurosurg. 2017;31(1):5–9.
10. Tian RF, Hao SY, Hou ZG, Gao ZX, Liu BY. The characteristics of post-neurosurgical bacterial meningitis in elective neurosurgery in 2012: a single institute study. Clin Neurol Neurosurg. 2015;139:41–5.
11. Wang JH, Lin PC, Chou CH, Ho CM, Lin KH, Tsai CT, et al. Intraventricular antimicrobial therapy in postneurosurgical gram-negative bacillary meningitis or ventriculitis: a hospital-based retrospective study. J Microbiol Immunol Infect. 2014;47(3):204–10.
12. Zhan R, Zhu Y, Shen Y, Shen J, Tong Y, Yu H, et al. Post-operative central nervous system infections after cranial surgery in China: incidence, causative agents, and risk factors in 1,470 patients. Eur J Clin Microbiol Infect Dis. 2014;33(5):861–6.
13. Gao L, Guo X, Tian R, Wang Q, Feng M, Bao X, et al. Pituitary abscess: clinical manifestations, diagnosis and treatment of 66 cases from a large pituitary center over 23 years. Pituitary. 2017;20(2):189–94.
14. Tunkel AR, Hasbun R, Bhimraj A, Byers K, Kaplan SL, Scheld WM, et al. 2017 Infectious Diseases Society of America's clinical practice guidelines for healthcare-associated ventriculitis and meningitis. Clin Infect Dis. 2017;64(6):701–6.
15. Clinical and Laboratory Standards Insitute. Performance standards for antimicrobial susceptebility testing: nineteenth informational supplement M100-S19. Wayne: CLSI; 2009.
16. Weinstein MP. Blood culture contamination: persisting problems and partial progress. J Clin Microbiol. 2003;41(6):2275–8.
17. Lai WA, Lu CH, Chang WN. Mixed infection in adult post-neurosurgical bacterial meningitis: a hospital-based study. Biom J. 2013;36(6):295–303.
18. Rolston KV, Nesher L, Tarrand JT. Current microbiology of surgical site infections in patients with cancer: a retrospective review. Infect Dis Ther. 2014;3(2):245–56.
19. Kourbeti IS, Vakis AF, Ziakas P, Karabetsos D, Potolidis E, Christou S, et al. Infections in patients undergoing craniotomy: risk factors associated with post-craniotomy meningitis. J Neurosurg. 2015;122(5):1113–9.
20. Cassir N, De La Rosa S, Melot A, Touta A, Troude L, Loundou A, et al. Risk factors for surgical site infections after neurosurgery: a focus on the postoperative period. Am J Infect Control. 2015;43(12):1288–91.
21. Korinek AM, Golmard JL, Elcheick A, Bismuth R, van Effenterre R, Coriat P, et al. Risk factors for neurosurgical site infections after craniotomy: a critical reappraisal of antibiotic prophylaxis on 4,578 patients. Br J Neurosurg. 2005; 19(2):155–62.
22. Ivan ME, Iorgulescu JB, El-Sayed I, McDermott MW, Parsa AT, Pletcher SD, et al. Risk factors for postoperative cerebrospinal fluid leak and meningitis after expanded endoscopic endonasal surgery. J Clin Neurosci. 2015;22(1):48–54.
23. Wang KW, Chang WN, Huang CR, Tsai NW, Tsui HW, Wang HC, et al.

Post-neurosurgical nosocomial bacterial meningitis in adults: microbiology, clinical features, and outcomes. J Clin Neurosci. 2005;12(6):647–50.
24. Kumar V, Shah AS, Singh D, Loomba PS, Singh H, Jagetia A. Ventriculoperitoneal shunt tube infection and changing pattern of antibiotic sensitivity in neurosurgery practice: alarming trends. Neurol India. 2016; 64(4):671–6.
25. Chang CJ, Chang BL, Tsai KC, Lai YJ, Fan CM. Acinetobacter baumannii Post-Operative Meningitis. Surg Infect. 2012;13(5):338–9.
26. Ni S, Li S, Yang N, Zhang S, Hu D, Li Q, et al. Post-neurosurgical meningitis caused by acinetobacter baumannii: case series and review of the literature. Int J Clin Exp Med. 2015;8(11):21833–8.
27. Nahaei MR, Shahmohammadi MR, Ebrahimi S, Milani M. Detection of methicillin-resistant coagulase-negative staphylococci and surveillance of antibacterial resistance in a multi-center study from Iran. Jundishapur J Microbiol. 2015;8(8):e19945.
28. Iyamba JM, Wambale JM, Lukukula CM, za Balega Takaisi-Kikuni N. High prevalence of methicillin resistant staphylococci strains isolated from surgical site infections in Kinshasa. Pan Afr Med J. 2014;18:322.
29. Sipahi OR. Economics of antibiotic resistance. Expert Rev Anti-Infect Ther. 2008;6(4):523–39.
30. Bardak-Ozcem S, Sipahi OR. An updated approach to healthcare-associated meningitis. Expert Rev Anti-Infect Ther. 2014;12(3):333–42.
31. Sader HS, Farrell DJ, Flamm RK, Jones RN. Antimicrobial susceptibility of gram-negative organisms isolated from patients hospitalized in intensive care units in United States and European hospitals (2009-2011). Diagn Microbiol Infect Dis. 2014;78(4):443–8.
32. Guo H, Qin J, Xiang J. Surveillance for and susceptibility of Acinetobacter baumannii in a large hospital and burn center in Shanghai, China, 2007-2013. Am J Infect Control. 2016;44(12):1718–9.
33. Talbot GH, Bradley J, Edwards JE Jr, Gilbert D, Scheld M, Bartlett JG. Bad bugs need drugs: an update on the development pipeline from the Antimicrobial Availability Task Force of the Infectious Diseases Society of America. Clin Infect Dis. 2006;42(5):657–68.
34. Shrestha S, Tada T, Miyoshi-Akiyama T, Ohara H, Shimada K, Satou K, et al. Molecular epidemiology of multidrug-resistant Acinetobacter baumannii isolates in a university hospital in Nepal reveals the emergence of a novel epidemic clonal lineage. Int J Antimicrob Agents. 2015;46(5):526–31.
35. Duarte A, Ferreira S, Almeida S, Domingues FC. Clinical isolates of Acinetobacter baumannii from a Portuguese hospital: PFGE characterization, antibiotic susceptibility and biofilm-forming ability. Comp Immunol Microbiol Infect Dis. 2016;45:29–33.

Emerging antimicrobial resistance in early and late-onset neonatal sepsis

Lamiaa Mohsen[1,4], Nermin Ramy[1,4*], Dalia Saied[1,4], Dina Akmal[1,4], Niveen Salama[1,4], Mona M. Abdel Haleim[2,4] and Hany Aly[3]

Abstract

Background: Compared to developed countries, the use of antimicrobials in Egypt is less regulated and is available over the counter without the need for prescriptions. The impact of such policy on antimicrobial resistance has not been studied. This study aimed to determine the prevalence of early and late onset sepsis, and the frequency of antimicrobial resistance in a major referral neonatal intensive care unit (NICU).

Methods: The study included all neonates admitted to the NICU over a 12-month period. Prospectively collected clinical and laboratory data were retrieved, including blood cultures and endotracheal aspirate cultures if performed.

Results: A total of 953 neonates were admitted, of them 314 neonates were diagnosed with sepsis; 123 with early onset sepsis (EOS) and 191 with late onset sepsis (LOS). A total of 388 blood cultures were obtained, with 166 positive results. Total endotracheal aspirate samples were 127; of them 79 were culture-positive. The most frequently isolated organisms in blood were *Klebsiella pneumoniae* (42%) and *Coagulase negative staphylococcus* (19%) whereas in endotracheal cultures were *Klebsiella pneumoniae* (41%) and *Pseudomonas aeruginosa* (19%). Gram negative organisms were most resistant to ampicillins (100%), cephalosporins (93%–100%) and piperacillin-tazobactam (99%) with less resistance to aminoglycosides (36%–52%). Gram positive isolates were least resistant to vancomycin (18%). Multidrug resistance was detected in 92 (38%) cultures, mainly among gram negative isolates (78/92).

Conclusions: Antibiotic resistance constitutes a challenge to the management of neonatal sepsis in Egypt. Resistance was predominant in both early and late onset sepsis. This study supports the need to implement policies that prohibits the non-prescription community use of antibiotics.

Keywords: Blood cultures, Tracheal aspirate, *Klebsiella pneumoniae*, Gram positive cocci, Antibiotic susceptibility, Early onset sepsis, Late onset sepsis, Multidrug resistance, Neonatal sepsis

Background

Neonatal sepsis is a major health problem worldwide [1]. Neonates are more at risk for bacterial sepsis, with a global prevalence of 1 to 10 per 1000 live births [2]. Sepsis problem is much higher in the developing than in the developed countries, with sepsis-related mortality rate as high as 50% for untreated newborns.

Neonatal sepsis is a clinical syndrome in an infant 28 days of life or younger, manifesting with a diversity of non-specific systemic signs and symptoms and isolation of a pathogen from the bloodstream [3]. According to inception, early onset sepsis (EOS) refers to infections during the first 72 h of life that is usually related to intrapartum transmission from mothers; whereas late onset sepsis (LOS) refers to postnatal acquisition of infections after the first 3 days of life [4]. Pathogens encountered in neonatal sepsis vary worldwide; reports from developing countries more commonly show Gram negative organisms [5, 6], although Gram positive organisms have been also reported [6–8]. The susceptibility patterns for early neonatal sepsis typically differs from late neonatal sepsis; more resistant organisms are expected from hospital acquired late sepsis when compared to vertically transmitted, community acquired,

* Correspondence: nerminramy74@gmail.com
[1]Department of Pediatrics, Faculty of Medicine, Cairo University, Cairo, Egypt
[4]New Children Hospital, (Abu El Rish), Cairo University Hospitals, Ali Basha Ebrahim, PO Box 11562, Cairo, Egypt
Full list of author information is available at the end of the article

early sepsis. However, a report from a developing country showed some resistant organisms to cause early neonatal sepsis [9]. Resistant organisms can potentially grow in the community with inappropriate use of antibiotics that is typical in some developing countries. Therefore, in this current study, investigators aimed to examine the microbiological patterns of early and late neonatal sepsis and to specify their antibiotic susceptibility.

Methods

Patients

This is a retrospective study of a prospectively collected data at the neonatal intensive care unit (NICU) of Cairo University Children's Hospital in Egypt, conducted over a 12-month- period. The study was approved by the Ethical Committee of the hospital. Infants were included if they were diagnosed with microbiological bacteremia, and/or clinical sepsis that was accompanied by non-microbiological laboratory values suggestive of infections. Infants were considered to have sepsis if they had a score of 3 or more of the following hematologic findings: i) abnormal total leucocyte count, ii) abnormal total neutrophil (PMN) count, iii) increased immature PMN count, iv) increased immature to total PMN ratio, v) immature to mature PMN ratio ≥ 0.3, vi) platelets count ≤150,000/mm3, and vii) pronounced degenerative changes in PMNs [10]. Infants were classified into two groups according to the timing of sepsis diagnosis: EOS diagnosed ≤72 h of life and LOS diagnosed >72 h of life. Demographic, clinical, and laboratory data were retrieved for all included infants.

Infectious control management

All admitted infants received a limited sepsis work up that included complete blood count, C-reactive protein, and blood culture. Empiric parenteral antibiotics were initiated for 3 days while awaiting blood culture results. Sepsis work ups were repeated during hospital stay whenever an infant displayed clinical signs suggestive for sepsis. Infants were considered to have bloodstream infection if they had at least one blood culture positive for organisms known to cause bacteremia [11]. For other organisms that may cause true bacteremia or may represent skin contamination, infection was considered if the same organism was recorded from at least two blood cultures. Endotracheal aspirate (ETA) cultures were occasionally obtained from mechanically ventilated cases if they displayed clinical signs suggestive of ventilator associated pneumonia such as increased oxygen requirement, increased ventilator support settings, worsening radiographic findings, and changes in tracheal aspirate volume, color or consistency.

Microbiological sampling

For blood cultures, at least 1 ml of blood sample was obtained from a peripheral vein under aseptic precautions. Blood samples were incubated in blood culture incubator (BACTEC- 9050, Beckton-Dickenson, Franklin Lakes, New Jersey, USA). ETA samples were obtained by direct endotracheal suction of respiratory secretions using sterile endotracheal suction catheters into sterile suction trap.

Sample processing

Specimens were processed on arrival to the laboratory. Enriched media used included: blood, MacConkey and chocolate agar plates. These were inoculated, incubated at 37 °C, and examined for growth at 24–48 h. Isolates, if any, were identified by: Gram staining, colony characteristics, and biochemical properties including catalase, DNAse agar, mannitol salt agar, and hemolysis on blood agar plates, for Gram positive isolates, and triple sugar iron (TSI), lysine iron agar (LIA), motility indole, ornithine (MIO), citrate, urease and oxidase for Gram negative bacilli [12]. All media and biochemical reactions were systematically quality controlled according to the standards by the American Type Culture Collection. Antibiotic susceptibility tests were performed by Kerby-Bauer disc diffusion method according to the standards of Clinical and Laboratory Standards Institute (CLSI). The antibiotic discs used represented different groups of antibiotics. The inhibition zones were measured and interpreted according to the CLSI recommendations [13]. Multi drug resistant (MDR) bacteria were defined by resistance to three or more antimicrobial classes [14].

Statistical analysis

All statistical procedures were performed using the Statistical Package for Social Science (SPSS) for windows version 16.0 (SPSS Inc., Chicago, Illinois, USA). Descriptive analyses were expressed as mean ± standard deviation (SD) for quantitative variables, and percentages (%) for categorical variables. Differences in distribution for categorical variables were done using the Chi square test.

Results

Nine hundred fifty three cases were admitted during the study period; of them 314 (32.9%) neonates were diagnosed with sepsis based on clinical signs and/or microbiological laboratory. Early onset sepsis was detected in 123 cases and late onset sepsis in 191 cases. The characteristics of the study population are presented in Table 1. Seventy-seven cases were admitted solely for sepsis whereas 237 had other associated morbidities as shown in Table 2. Sepsis presented more frequently in males than females (178 vs. 136).

Table 1 Demographic characteristics of the study population

Variable	Early onset sepsis (*n* = 123)	Late onset sepsis (*n* = 191)
- Gestational age (weeks)		
≤ 28 weeks (n) (%)	10 (8.13%)	12 (6.28%)
> 28–32 weeks (n) (%)	40 (32.52%)	21 (10.99%)
> 32–36 weeks (n) (%)	32 (26.01%)	43 (22.51%)
> 36 weeks (n) (%)	41 (33.33%)	115 (60.20%)
- Male/Female (n)	72/51	106/85
- Age on admission (days) (mean ± SD)	2.41 ± 4.1	9.96 ± 9.2
- Length of hospital stay(days) (mean ± SD)	16.46 ± 16.48	18.68 ± 16.61
- Outcome (deaths) (n) (%)	38 (30.8%)	32 (16.8%)

A total of 388 blood specimens were cultured from our 314 septic neonates, with more than one culture obtained from the same case in some occasions, with 166 microbiologically positive cultures; of them 49 cultures for cases with EOS and 117 cultures for cases with LOS. The most common organisms for EOS and LOS were gram negative bacilli (31/49 and 87/117 respectively), mainly *Klebsiella pneumoniae spp. (n* = 20 for EOS, and 49 for LOS). Table 3 represents the isolated organisms in the studied population.

A total of 127 endotracheal aspirates (ETA) were obtained during the study period from 58 patients with 79 positive cultures; of them 24 cultures belonged to cases with EOS and 55 with LOS. The most prominent organisms in ETA cultures were *Klebsiella pneumoniae* in cases with EOS (22/24) and *Pseudomonas aeruginosa* (21/55) in LOS cases (Table 4). Organisms isolated from ETA cultures differed from those in blood cultures in 29% of cases.

Antimicrobial sensitivity and resistance patterns were assessed for all 245 isolated bacteria; 166 blood cultures and 79 ETA cultures. Tables 5 and 6 present the susceptibility patterns of gram negative bacilli and gram positive cocci respectively. Gram negative bacilli showed highest resistance to ampicillins (ampicillin- sulbactam, 100% and amoxicillin-clavulanate, 97%), cephalosporins (cefotaxime, 93%, ceftazidime, 96%, cefoperazone, 95%, ceftriaxone, 99%, cefuroxime, 100%), and piperacillin-

Table 2 Clinical presentations and diagnoses among studied cases with suspected sepsis

Clinical manifestation/ diagnosis	Number (%)
- Poor suckling & sluggish reflexes	77 (24.5%)
- Respiratory distress	91 (29.0%)
- Pulmonary hypertension	3 (1.0%)
- Meconium aspiration syndrome	4 (1.3%)
- Apnea	35 (11.2%)
- Congenital heart disease	6 (1.9%)
- Neonatal jaundice	19 (6.1%)
- Neonatal convulsions	12 (3.8%)
- Hypoxic ischemic encephalopathy	11 (3.5%)
- Neonatal hypoglycemia	7 (2.2%)
- Multiple congenital anomalies	10 (3.2%)
- Low birth weight	10 (3.2%)
- Neonatal Pneumonia	15 (4.8%)
- Bleeding tendency or hemorrhage	14 (4.5%)
- Total	314(100%)

Table 3 Organisms in blood cultures of infants with early and late onset sepsis (*n* = 166)

Isolated organism	Blood culture		
	Early onset sepsis	Late onset sepsis	Total
-Klebsiella pneumoniae	20	49	69 (41.56%)
-Pseudomonas aeruginosa	7	14	21 (12.65%)
-Acinetobacter	3	10	13 (7.83%)
-CONS	15	16	31 (18.67%)
-MRSA	2	7	9 (5.42%)
-B streptococci	0	4	4 (2.40%)
-Streptococcus pneumoniae	1	0	1 (0.60%)
-Staphylococcus aureus	0	3	3 (1.80%)
-Escherichia coli	0	4	4 (2.40%)
-Enterobacter	1	7	8 (4.81%)
-Salmonella	0	1	1 (0.60%)
-Stenotrophomonaes	0	2	2 (1.20%)
-Total			166

CONS coagulase negative staphylococci, *MRSA* methicillin resistant staphylococcus aureus

Table 4 Organisms isolated in endotracheal aspirate cultures of infants (*n* = 79)

Isolated organism	ETA culture Total
-Klebsiella Pneumoniae	36 (45.6%)
-Pseudomonas aeruginosa	23 (29.1%)
-Acinetobacter	11 (13.9%)
-Escherichia coli	2 (2.5%)
-Enterobacter	4 (5.1%)
-CONS	2 (2.5%)
-Staphylococcus aureus	1 (1.3%)
Total	79

CONS coagulase negative staphylococci

Table 5 Resistance of gram negative bacilli to various antimicrobials

Organism (number)	Ampicillin-sulbactam	Amikacin	Cefotaxime	Ceftazidime	Imipenem	Vancomycin	Ciprofloxacin	Clindamycin		Rifampicin	Piperacillin-tazobactam
Kl(105)	105(100%)	45(43%)	103(98.1%)	105(100%)	22(21%)	ND	48(45.7%)	ND		ND	103(98.1%)
Pseudomonas (44)	44(100%)	12(27.3%)	39(88.6%)	41(93.2%)	17(38.6%)	ND	22(50%)	ND		ND	44(100%)
Acinetobacter (24)	24(100%)	8(33.3%)	20(83.3%)	21(87.5%)	9(37.5%)	ND	8(33.3%)	ND		ND	24(100%)
Salmonella (1)	1(100%)	1(100%)	1(100%)	1(100%)	0	ND	0	ND		ND	1(100%)
E coli (6)	6(100%)	1(16.7%)	4(66.7%)	5(83.3%)	0	ND	2(33.3%)	ND		ND	6(100%)
Enterobacter (12)	12(100%)	3(25%)	12(100%)	12(100%)	2(16.7%)	ND	5(41.7%)	ND		ND	12(100%)
Stenotrophomonas(2)	2(100%)	0	2(100%)	2(100%)	1(50%)	ND	2(100%)	ND		ND	2(100%)
	Gentamicin	Meropenem	Cefoperazone	Cefepime	Amoxicillin-clavulanate	Ceftriaxone	Cotrimoxazole	Erythromycin	Cefoxitin	Levofloxacin	Cefuroxime
Kl (105)	63(60%)	34(32.4%)	103(98.1%)	86(81.9%)	101(96.2%)	103(98.1%)	86(81.9%)	ND	82(78.1%)	25(24%)	105(100%)
Pseudomonas (44)	21(47.7%)	20(45.5%)	39(88.6%)	28(63.6%)	43(97.7%)	44(100%)	37(84.1%)	ND	38(86.4%)	8(18%)	44(100%)
Acinetobacter (24)	7(29.2%)	10(41.7%)	21(87.5%)	14(58.3%)	24(100%)	24(100%)	19(79.2%)	ND	16(66.7%)	7(29%)	24(100%)
Salmonella (1)	1(100%)	0	1(100%)	1(100%)	1(100%)	1(100%)	0	ND	1(100%)	0	1(100%)
E coli (6)	1(16.7%)	0	6(100%)	5(83.3%)	6(100%)	6(100%)	2(33.3%)	ND	2(33.3%)	1(17%)	6(100%)
Enterobacter(12)	8(66.7%)	4(33.3%)	12(100%)	8(66.7%)	11(91.7%)	12(100%)	10(83.3%)	ND	11(91.7%)	3(25%)	12(100%)
Stenotrophomonas(2)	0	1(50%)	2(100%)	2(100%)	2(100%)	2(100%)	2(100%)	ND	1(50%)	2(100%)	2(100%)

ND* Sensitivity was not done, *E coli Escherichia coli, Klebsiella Klebsiella pneumoniae, Pseudomonas Pseudomonaas aeruginosa

Table 6 Resistance of gram positive cocci to various antimicrobials

Organism (number)	Ampicillin-sulbactam	Amikacin	Cefotaxime	Ceftazidime	Imipenem	Vancomycin	Ciprofloxacin	Clindamycin	Polymyxin	Rifampicin	Piperacillin-tazobactam
CONS (33)	33(100%)	16(48.5%)	31(93.9%)	31(93.9%)	28(84.8%)	8(24.2%)	25(75.8%)	18(55%)	ND	15(46%)	33(100%)
MRSA (9)	9(100%)	3(33.3%)	9(100%)	9(100%)	8(88.9%)	0	8(88.9%)	3(33%)	ND	3(33%)	9(100%)
B streptococcus (4)	4(100%)	2(50%)	3(75%)	3(75%)	2(50%)	1(25%)	3(75%)	3(75%)	ND	4(100%)	4(100%)
St. pneumonie (1)	1(100%)	1(100%)	1(100%)	1(100%)	1(100%)	0	0	1(100%)	ND	1(100%)	1(100%)
Staph aureus (4)	4(100%)	3(75%)	4(100%)	4(100%)	4(100%)	0	3(75%)	2(50%)	ND	2(50%)	4(100%)
	Gentamicin	Meropenem	Cefoperazone	Cefepime	Amoxicillin-clavulanate	Ceftriaxone	Cotrimoxazole	Erythromycin	Cefoxitin	Levofloxacin	Cefuroxime
CONS (33)	18(55%)	28(85%)	33(100%)	29(88%)	26(79%)	33(100%)	27(82%)	28(85%)	25(76%)	22(67%)	33(100%)
MRSA (9)	7(77.8%)	9(100%)	9(100%)	9(100%)	9(100%)	9(100%)	8(89%)	7(78%)	9(100%)	7(78%)	9(100%)
B streptococcus (4)	0	2(50%)	4(100%)	2(50%)	3(75%)	4(100%)	4(100%)	4(100%)	3(75%)	4(100%)	4(100%)
St. pneumonie (1)	0	1(100%)	1(100%)	0	0	1(100%)	1(100%)	1(100%)	1(100%)	1(100%)	1(100%)
Staph aureus (4)	4(100%)	4(100%)	4(100%)	4(100%)	0	4(100%)	4(100%)	4(100%)	3(75%)	4(100%)	4(100%)

ND sensitivity was not done, *CONS coagulase negative staphylococci, MRSA methicillin resistant staphylococcus aureus, St streptococcus, Staph. aureus Staphylococcus aureus*

tazobactam, 99%. Less resistance was evident to aminoglycosides, mainly amikacin (36%) and gentamicin (52%), as well as carbapenems (imipenem, 26% and meropenem, 64%). Least resistance to quinolones (levofloxacin, 24%). Gram positive cocci showed highest resistance to ampicillins (amoxicillin-sulbactam, 100% and amoxicillin-clavulanate, 75%), cephalosporins (ceftazidime, 94%, cefoperazone, 100%, cefepime, 86%, ceftriaxone, 100%, cefuroxime, 100%, cefoxitin, 80%), carbapenems (imipenem, 84%, meropenem, 86%), piperacillin-tazobactam (100%), and erythromycin (86%). Less resistance was evident to aminoglycosides (amikacin, 49%, gentamicin, 57%), quinolones (ciprofloxacin, 77%, levofloxacin, 75%), clindamycin (53%), and rifampicin (49%). Least resistance among gram positive bacteria was found to vancomycin (18%). Multidrug resistance was detected in 67 cases; 18 with EOS and 49 with LOS, and in 92 (37.6%) cultures, mainly among gram negative isolates (78/92).

Discussion

Neonatal sepsis, a life-threatening condition, needs immediate empirical antimicrobial therapy. It is important to choose an antibiotic combination that covers the most common pathogens [15]. Blood culture remains the gold standard for diagnosis of neonatal sepsis, despite its low sensitivity which may be due to small volume of blood sample, or empirical antibiotics prior to sampling [16].

We observed the emergence of multi drug resistance among cases of EOS, which has not been frequently mentioned. A previous study from India stated that multidrug resistant organisms were leading causes of early as well as late onset sepsis [17]. Even studies from Egypt addressing this problem studied multi drug resistance either collectively [18] or in relation to late onset sepsis only [19]. The worrisome rise in levels of antimicrobial resistance among pathogens retrieved from NICUs highlight the needs for better understanding of the problem of early onset sepsis and implementing strategies to combat, especially in countries with limited resources [20].

In the current study, the overall incidence of suspected sepsis was 32.9%. These results are comparable to other studies from Egypt [21, 22], but are better than a previous report in 2001 wherein the rate of sepsis exceeded 50% [23], which may be due to better awareness and adherence to infection control measures.

In this study, the overall mortality in septic neonates was 22.3%. This value is lower than sepsis related deaths reported in other studies from Egypt [21, 23], however, several studies reviewed from different developing countries showed a wide range of infection related neonatal mortality ranging between 8 and 80% [24]. A sepsis related mortality of 19% was reported in studies from east Africa [25, 26].

In this work, the incidence of LOS was higher than that of EOS. Comparable findings were reported in other studies from Egypt and South Africa [21, 27]. The opposite was found in studies from Nepal [28] and Iran [29].

Suspected sepsis was confirmed by blood culture, yielding different bacterial growths in only 166/388 cultures (42.8%). This rate is in the vicinity to those of other studies from Egypt [21] and other developing African and Asian countries [25, 30]. Despite being the gold standard for diagnosing sepsis, blood cultures suffer from low sensitivity, postulated reasons include prior use of antibiotics, insufficient or wrong sampling, poor transport conditions, and slow-growing or fastidious bacteria [31]. Also, some culture negative patients might be due to non-bacterial causes as fungi, viruses and parasites [32]. ETA cultures yielded matching results to blood cultures in 38% of simultaneous cultures and grew different organisms in 29% of cases. Authors showed ETA cultures to be of no value in predicting pathogens causing septicemia in ventilated infants [33]. Higher percentages of matching cultures in this study may be explained by higher simultaneous negative cultures.

Gram negative bacilli were more frequently encountered than gram positive cocci, with *Klebsiella pneumoniae* being the most commonly isolated organism both in blood and ETA cultures (42% and 41% respectively),. These results were consistent in multiple reports from Egypt over two decades [22, 34, 35]. However, other reports from Egypt showed *CONS* as the leading cause of sepsis in 2006 [36], 2010/2011 [37], and 2011/2012 [21]. These results support the fact that the diversity of organisms causing sepsis varies from region to another and changes over time even in the same place [38].

The frequency of gram negative pathogens varied from 31% to 63% with *Klebsiella pneumoniae, Pseudomonas aeruginosa* and *Escherichia coli* being the predominant organisms in almost all countries of Latin America [39]. Several other studies in a diversity of developing countries showed that gram negative bacteria were responsible for most cases of neonatal sepsis [29, 30, 40, 41]. Although some authors state that gram-positive bacteria are the most commonly encountered in NICU patients [42, 43], yet case fatalities are highest for gram-negatives [44]. Others have indicated increasing incidence of gram-negative bacterial infections in NICUs [45].

Among gram negative organisms, *Klebsiella pneumoniae* is increasingly emerging as a common bacteria in hospital settings [46].

The first line of empirical treatment in this NICU is Ampicillin-sulbactam combined with cephalosporins or aminoglycosides. In the absence of clinical improvement, antibiotics are changed to carbapenems and vancomycin until the blood culture results are available. Quinolones are used in culture-proven sepsis with multidrug resistant organisms. In this study, gram negative organisms were most resistant to ampicillins, cephalosporins, and piperacillin- tazobactam. Less resistance was observed to aminoglycosides and carbapenems with least resistance to levofloxacin. Several studies showed high resistance to ampicillin and amoxicillin, aminoglycosides, and different classes of cephalosporins [41, 47]. Even within the aminoglycoside spectrum, some authors found amikacin (which was less used in their units) more sensitive than gentamicin (which was more commonly used) [47]. Two studies in sub-Saharan Africa and Asia revealed resistance of the two common pathogens *Klebsiella* and *Staphylococcus aureus* to almost all commonly used antibiotics in one study [48], and *Klebsiella pneumoniae* median resistance to ampicillins and cephalosporins in 94 and 84% of cases in Asia and 100 and 50% in Africa [49] in the other study. Although short courses of antimicrobials as carbapenems and cephalosporins especially third generation cover a broad spectrum of bacteria, yet their extended use caused the emergence of extended spectrum β lactamase producing gram negative bacteria. This confers resistance to penicillins and cephalosporins and often coexisting with resistance to other categories of antibiotics as quinolones and aminoglycosides [50–53]. In Egypt, gram negative bacteria were resistant to ampicillin, amoxicillin clavulanate and cephalosporins, with highest sensitivity to either or both carbapenems and quinolones [21, 35, 37].

The increasing multidrug resistant gram negative bacteria with relative deficiency of new antibiotics to combat led to the revival of other classes of drugs as polymyxins, which are active against *Acinetobacter* species, *Pseudomonas aeruginosa*, *Klebsiella* species, and *Enterobacter* species [54].

In this work, gram positive organisms were most resistant to ampicillins (mainly ampicillin-sulbactam), a wide variety of cephalosporins (ceftazidime, cefoperazone, cefepime, ceftriaxone, cefoxitime, cefuroxime), carbapenems, piperacillin-tazobactam, and erythromycin. They were less resistant to aminoglycosides, quinolones, clindamycin, and rifampicin and least resistant to vancomycin.

In one study in India, rifampicin was effective against *Staphylococcus aureus* [55]. Other drugs as erythromycin show rising resistance among streptococci species (mainly *group B streptococci, group A streptococci, Streptococcus pyogenes*, and *Streptococcus pneumoniae*) and *Staphylococcus aureus* [56]. Similarly, in current work, erythromycin resistance was highest against *Streptococcus pneumoniae, group B streptococci.* There is an increasing incidence of multi drug resistant gram positive organisms [57], as well as increasing vancomycin resistant isolates [58], however; vancomycin still is an important first-line antimicrobial for treatment of serious infections as *Methicillin-Resistant Staphylococcus aureus* [59]. In our study, we found high resistance to fluoroquinolones among gram positive organisms. This resistance is emerging due to their extensive and increasing use in medical practice and was stated in the literature to be greatest in *Staphylococcus aureus* isolates especially methicillin resistant strains [60].

Conclusion

This study demonstrated a high prevalence of gram negative bacilli sepsis and tracheal colonization. Both gram negative bacilli and gram positive cocci were highly resistant to multiple broad-spectrum antimicrobials. Resistance was the highest against antibiotics used frequently in the NICU as the first line or the second line empirical treatment. It is worrisome to discover that pan drug resistance was not restricted to LOS; infants admitted from the community with early onset sepsis had a high resistance index to the multiple antibiotics. Of note, antibiotics in Egypt are available over the counter and do not require a physician's prescription. This study calls for global regulations to restrict the use of antimicrobials in the community as well as in the hospital setting.

Abbreviations

CLSI: Clinical and Laboratory Standards Institute; EOS: Early onset sepsis; ETA: Endotracheal aspirate; LIA: Lysine iron agar; LOS: Late onset sepsis; MDR: Multi drug resistance; MIO: Motility indole ornithine; NICU: Neonatal ntensive Care Unit; PMN: Polymorph nuclear leucocytes; spp.: Species; SPSS: Statistical Package for Social Science; TSI: Triple sugar iron

Funding

This work did not receive any funding from any source.

Authors' contributions

LM designed the study and reviewed the manuscript for important intellectual content. NR analyzed the data and wrote the manuscript. DS took part in data analysis and reviewed the manuscript. MMA performed experimental works. DA and NS were responsible for collecting the data. HA critically revised the manuscript and participated in writing. All authors read and approved the final manuscript.

Competing interests

The authors declare they have no competing interests.

Consent for publication

Not applicable.

Author details

[1]Department of Pediatrics, Faculty of Medicine, Cairo University, Cairo, Egypt. [2]Department of Clinical and Chemical Pathology, Cairo University, Cairo, Egypt. [3]Division of Neonatology, the George Washington University and Children's National Health System, 900 23rd Street, N.W. Suite G2092, Washington, DC 20037, USA. [4]New Children Hospital, (Abu El Rish), Cairo University Hospitals, Ali Basha Ebrahim, PO Box 11562, Cairo, Egypt.

References

1. Afroza S. Neonatal sepsis- a global problem: an overview. Mymensingh Med J. 2006;15(1):108–14.
2. Goldstein B, Giroir B, Randolph A. International consensus conference on pediatric sepsis. International pediatric sepsis consensus conference: definitions for sepsis and organ dysfunction in pediatrics. Pediatr Crit Care Med. 2005;6(1):2–8.
3. Edwards MS, Baker CJ. Sepsis in the newborn. In: Gershon AA, Hotez PJ, Katz SL, editors. Krugman's infectious diseases of children. Philadelphia: Mosby; 2004. p. 545.
4. Bizzarro MJ, Dembry LM, Baltimore RS, Gallagher PG. Changing patterns in neonatal *Escherichia coli* sepsis and ampicillin resistance in the era of intrapartum antibiotic prophylaxis. Pediatrics. 2008;121(4):689–96.
5. Tallur SS, Kasturi AV, Nadgir SD, Krishna BV. Clinico-bacteriological study of neonatal septicemia in Hubli. Indian J Pediatr. 2000;67(3):169–74.
6. Karunasekera KA, Pathirana D. A preliminary study on neonatal septicaemia in a tertiary referral hospital paediatric unit. Ceylon Med J. 1999;44(2):81–6.
7. Karthikeyan G, Premkumar K. Neonatal sepsis: *Staphylococcus aureus* as the predominant pathogen. Indian J Pediatr. 2001;68(8):715–7.
8. Malik AS, Pennie RA. Early onset neonatal septicaemia in a level II nursery. Med J Malaysia. 1994;49(1):17–23.
9. Mahmood A, Karamat KA, Butt T. Neonatal sepsis: high antibiotic resistance of the bacterial pathogens in a neonatal intensive care unit in Karachi. J Pak Med Assoc. 2002;52(8):348–50.
10. Rodwell RL, Leslie AL, Tudehope DI. Early diagnosis of neonatal sepsis using a hematologic scoring system. J Pediatr. 1988;112(5):761–7.
11. Villari P, Sarnataro C, Lacuzio L. Molecular epidemiology of *Staphylococcus epidermidis* in a neonatal intensive care unit over a three year period. J Clin Microbiol. 2000;38(5):1740–6.
12. Miller M, Holmes HT, Krisher K. Susceptibility test methods: dilution and disc diffusion methods. In: Murray PR, Pfaller MA, Jorgensen JH, Yolken RH, editors. Manual of clinical microbiology, vol. 118. 8th ed; 2003. p. 1526–43.
13. Clinical and Laboratory Standards Institute. Performance standards for antimicrobial susceptibility testing; twenty- fifth informational supplement (M100-S25). Wayne: Clinical and Laboratory Standards Institute; 2015.
14. Magiorakos AP, Srinivasan A, Carey RB, Carmeli Y, Falagas ME, Giske CG, et al. Multi drug-resistant, extensively drug-resistant and pan drug-resistant bacteria: an international expert proposal for interim standard definitions for acquired resistance. Clin Microbiol Infect. 2012;18(3):268–81.
15. Taheri PA, Eslamieh H, Salamati P. Is ceftizoxime an appropriate surrogate for amikacin in neonatal sepsis treatment? A randomized clinical trial. Acta Med Iran. 2011;49(8):499–503.
16. Kalathia MB, Shingala PA, Parmar PN, Parikh YN, Kalathia IM. Study of umbilical cord blood culture in diagnosis of early-onset sepsis among newborns with high-risk factors. J Clin Neonatol. 2013;2(4):169–72.
17. Viswanathan R, Singh AK, Basu S, Chatterjee S, Sardar S, Isaacs D. Multi-drug resistant gram negative bacilli causing early neonatal sepsis in India. Arch Dis Child Fetal Neonatal Ed. 2012;97(3):F182–7.
18. Awad HA, Mohamed MH, Badran NF, Mohsen M, Abd-Elrhman AS. Multidrug-resistant organisms in neonatal sepsis in two tertiary neonatal ICUs, Egypt. J Egypt Public Health Assoc. 2016;91(1):31–8.
19. Aamir MM, Abu El Wafa WM, Ali AE, Hamouda HM, Mourad FE. Prevalence of multidrug resistant bacteria causing late-onset neonatal sepsis. Int J Curr Microbiol App Sci. 2015;4(5):172–90.
20. Chaurasia S, Sankar MJ, Agarwal R, Yadav CP, Arya S, Investigators of the Delhi Neonatal Infection Study (DeNIS) collaboration. Characterization and antimicrobial resistance of sepsis pathogens in neonates born in tertiary care centres in Delhi, India: a cohort study. Lancet Glob Health. 2016;4:e752–60.
21. Moore KL, Kainer MA, Badrawi N, Afifi S, Wasfy M, Bashir M, et al. Neonatal sepsis in Egypt associated with bacterial contamination of glucose-containing intravenous fluids. Pediatr Infect Dis J. 2005;24(7):590–4.
22. Shehab El-Din ER, El-Sokkary MA, Bassiouny MR, Hassan R. Epidemiology of neonatal sepsis and implicated pathogens: a study from Egypt. Biomed Res Int. 2015; doi:10.1155/2015/509484.
23. Mohammed D, El Seifi OS. Bacterial nosocomial infections in neonatal intensive care unit, Zagazig university hospital, Egypt. Egyptian Pediatric Association Gazette. 2014;62:72–9.
24. Thaver D, Zaidi AK. Burden of neonatal infections in developing countries: a review of evidence from community-based studies. Pediatr Infect Dis J. 2009;28(1):3–9.
25. Mugalu J, Nakakeeto MK, Kiguli S, Kaddu-Mulindwa DH. Aetiology, risk factors and immediate outcome of bacteriologically confirmed neonatal septicaemia in Mulago hospital, Uganda. Afr Health Sci. 2006;6(2):120–6.
26. Singh SA, Dutta S, Narang A. Predictive clinical scores for diagnosis of late onset neonatal septicemia. J Trop Pediatr. 2003;49(4):235–9.
27. Motara F, Ballot DE, Perovic O. Epidemiology of neonatal sepsis at Johannesburg hospital. S Afr J Epidemiol Infect. 2005;20(3):90–3.
28. Jain NK, Jain VM, Maheshwari S. Clinical profile of neonatal sepsis. Kathmandu Univ Med J. 2003;1(2):117–20.
29. Movahedian AH, Moniri R, Mosayebi Z. Bacterial culture of neonatal sepsis. Iranian J Public Health. 2006;35(4):84–9.
30. Ahmed AS, Chowdhury MA, Hoque M, Darmstadt GL. Clinical and bacteriological profile of neonatal septicemia in a tertiary level pediatric hospital in Bangladesh. Indian Pediatr. 2002;39(11):1034–9.
31. Lever A, Mackenzie I. Sepsis: definition, epidemiology, and diagnosis. BMJ. 2007;335(7625):879–83.
32. Blanco J, Muriel-Bombin A, Sagredo V, Taboada F, Gandia F, Tamayo L, et al. Incidence, organ dysfunction and mortality in severe sepsis: a Spanish multicentre study. Crit Care. 2008;12(6):R158.
33. Slagle TA, Bifano EM, Wolf JW, Gross SJ. Routine endotracheal cultures for the prediction of sepsis in ventilated babies. Arch Dis Child. 1989;64(1 Spec No):34–8.
34. El Badawy A, El Sebaie D, Khairat S, Fouad S. A study of microbiological pattern of neonatal sepsis. Alexandria J Pediatr. 2005;19(2):357–67.
35. Fahmey SS. Early-onset sepsis in a neonatal intensive care unit in Beni Suef, Egypt: bacterial isolates and antibiotic resistance pattern. Korean J Pediatr. 2013;56(8):332–7.
36. Abd el Haleim MM, Nawar NN, Abd el Rahman EM, Abo Hussein HH, Kamel NR. Epidemiologic and microbacteriologic study of neonatal septicaemia in Cairo University neonatal intensive care units. Res J Med Med Sci. 2009;4(1):67–77.
37. El Feky EA. Abd el Rahman Z, Mansi YA. Retrospective analysis of neonatal bacteremia and antimicrobial resistance pattern in neonatal intensive care unit. Res J Med Med Sci. 2011;6(2):62–8.
38. Shrestha S, Adhikari N, Rai BK, Shreepaili A. Antibiotic resistance pattern of bacterial isolates in neonatal care unit. J Nepal Med Assoc. 2010;50(180):277–81.
39. Berezin EN. Solorzano F; Latin America working group on bacterial resistance. Gram negative infections in pediatric and neonatal intensive care units in Latin America. J Infect Dev Ctries. 2014;8(8):942–53.
40. Aftab R, Iqbal I. Bacteriological agents of neonatal sepsis in NICU at Nishtar Hospital Multan. J Coll Physicians Surg Pak. 2006;16(3):216–9.
41. Rahman S, Hameed A, Roghani MT, Ullah Z. Multidrug resistant neonatal sepsis in Peshawar, Pakistan. Arch Dis Child Fetal Neonatal Ed. 2002;87(1):F52–4.
42. Anwer SK, Mustafa S, Pariyani S, Ashraf S, Taufiq KM. Neonatal sepsis: an etiologic study. J Pak Med Assoc. 2000;50(3):91–4.
43. Robillard PY, Nabeth P, Hulsey TC, Sergent MP, Perianin J, Janky E. Neonatal bacterial septicemia in a tropical area. Four-year experience in Guadeloupe (French West Indies). Acta Paediatr. 1993;82(8):687–9.
44. Stoll BJ, Hansen N, Fanaroff AA, Wright LL, Carlo WA, Ehrenkranz RA, et al. Late onset sepsis in very low birth weight neonates: the experience of the NICHD Neonatal Research Network. Pediatrics. 2002;110(2Pt1):285–91.
45. Nambiar S, Singh N. Change in epidemiology of health care associated infections in a neonatal intensive care unit. Pediatr Infect Dis J. 2002;21(9):839–42.
46. Mannan MA, Shahidullah M, Noor MK, Dey AC, Nasrin N, Marma U. Nosocomial infections in a newborn intensive care unit of a tertiary care health. Bangladesh J Child Health. 2008;32:92–6.
47. Muhammad Z, Ahmed A, Hayat U, Wazir MS, Rafiyatullah, Waqas H. Neonatal sepsis: causative bacteria and their resistance to antibiotics. J Ayub Med Coll Abbottabad. 2010;22(4):33–6.
48. Sivanandan S, Soraisham AS, Swarnam K. Choice and duration of antimicrobial therapy for neonatal sepsis and meningitis. Int J Pediatr. 2011; doi:10.1155/2011/712150.
49. Le Doare K, Bielicki J, Heath PT, Sharland M. Systematic review of antibiotic resistance rates among gram negative bacteria in children with sepsis in resource limited countries. J Ped Infect Dis. 2014;4(1):11–20.
50. Patel SJ, Saiman L. Antibiotic resistance in neonatal intensive care unit pathogens: mechanisms, clinical impact, and prevention including antibiotic stewardship. Clin Perinatol. 2010;37(3):547–63.
51. Polin RA, Denson S. Brady MT; Committee on Fetus and Newborn;

Committee on Infectious Diseases. Strategies for prevention of health care associated infections in the NICU. Pediatrics. 2012;129(4):e1085–93.
52. Gray JW, Ubhi H, Milner P. Antimicrobial treatment of serious gram negative infections in newborns. Curr Infect Dis Rep. 2014;16(2):400.
53. Isaacs D. Unnatural selection: reducing antibiotic resistance in neonatal units. Arch Dis Child Fetal Neonatal Ed. 2006;91(1):F72–4.
54. Falagas ME, Kasiakou SK. Colistin: the revival of Polymyxins for the management of multidrug resistant gram negative bacterial infections. Clin Infect Dis. 2005;40(9):1333–41.
55. Goswami NN, Trivedi HR, Goswami AP, Patel TK, Tripathi CB. Antibiotic sensitivity profile of bacterial pathogens in postoperative wound infections at a tertiary care hospital in Gujarat, India. J Pharmacol Pharmacother. 2011;2(3):158–64.
56. Desjardins M, Delgaty KL, Ramotar K, Seetaram K, Toye B. Prevalence and mechanisms of erythromycin resistance in group a and group B streptococcus: implications for reporting susceptibility results. J Clin Microbiol. 2004;42(12):5620–3.
57. Rice LB. Antimicrobial resistance in gram-positive bacteria. Am J Med. 2006; 119(6 Suppl 1):S11–9.
58. Courvalin P. Vancomycin resistance in gram positive cocci. Clin Infect Dis. 2006;42(Suppl 1):S25–34.
59. Chua K, Howden BP. Treating gram-positive infections: vancomycin update and the whys, wherefores and evidence base for continuous infusion of anti-gram-positive antibiotics. Curr Opin Infect Dis. 2009;22(6):525–34.
60. Hooper DC. Fluoroquinolone resistance among Gram positive cocci. Lancet Infect Dis. 2002;2(9):530–8.

11

Bacterial etiology of bloodstream infections and antimicrobial resistance in Dhaka, Bangladesh, 2005–2014

Dilruba Ahmed*, Md Ausrafuggaman Nahid, Abdullah Bashar Sami, Farhana Halim, Nasrin Akter, Tuhin Sadique, Md Sohel Rana, Md Shahriar Bin Elahi and Md Mahbubur Rahman

Abstract

Background: Bloodstream infections due to bacterial pathogens are a major cause of morbidity and mortality in Bangladesh and other developing countries. In these countries, most patients are treated empirically based on their clinical symptoms. Therefore, up to date etiological data for major pathogens causing bloodstream infections may play a positive role in better healthcare management. The aim of this study was to identify the bacterial pathogens causing major bloodstream infections in Dhaka, Bangladesh and determine their antibiotic susceptibility pattern.

Methods: From January 2005 to December 2014, a total of 103,679 single bottle blood samples were collected from both hospitalized and domiciliary patients attending Dhaka hospital, icddrb, Bangladesh All the blood samples were processed for culture using a BACT/Alert blood culture machine. Further identification of bacterial pathogens and their antimicrobial susceptibility test were performed using standard microbiological procedures.

Results: Overall, 13.6% of the cultured blood samples were positive and Gram-negative (72.1%) bacteria were predominant throughout the study period. *Salmonella* Typhi was the most frequently isolated organism (36.9% of samples) in this study and a high percentage of those strains were multidrug-resistant (MDR). However, a decreasing trend in the *S.* Typhi isolation rate was observed and, noticeably, the percentage of MDR *S. Typhi* isolated declined sharply over the study period. An overall increase in the presence of Gram-positive bacteria was observed, but most significantly we observed the percentage of MDR Gram-positive bacteria to double over the study period. Overall, Gram positive bacteria were more resistant to most of the commonly used antibiotics than Gram-negative bacteria, but the MDR level was high in both groups.

Conclusions: This study identified the major bacterial pathogens involved with BSI in Dhaka, Bangladesh and also revealed their antibiotic susceptibility patterns. We expect our findings to help healthcare professionals to make informed decisions and provide better care for their patients. Also, we hope this study will assist researchers and policy makers to prioritize their research options to face the future challenges of infectious diseases.

Keywords: Bloodstream infection, BSI, Antimicrobial resistance, Multidrug-resistance (MDR), Epidemiology, Gram-positive bacteria, Gram-negative bacteria, Dhaka, Bangladesh

* Correspondence: dahmed@icddrb.org
International Centre for Diarrhoeal Disease Research, Bangladesh (icddr,b), Dhaka 1212, Bangladesh

Background

Bloodstream infection (BSI) due to bacterial pathogens is a global concern. It is often associated with increased length of hospital stay, a significant amount of health-care related costs and most significantly, a high rate of morbidity and mortality [1]. Depending on the age, severity of infection and other risk factors, the mortality rate for BSI varies between 4.0 and 41.5% [2–7]. Recent studies have reported a rapid increase in the number of bloodstream infections from both community and nosocomial sources [8, 9]. *Staphylococcus aureus*, *Streptococcus pneumoniae* and *Escherichia coli* have been found to be the most commonly isolated pathogens associated with BSI worldwide [3, 6].

The epidemiology of BSI varies depending on the geographic location, age and co-morbid illnesses. As an example, *Salmonella enterica* is a frequently isolated pathogen from blood samples in both African and Asian regions, however their serotypes differ substantially [10]. *S.* Paratyphi is the predominant organism in the *Salmonella* group in Africa whereas *S.* Typhi is the most frequently isolated organism in Asia. Besides their isolation rate, their antibiotic susceptibility pattern varies substantially [10]. So, understanding of local epidemiology may play an important role in making proper empirical treatment choices before laboratory test results are available. This is especially true for Bangladesh and other developing countries where healthcare systems operate on poor hygiene system and lack proper facilities to contain infections. In these countries, early treatment is usually based on the patient's clinical symptoms rather than diagnostic results. Therefore, patient's early prognosis to final outcome might be much improved by available epidemiologic data for the most frequently isolated pathogenic organisms. However, complete data on BSI causing organisms from Dhaka, Bangladesh is scarce.

In this study, we aimed to identify the most prevalent bacterial pathogens involved in BSI in hospital and domiciliary patients from Dhaka, Bangladesh. We also determined pathogen antibiotic susceptibility patterns to evaluate the changing trend of antimicrobial susceptibility in this region.

Methods

In this retrospective study, blood samples were obtained from patients attending out-patient and in-patient services at Dhaka hospital, icddrb, Bangladesh which is a primary care hospital with 200 in-patient beds. A total of 103679 blood samples were processed from January 2005 to December 2014. In the consecutive ten years of the study 9600, 9364, 9189, 9523, 9523, 11578, 11179, 10822, 10161 and 12740 samples were received and processed from 2005 to 2014 respectively. All the blood samples were processed for culture using a BACT/Alert blood culture machine to identify the presence of bacterial pathogens. Antimicrobial susceptibility tests were performed on the isolated pathogens using standard microbiological procedures [11].

Bacterial isolation

Collected blood samples were directly inoculated into adult (more than 12 years of age) and pediatric (up to 12 years of age) FAN blood culture bottle. Bottles were incubated in the BACT/Alert machine for up to 5 days. Positive culture samples were directly inoculated onto MacConkey (MC) agar, chocolate agar and blood agar (5% sheep blood) plates. MC plates were then incubated at 35 °C in aerobic condition. Chocolate and blood agar plates were incubated at 35 °C in microaerophilic condition (containing 5% CO_2). Bacterial pathogens were identified using standard bacteriological procedures [11]. API identification strips (bioMérieux, France) were used as supportive tests for further identification.

Antimicrobial susceptibility testing

Antimicrobial susceptibility tests were performed by using the disk diffusion method and susceptibility patterns were determined following CLSI guidelines [11–14]. The study was begun following CLSI, 2004 guidelines [14] and later the relevant changes made in 2010, 2012 and 2013 by CLSI were incorporated. Breakpoint changes made in 2010 and 2013 for carbapenems in the case of *Enterobacteriaceae* [12, 13] were adapted, and also the revised ciprofloxacin breakpoint for *Salmonella* in 2012 [11]. Antibiotic susceptibility was tested for CN (10 μg), SXT (25 μg), Cip (5 μg), CRO (30 μg), AMP (10 μg), Caz (30 μg), Imp (10 μg), Net (30 μg), Ak (30 μg), CFM (5 μg), Azi (15 μg), Pen G (10 μg), E (15 μg), C (30 μg), Van (30 μg) and Tet (30 μg). All the antibiotic disks were obtained from Oxoid, UK. *E. coli* ATCC 25922 and *Pseudomonas aeruginosa* ATCC 27853 were used as quality control strains.

We were not able to find any standard definition of multidrug-resistance (MDR) and observed that many previous studies have used the definition of MDR as resistance against three or more classes of antibiotics both for Gram-positive [15–17] and Gram-negative [18–21] bacteria. Consequently, the definition of MDR as acquired non-susceptibility against at least three classes of antibiotics was adopted. *Salmonella* species were tested against six classes of antibiotics; penicillin and cephalosporin (AMP, CRO, CFM), aminoglycosides (CN), fluor/quinolones (Cip, NA), sulfonamides (SXT), macrolides (Azi) and chloramphenicol. Other Gram-negative bacteria were tested against seven classes of antibiotics; penicillin and cephalosporin (AMP, CRO, CFM, Caz), carbapenems (Imp, Mem), aminoglycosides (CN, Net, Ak), fluoro/quinolones (Cip, NA), sulfonamides (SXT), macrolides (Azi) and chloramphenicol. Gram-positive bacteria were tested against seven classes of antibiotics; penicillin and cephalosporin (AMP, Pen G, Oxa, CRO, CFM), carbapenems (Imp), aminoglycosides (CN), fluor/quinolones (Cip), sulfonamides (SXT), macrolides (Azi, E) and others (C, Van, Rif).

Statistical analysis

Blood-borne pathogen trends for isolation and antimicrobial susceptibility over the last ten years was determined using χ^2 (chi-square) test for trend in SPSS version 16.0. P value ≤ 0.05 was considered significant. Standard error of the mean (SEM) was calculated for mean isolation rates. Odd ratios for age and sex were calculated to show their association with infection by particular organisms, and SPSS version 16.0 was used for this purpose. For age, an odds ratio greater than 1.0 indicated the association of a pathogen with age group of less than five years old, and an odds ratio of less than 1.0 indicated the association of a pathogen with age group of more than five years old. For sex, an odds ratio of less than 1.0 indicated the association of a pathogen with female patient group and an odds ratio of more than 1.0 indicated an association of that pathogen with male patient group.

Results

From January 2005 to December 2014, a total of 103,679 blood samples were received from both hospitalized and domiciliary patients and among them 14015 samples were found to be culture positive. Over these past ten years 11.9, 12.2, 13.9, 16.5, 16.0, 17.3, 12.7, 12.9, 10.7 and 11.9% of the samples were found to be culture positive ($P < 0.001$) respectively. The mean culture positive rate was $13.6 \pm 0.7\%$. Table 1 shows the distribution of organisms found throughout this study period. Blood samples were received from patients with age range of 1 day to 115 years and the mean age was 18 years. *S.* Typhi was the most frequently isolated blood-borne bacterial pathogen in this study, accounting for 36.9% of the total isolates. Other frequently isolated pathogens included coagulase-negative *Staphylococcus* species (21.5%), *Pseudomonas* species (12.5%), *S.* Paratyphi A, B (8.9%) and *Acinetobacter* species (5.1%).

Pseudomonas species and *Acinetobacter* species were the two major non-fermenter bacteria isolated between 2005 and 2014. *Pseudomonas* species showed a sharp increase in isolation rate, from 40.6 to 79.2% ($\chi^2 = 105.1$, $P < 0.001$) of the total non-fermenter bacteria, between 2005 and 2010. However, for the next four years their isolation rate decreased slightly and reached 74.3% in 2014. *Acinetobacter* species showed a decreasing trend in their isolation rate over this study period, from 49.8 to 24.4% ($\chi^2 = 95.5$, $P < 0.001$). *Salmonella* species accounted for 46.7% of the total blood-borne pathogens. We observed an overall decreasing trend in their isolation rate from 2005 to 2014 ($\chi^2 = 306.5$, $P < 0.001$). Besides non-fermenter and *Salmonella* species, other Gram-negative bacteria constituted only 7.7% ($\chi^2 = 72.0$, $P < 0.001$) of the total blood-borne pathogens. *E. coli*, *Enterobacter* species and *Serratia* species had a steady isolation rate over the ten year period, while *Klebsiella* species showed an increasing trend in their isolation rate, from 22.6 to 50.9% ($\chi^2 = 29.1$, $P < 0.01$) of the total Gram-negative bacterial group (excluding *Salmonella* species). Gram-positive bacteria accounted for 27.7% of the total blood-borne pathogens. Their isolation rate increased from 20.6 to 30.8% ($\chi^2 = 351.7$, $P < 0.001$) over study period. From 2005 to 2014, *Streptococcus pneumoniae* showed a decreasing trend in their isolation rate, from 20.8 to 5.6% ($\chi^2 = 158.7$, $P < 0.001$) of the total Gram-positive bacteria.

We observed significant associations between different age groups and infection from specific pathogenic organisms (Additional file 1: Table S7). *Pseudomonas* species (OR: 0.383, 0.341- 0.430, $P < 0.001$), *S.* Paratyphi A, B (0.510, 0.449-0.579, $P < 0.001$) and *Serratia* species (0.592, 0.373-0.941, $P < 0.05$) had significant associations with age group of more than five years old. On the other hand, non-typhoidal *Salmonella* species (5.082, 3.171-8.146, $P < 0.001$) and *S. pneumoniae* (3.827, 2.922-5.012, $P < 0.001$) had significant association with age group of less than five years old. We also observed the association of sex with infection from different pathogenic bacteria (Additional file 2: Table S8). *S. aureus* (1.348, 1.019-1.783, $P < 0.05$) infection was significantly associated with the male patient group, while *E. coli* (0.705, 0.581-0.855, $P < 0.001$) was more associated with the female patient group. Seasonal fluctuation was also observed in the incidence rate of a few pathogens (Fig. 1). *Acinetobacter* species (April-May), *Enterobacter* species (July), *S. aureus* (March and November) and *S. pneumoniae* (March) showed distinct seasonal peaks.

Acinetobacter species showed an increasing trend of resistance against gentamicin ($\chi^2 = 101.6$, $P < 0.001$), ceftriaxone ($\chi^2 = 51.8$, $P < 0.001$) and ciprofloxacin ($\chi^2 = 135.2$, $P < 0.001$) (Additional file 3: Table S1). *Pseudomonas* species also showed an increasing trend of resistance against gentamicin ($\chi^2 = 127.5$, $P < 0.001$), and ciprofloxacin ($\chi^2 = 141.7$, $P < 0.001$) (Additional file 4: Table S2). Additionally, *Acinetobacter* species and *Pseudomonas* species showed an overall 56.2, 47.6, 32.8, 51.4 and 23.0, 17.4, 56.2, 50.8% resistance against ceftazidime, imipenem, netilmicin and amikacin respectively. Table 2 shows the distribution of their MDR strains over this study period.

S. Typhi was found to be consistently sensitive to ceftriaxone and cefixime over this study period; however, a strain of ESBL *S.* Typhi was reported [22]. At the same time, decreasing trends of resistance against ampicillin

Table 1 Bacterial pathogens isolated from blood cultures in Dhaka, Bangladesh from 2005 to 2014

Organisms	Year										Total (14015)
	2005 (1126)	2006 (1132)	2007 (1266)	2008 (1566)	2009 (1522)	2010 (2003)	2011 (1418)	2012 (1391)	2013 (1077)	2014 (1514)	
Salmonella	**566[a] (50.3)[b]**	**747 (66.0)**	**707 (55.8)**	**755 (48.2)**	**593 (39.0)**	**828 (41.3)**	**592 (41.7)**	**663 (47.7)**	**474 (44.0)**	**623 (41.1)**	**6548 (46.7)**
Salmonella Typhi	457 (40.6)	595 (52.6)	571 (45.1)	600 (38.3)	483 (31.7)	643 (32.1)	451 (31.8)	527 (37.9)	355 (33.0)	509 (33.6)	5191 (37.0)
Salmonella Paratyphi A, B	85 (7.5)	133 (11.7)	127 (10.0)	146 (9.3)	102 (6.7)	179 (8.9)	135 (9.5)	129 (9.3)	107 (9.9)	110 (7.3)	1253 (8.9)
Non-typhoidal *Salmonella* species	24 (2.1)	19 (1.7)	9 (0.7)	9 (0.6)	8 (0.5)	6 (0.3)	6 (0.4)	7 (0.5)	12 (1.1)	4 (0.3)	104 (0.7)
Non-fermenter	**178 (15.8)**	**196 (17.3)**	**232 (18.3)**	**290 (18.5)**	**276 (18.1)**	**338 (16.9)**	**248 (17.5)**	**232 (16.7)**	**187 (17.4)**	**307 (20.3)**	**2484 (17.7)**
Acinetobacter species	98 (8.7)	45 (4.0)	101 (8.0)	86 (5.5)	82 (5.4)	68 (3.4)	55 (3.9)	55 (4.0)	56 (5.2)	76 (5.0)	722 (5.2)
Pseudomonas species	80 (7.1)	151 (13.3)	131 (10.3)	204 (13.0)	194 (12.7)	270 (13.5)	193 (13.6)	177 (12.7)	131 (12.2)	231 (15.3)	1762 (12.6)
Gram Negative	**146 (13.0)**	**66 (5.8)**	**78 (6.2)**	**85 (5.4)**	**130 (8.5)**	**138 (6.9)**	**114 (8.0)**	**128 (9.2)**	**74 (6.9)**	**116 (7.7)**	**1075 (7.7)**
Escherichia coli	35 (3.1)	29 (2.6)	34 (2.7)	46 (2.9)	51 (3.4)	64 (3.2)	48 (3.4)	45 (3.2)	39 (3.6)	36 (2.4)	427 (3.0)
Klebsiella species	33 (2.9)	27 (2.4)	31 (2.4)	27 (1.7)	37 (2.4)	51 (2.5)	35 (2.5)	46 (3.3)	29 (2.7)	59 (3.9)	375 (2.7)
Enterobacter species	30 (2.7)	8 (0.7)	11 (0.9)	8 (0.5)	42 (2.8)	17 (0.8)	24 (1.7)	27 (1.9)	4 (0.4)	17 (1.1)	188 (1.3)
Serratia species	48 (4.3)	2 (0.2)	2 (0.2)	4 (0.3)	0 (0.0)	6 (0.3)	7 (0.5)	10 (0.7)	2 (0.2)	4 (0.3)	85 (0.6)
Gram Positive	**236 (21.0)**	**123 (10.9)**	**249 (19.7)**	**436 (27.8)**	**523 (34.4)**	**699 (34.9)**	**464 (32.7)**	**368 (26.5)**	**342 (31.8)**	**468 (30.9)**	**3908 (27.9)**
Coagulase-negative *Staphylococci*	147 (13.1)	54 (4.8)	179 (14.1)	350 (22.2)	416 (27.3)	591 (29.5)	364 (25.7)	271 (19.5)	248 (23.0)	372 (24.6)	2992 (21.3)
Staphylococcus aureus	14 (1.2)	10 (0.9)	15 (1.2)	23 (1.5)	26 (1.7)	30 (1.5)	25 (1.8)	23 (1.7)	23 (2.1)	30 (2.0)	219 (1.6)
Streptococcus pneumoniae	49 (4.4)	32 (2.8)	23 (1.8)	23 (1.5)	25 (1.6)	25 (1.2)	29 (2.0)	23 (1.7)	21 (1.9)	26 (1.7)	276 (2.0)
Streptococcus species	21 (1.9)	22 (1.9)	17 (1.3)	23 (1.5)	30 (2.0)	27 (1.3)	29 (2.0)	29 (2.1)	35 (3.2)	23 (1.5)	256 (1.8)
Enterococcus faecalis	5 (0.4)	5 (0.4)	15 (1.2)	17 (1.1)	26 (1.7)	26 (1.3)	17 (1.2)	22 (1.6)	15 (1.4)	17 (1.1)	165 (1.2)

[a]Values in parentheses indicate the number of isolates found in each year; [b]Values in parentheses indicate the percentage of isolates found in each year
The bolded data indicates the total number and percentage of that group

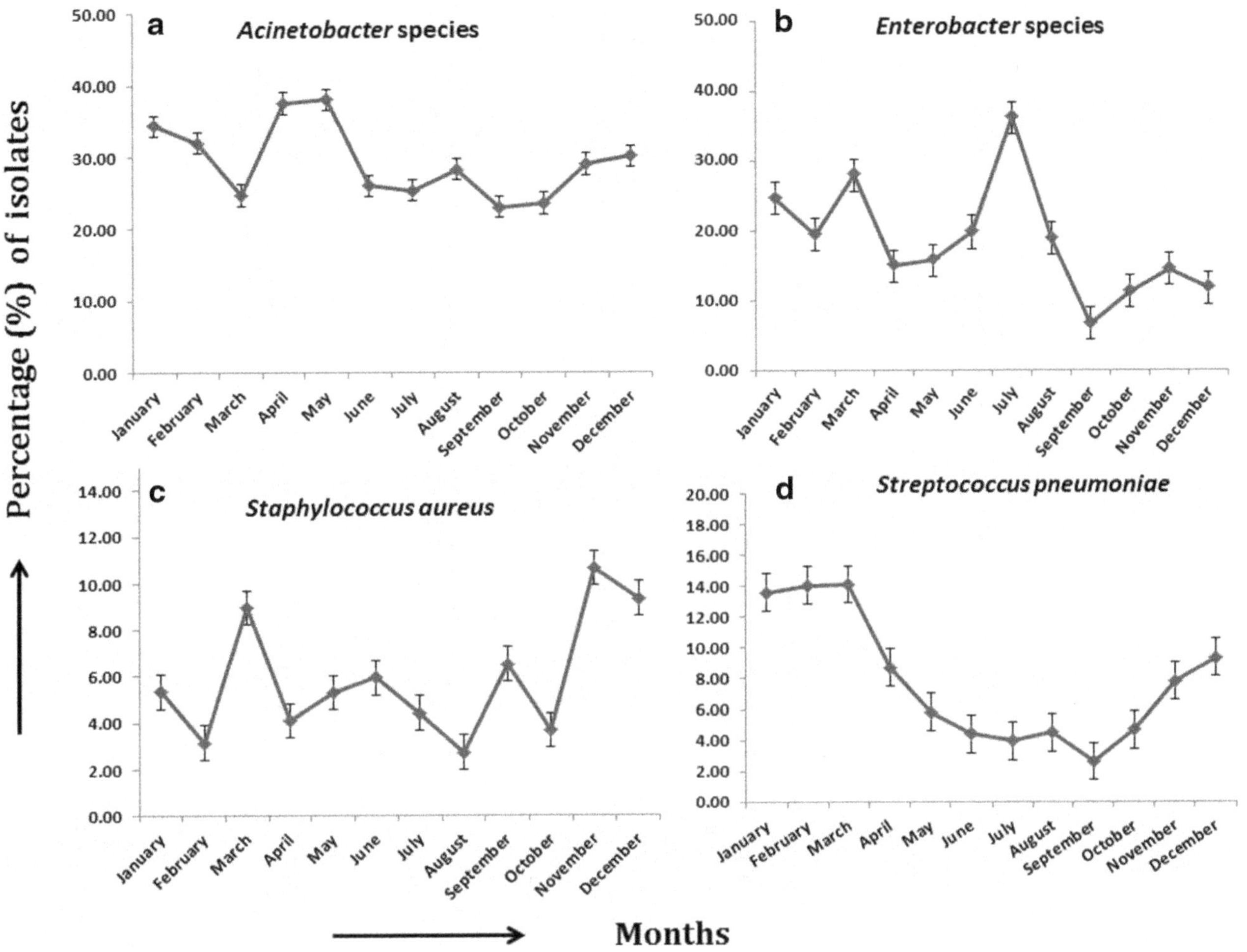

Fig. 1 Seasonal variability of BSI causing pathogens- **a** *Acinetobacter* species, **b** *Enterobacter* species, **c** *Staphylococcus aureus*, **d** *Streptococcus pneumoniae*

($\chi^2 = 540.4$, $P < 0.001$) and co-trimoxazole ($\chi^2 = 740.3$, $P < 0.001$) were observed. *S.* Paratyphi A, B was found to be consistently susceptible to ampicillin, co-trimoxazole, ceftriaxone and cefixime over the ten year period. Noticeably, both *S.* Typhi and *S.* Paratyphi A, B showed a trend of increasingly reduced susceptibility against ciprofloxacin ($\chi^2 = 24.3$ and 66.1 respectively, $P < 0.001$) throughout this study period (Table 3).

E. coli and *Enterobacter* species showed an increasing trend of resistance against gentamicin ($\chi^2 = 52.44$ and statistically insignificant respectively, $P < 0.001$) and ceftriaxone ($\chi^2 = 52.4$ and 16.5 respectively, $P < 0.001$). A reducing trend of susceptibility against ciprofloxacin ($\chi^2 = 89.9$ and 86.8 respectively, $P < 0.001$) was also observed (Table 4 and Additional file 5: Table S4). Additionally, *E. coli* showed an overall increase in resistance, from 69.0 to 90.0%, against co-trimoxazole and ampicillin between 2005 and 2014. *Klebsiella* species showed an increasing trend of resistance against imipenem ($\chi^2 = 79.6$, $P < 0.001$), and a reducing trend of susceptibility against ciprofloxacin ($\chi^2 = 36.1$, $P < 0.001$) (Additional file 6: Table S3). Over the same time period an overall increase in resistance, from 62.0 to 76.0%, was observed against gentamicin and ceftriaxone respectively for *Klebsiella species*. Additionally, *Klebsiella species* showed an overall 86.0, 33.0 and 70.0% resistance against cefixime, meropenem and azithromycin respectively from 2010 to 2014.

S. pneumoniae was found to be consistently susceptible to ampicillin and ceftriaxone between 2005 and 2014 (Table 5). Over this period, their resistance to co-trimoxazole reduced ($\chi^2 = 92.5$, $P < 0.001$). However, it increased against penicillin G ($\chi^2 = 195.3$, $P < 0.001$) and erythromycin ($\chi^2 = 293.2$, $P < 0.001$). Also, a trend of increased susceptibility was observed against ciprofloxacin ($\chi^2 = 79.2$, $P < 0.001$). Other *Streptococcus* species showed an increasing trend of resistance against gentamicin ($\chi^2 = 44.9$, $P < 0.001$) and erythromycin ($\chi^2 = 70.0$, $P < 0.001$), while there was a reducing trend in susceptibility against ciprofloxacin ($\chi^2 = 67.3$, $P < 0.001$) (Additional file 7: Table S5). *S. aureus* was found to be highly resistant to ampicillin (up to 100%) throughout

Table 2 Percentage of MDR strains isolated from blood cultures in Dhaka, Bangladesh from 2005 to 2014

Organisms	Year									
	2005	2006	2007	2008	2009	2010	2011	2012	2013	2014
Salmonella	**286[a] (50.5)[b]**	**383 (51.3)**	**308 (43.6)**	**269 (35.7)**	**189 (31.9)**	**219 (26.4)**	**131 (22.1)**	**109 (16.4)**	**87 (18.4)**	**120 (19.3)**
Salmonella Typhi	282 (61.7)	379 (63.7)	307 (53.8)	268 (44.7)	188 (38.9)	219 (34.1)	130 (28.8)	109 (20.7)	87 (24.5)	120 (23.6)
Salmonella Paratyphi A, B	1 (1.2)	0 (0.0)	0 (0.0)	0 (0.0)	0 (0.0)	0 (0.0)	1 (0.7)	0 (0.0)	0 (0.0)	0 (0.0)
Non-typhoidal *Salmonella* species	3 (12.5)	4 (21.1)	1 (11.1)	1 (12.5)	1 (12.5)	0 (0.0)	0 (0.0)	0 (0.0)	0 (0.0)	0 (0.0)
Non-Fermenter	**67 (37.6)**	**81 (41.3)**	**85 (36.6)**	**138 (47.6)**	**112 (40.6)**	**101 (29.9)**	**52 (21.0)**	**51 (22.0)**	**57 (30.5)**	**99 (32.2)**
Acinetobacter species	24 (24.5)	17 (37.8)	25 (24.8)	37 (43.0)	42 (51.2)	35 (51.5)	23 (41.8)	30 (54.5)	34 (60.7)	50 (65.8)
Pseudomonas species	43 (53.8)	64 (42.4)	60 (45.8)	101 (49.5)	70 (36.1)	66 (24.4)	29 (15.0)	21 (11.9)	23 (17.6)	49 (21.2)
Gram-Negative	53 (36.3)	40 (60.6)	45 (57.7)	47 (55.3)	79 (60.8)	98 (71.0)	57 (50.0)	76 (59.4)	53 (71.6)	86 (74.1)
Escherichia coli	**22 (62.9)**	**19 (65.5)**	**19 (55.9)**	**23 (50.0)**	**37 (72.5)**	**38 (59.4)**	**25 (52.1)**	**31 (68.9)**	**27 (69.2)**	**26 (72.2)**
Klebsiella species	24 (72.7)	18 (66.7)	16 (51.6)	20 (74.1)	21 (56.8)	43 (84.3)	19 (54.3)	24 (52.2)	22 (75.9)	48 (81.4)
Enterobacter species	6 (20.0)	3 (37.5)	8 (72.7)	1 (12.5)	21 (50.0)	12 (70.6)	9 (37.5)	12 (44.4)	3 (75.0)	12 (70.6)
Serratia species	1 (2.1)	0 (0.0)	2 (100)	3 (75.0)	-	5 (84.3)	4 (57.1)	9 (90.0)	1 (50.0)	0 (0.0)
Gram-Positive	**16 (18.0)**	**16 (23.2)**	**26 (37.1)**	**37 (43.0)**	**51 (47.7)**	**36 (33.3)**	**30 (30.0)**	**27 (27.8)**	**27 (28.7)**	**34 (35.4)**
Staphylococcus aureus	4 (28.6)	2 (20.0)	5 (33.3)	16 (69.6)	15 (57.7)	16 (53.3)	14 (56.0)	12 (52.2)	10 (43.5)	19 (63.3)
Streptococcus pneumoniae	3 (6.1)	3 (9.4)	3 (13.0)	1 (4.3)	4 (16.0)	4 (16.0)	2 (6.9)	3 (13.0)	6 (28.6)	4 (15.4)
Streptococcus species	6 (28.6)	10 (45.5)	6 (35.3)	8 (34.8)	13 (43.3)	10 (37.0)	8 (27.6)	9 (31.0)	9 (25.7)	7 (30.4)
Enterococcus faecalis	3 (60)	1 (20.0)	12 (80.0)	12 (70.6)	19 (73.1)	6 (23.1)	6 (35.3)	3 (13.6)	2 (13.3)	4 (23.5)

[a]Indicates the number of MDR strain isolated at that particular year; [b]indicates the percentage of MDR strains of that particular strain
The bolded data indicates the total number and percentage of that group

Table 3 Percentage of antimicrobial resistance in *Salmonella* Typhi and *Salmonella* Paratyphi A, B strains isolated from blood cultures

	Salmonella Typhi									
	2005 (457)[a]	2006 (595)	2007 (571)	2008 (600)	2009 (483)	2010 (643)	2011 (451)	2012 (527)	2013 (354)	2014 (509)
AMP	61	62	54	50	41	41	42	24	28	26
SXT	61	63	54	44	39	34	29	21	24	24
Cip^{R}	3	4	2	1	0	2	2	1	1	4
Cip^{I}	87	89	88	93	94	94	92	96	92	94
CRO	0	0	0	0	0	0	0	0	0	0
CFM	0	0	0	0	0	0	0	0	1	0

	Salmonella Paratyphi A, B									
	2005 (85)[a]	2006 (133)	2007 (127)	2008 (146)	2009 (102)	2010 (179)	2011 (135)	2012 (129)	2013 (107)	2014 (110)
AMP	1	1	0	1	0	0	1	0	1	0
SXT	1	0	0	0	0	0	0	0	1	2
Cip^{R}	1	0	0	0	0	0	0	0	0	1
Cip^{I}	91	93	97	99	100	99	98	100	98	99
CRO	0	0	0	0	0	0	0	0	0	0
CFM	0	0	1	0	0	0	1	0	0	0

AMP ampicillin, *SXT* cotrimoxazole, *Cip* ciprofloxacin, *CRO* ceftriaxone, *CFM* cefixime, [a]Values in parentheses indicate the number of isolates tested each year

this study (Table 6). For this species, resistance against erythromycin increased from 36.0% in 2005 to 75.0% in 2014 ($P < 0.09$) while susceptibility to ciprofloxacin reduced ($\chi^2 = 37.2$, $P < 0.001$). *S. aureus* remained consistently susceptible to vancomycin for the last five years of the study and during the same time period they showed an overall 42.0% resistance against ceftriaxone. *E. faecalis* was found consistently susceptible to vancomycin between 2010 and 2014, while this species showed an overall 31.0, 45.0, 60.0, 39.0 and 81.0% resistance against ampicillin, gentamicin (120), ciprofloxacin, penicillin G and cotrimoxazole respectively (Additional file 8: Table S6).

Discussion

In this retrospective study, we aimed to identify the most prevalent pathogenic organisms involved in bloodstream infections (BSI) over a ten year period (2005–14) in patients in Dhaka, Bangladesh. We also aimed to determine the antimicrobial susceptibility of the isolated pathogens against multiple antibiotics to achieve a clear outlook on the changing trend of their antibiotic susceptibility.

S. Typhi, the causative agent of typhoid fever, is a major public health concern in Bangladesh and other developing Asian countries. Several studies from Bangladesh have already identified *S.* Typhi as a common cause of bloodstream infection in this region [23–25]. We found *Salmonella* species to be responsible for almost half of the disease burden associated with BSI in Dhaka, Bangladesh and about 80% of these infections were due to *S.* Typhi. However, we have observed an overall decrease in *Salmonella* species isolation rate over this study period. This decrease may be attributed to the improved urban water management system and sanitation practices in Dhaka city over the past years.

A significant change in the epidemiology of *S.* Typhi was observed in early 1990's as those years experienced a dramatic rise of MDR strains in Dhaka, Bangladesh [26]. By mid-1990s, about half of the *S.* Typhi strains were MDR; these were resistant against three first line antibiotics - ampicillin, cotrimoxazole and chloramphenicol [26]. Noticeably, after a few years of an initial epidemic period, a decreasing trend in the isolation rate of MDR *S.* Typhi strains was observed [23]. Our study confirms this trend to continue; from 2005 to 2010, the percentage of MDR *S.* Typhi strains isolated declined from 61.7 to 23.7% (Fig. 2). As indicated by recent studies from Bangladesh, *S.* Typhi still shows a high level of resistance against first line antibiotics [23]. However, we have observed a steady decrease in resistance against ampicillin and cotrimoxazole over the ten year study period. Hopefully, if this trend continues, then using the cheaper, first line antibiotics again to treat *S.* Typhi infections might be a possibility in near future. Ciprofloxacin or ceftriaxone is

Table 4 Percentage of antimicrobial resistance in *E. coli* strains isolated from blood cultures

	E. coli									
	2005 (35)[a]	2006 (29)	2007 (34)	2008 (46)	2009 (51)	2010 (64)	2011 (48)	2012 (45)	2013 (39)	2014 (36)
Amp	88	96	71	79	97	96	93	94	92	92
SXT	74	75	76	61	73	70	68	73	56	67
CN	15	28	24	33	37	36	38	30	44	36
Cip^{R}	51	48	41	54	63	73	49	71	72	72
Cip^{I}	0	0	6	2	6	2	2	4	0	0
CRO	34	55	32	46	55	63	66	76	69	75

	2010 (64)	2011 (48)	2012 (45)	2013 (39)	2014 (36)
Net	8	7	7	8	14
Ak	7	4	4	8	14
Imp	3	2	4	8	11
Caz	35	30	38	36	56
CFM	69	70	79	68	78

AMP ampicillin, *SXT* cotrimoxazole, *CN* gentamicin, *Cip* ciprofloxacin, *CRO* ceftriaxone, *Net* netilmicin, *Ak* amikacin, *Imp* imipenem, *Caz* ceftazidime, *CFM* cefixime, [a]Values in parentheses indicate the number of isolates tested each year

Table 5 Percentage of antimicrobial resistance in *Streptococcus pneumoniae* strains isolated from blood cultures

	Streptococcus pneumoniae									
	2005 (49)[a]	2006 (32)	2007 (23)	2008 (23)	2009 (25)	2010 (25)	2011 (29)	2012 (23)	2013 (21)	2014 (26)
Amp	2	0	0	0	0	0	0	0	0	0
SXT	91	90	87	73	76	91	78	70	71	73
CipR	6	0	5	0	4	0	8	0	0	0
CipI	22	38	24	5	16	0	8	0	9	9
CRO	0	0	0	0	0	0	0	0	0	0
Pen G	2	0	0	0	9	8	3	4	5	8
E	4	0	0	0	8	5	24	23	48	31
Azi	-	-	-	-	-	7	39	14	55	31
CFM	-	-	-	-	-	17	0	7	0	8

AMP ampicillin, *SXT* cotrimoxazole, *Cip* ciprofloxacin, *CRO* ceftriaxone, *Pen G* penicillin G, *E* erythromycin, *Azi* azithromycin, *CFM* cefixime. [a]Values in parentheses indicate the number of isolates tested each year; – indicates absence of data in respective years

usually the choice of treatment against MDR *Salmonella* strains [27]. We found all *Salmonella* isolates were consistently susceptible to ceftriaxone, but a very high level of reduced susceptibility exists against ciprofloxacin. Studies suggest that the presence of a mutation in the quinolone resistance-determining region (QRDR) of the gyrA gene is responsible for the emergence of this reduced susceptibility [28].

Non-fermenter Gram-negative bacilli are well known for their ability to cause nosocomial infections [29, 30]. We identified *Pseudomonas* species and *Acinetobacter* species to be the third (12.6%) and fifth (5.2%) most prevalent organisms associated with BSI in Dhaka, Bangladesh. A gradual decrease in the presence of *Acinetobacter* species and a significant increase in the presence of *Pseudomonas* species were observed over the study period. This increase in BSI from *Pseudomonas* species was possibly from the patients increased access to the health care facilities over these years. Also noticeably, *Pseudomonas* species was found to be more associated with patients above five years of age; almost 70% of the infections occurring among adults (≥18 years of age). A recent study from Bangladesh also suggested that there is a very low amount of bacteremia cases due to *Pseudomonas* species among diarrheal children less than five years of age [31].

Acinetobacter species and *Pseudomonas* species are well known for their high degree of resistance against all classes of antibiotics, and the emergence of MDR strains makes it very difficult to treat them. An aminoglycosides combined with a β-lactamase-stable β-lactam is the typical choice of treatment for *Acinetobacter* species infection [32], and carbapenems are known to be most effective against their MDR strains [33]. We observed *Acinetobacter* species to develop increasingly high levels of antibiotic resistance against all aminoglycosides, and noticeably, very high levels of resistance against imipenem (64%). Usually, in the case of resistance against carbapenems, the expert's choice of treatment for *Acinetobacter* species infections entails colistin and tigecycline [34]. We found only 3.73% of the MDR *Acinetobacter* species strains to be resistant against polymyxin B (300 u), therefore it might be considered as a good treatment choice against MDR *Acinetobacter* species. Colistin and polymyxin B (300 u) are usually considered as the last resort for treatment of infections due to MDR *Pseudomonas* species [35], but we observed high levels of resistance against them. In contrast, we found imipenem to be consistently effective against all *Pseudomonas* species so it might be considered as a good choice of treatment.

Besides non-fermenter and *Salmonella* species, other clinically important Gram-negative bacteria were *E. coli*, *Enterobacter* species, *Klebsiella* species and *Serratia* species. *E. coli* has been reported as the leading cause of BSI in developed countries [1]; however, data is relatively unavailable for Bangladesh. We found *E. coli* to be responsible for only 3.05% of the total BSI cases. It is likely that the presence of *E. coli* is overshadowed by the overwhelming presence of *Salmonella* species in Dhaka, Bangladesh, so it would be unwise to ignore them as clinically insignificant.

A recent study from Bangladesh has shown a very high level of antibiotic resistance and MDR level among *E. coli* isolates from environmental samples [36]. In this study we identified a much higher level of antibiotic resistance and MDR level (36% MDR in environment samples vs. 62.38% MDR in our clinical samples) among BSI causing *E. coli* strains. We found carbapenems to be the

Table 6 Percentage of antimicrobial resistance in *Staphylococcus aureus* strains isolated from blood cultures

	Staphylococcus aureus									
	2005 (14)[a]	2006 (10)	2007 (15)	2008 (23)	2009 (26)	2010 (30)	2011 (25)	2012 (23)	2013 (23)	2014 (30)
Amp	100	100	88	90	88	67	100	100	100	71
SXT	29	20	20	52	35	33	36	23	17	38
C	7	0	7	4	4	4	0	13	4	17
E	36	20	33	78	81	67	72	73	64	75
CipR	25	20	40	65	54	57	64	48	39	67
CipI	8	0	0	0	4	3	4	9	13	0
CN	25	11	20	26	27	33	24	13	22	27
CRO	-	-	-	-	-	43	29	50	41	45
Van	-	-	-	-	-	4	0	0	0	0

AMP ampicillin, *SXT* cotrimoxazole, *C* chloramphenicol, *E* erythromycin, *Cip* ciprofloxacin, *CN* gentamicin, *CRO* ceftriaxone, *Van* vancomycin, [a]Values in parentheses indicate the number of isolates tested each year; – indicates absence of data in respective years

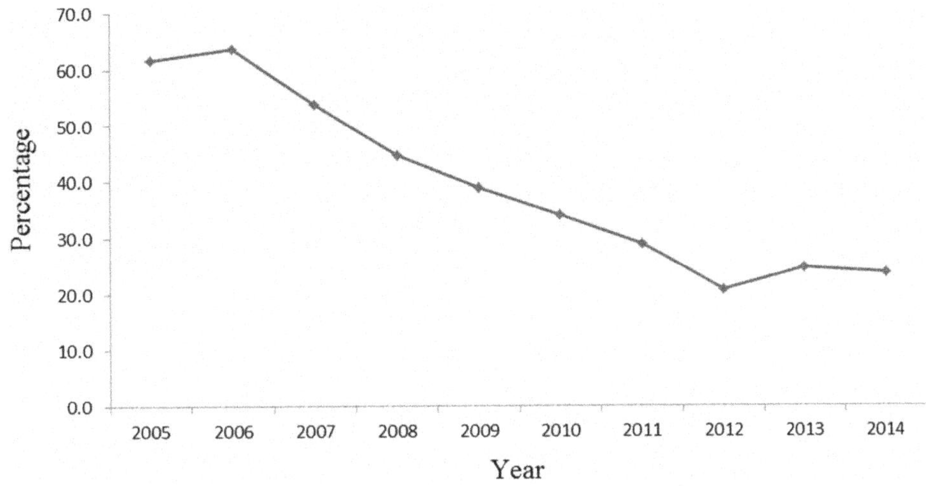

Fig. 2 Decrease of multidrug-resistant (MDR) *Salmonella* Typhi isolation rate from blood cultures

most active antibiotics against *E. coli*. Overall, 3.2% (including MDR strains) of the *E. coli* strains showed resistance against them. So, carbapenems may be considered as a good choice of treatment for BSI caused by *E. coli*. *Klebsiella* species showed the highest level of resistance against β-lactams, especially penicillins and third generation cephalosporins. Previous studies suggested that carbapenems were highly effective against *Klebsiella* species until the early years of 2000s. According to Centers for Disease Control and Prevention (CDC) in the USA, *Klebsiella* species acquired the highest amount of carbapenem resistance (from 1.6 to 10.4%) in the decade from 2001–2011. In accordance with this finding, we observed a very dramatic rise in *Klebsiella* species resistance against imipenem (0 to 46%) and meropenem (0 to 46.5%) from 2005 to 2014. In fact, we found *Klebsiella* species to show the highest level of MDR (68%) among all the isolated pathogens. Overall, *E. coli*, *Klebsiella* species and *Enterobacter* species had relatively low prevalence throughout this study period. However, they should be considered important as they had the highest amount of MDR strains and thus the potential to cause serious health threats.

Gram-positive bacteria also pose serious threats as their incidence in BSI is increasing steadily worldwide. The problem is particularly acute in nosocomial settings where methicillin-resistant *S. aureus* (MRSA) and vancomycin resistant *Enterococcus* (VRE) are considered serious health threats [37, 38]. In this study, we observed an increasing trend in the isolation rate of Gram-positive bacteria. This trend may be attributed to the patient's increased access to the health care facilities where BSI from Gram-positive bacteria is common. We identified *S. aureus* and *S. pneumoniae* as the two major Gram-positive pathogenic bacteria associated with BSI in Dhaka, Bangladesh. *S. pneumoniae* reportedly kills about 0.7 to 1 million children under five years of age every year worldwide and 90% of these deaths occur in developing countries [39]. Pneumonia is the primary cause of childhood death in Bangladesh [40] and studies suggest that the incidence of pneumonia among preschool children in Bangladesh is surprisingly higher than in developed countries [41, 42]. We found almost 75% of the BSI cases from *S. pneumoniae* to occur among children less than five years of age. However, a decreasing trend in their isolation rate was observed throughout this study period.

Increasing levels of antibiotic resistance are a big concern for *S. pneumoniae*, especially their resistance against macrolides and β-lactams, which are the first choice of treatment for most pneumonia cases. One recent review indicates a very high level of penicillin resistance among *S. pneumoniae* strains in different Asian countries [43]. However, we observed only a small increase in penicillin resistance in Dhaka, Bangladesh. Another study from Dhaka indicates the presence of high level of resistance against ciprofloxacin. However our study found a much lower level of resistance against ciprofloxacin and also we observed a decreasing trend in their susceptibility pattern [44]. Ampicillin and ceftriaxone were found to be consistently active against *S. pneumoniae*, so they might be considered as good treatment choices for them. Emergence of MRSA strain marks another very important epidemiological change for the past few decades [45]. Naturally, *S. aureus* are susceptible to commonly used antibiotics. However methicillin resistance is associated with resistance against a broad range of antibiotics [46]. Over the study period, we found overall 50.2% of *S. aureus* strains to be MDR. In the first five years of our study, we identified 34.4% of the *S. aureus* strains to be oxacillin (a synthetic form of methicillin) resistant; however, the percentage was much higher (58.7%) amongst the MDR strains. Vancomycin has been widely used as the preferred choice of treatment for MRSA strains [47], and we also found vancomycin to be highly effective against all *S. aureus* strains; only 2.1% strains were resistant. Linezolid was also found to be very effective against *S. aureus*; only one resistant strain was detected over the study period. Therefore, both vancomycin and linezolid might be considered as a good treatment choices against *S. aureus* which are resistant to commonly used antibiotics.

Limitations of the study

Due to the lack of resources, we were not able to differentiate the samples received from our hospital patients and from domiciliary patients. As a result we could not show the difference in epidemiology between nosocomial and community acquired BSI. Also due to lack of resources, we were not able to collect patient data on the clinical manifestations or any other patient characteristics, other than age and sex, which could be considered as risk factors for BSI. However, we confirm that each patient was diagnosed with signs of bacteremia by their respective physicians. Also, we were not able to perform any molecular tests on received samples due to lack of required resources.

Conclusion

This study clearly identifies the bacterial pathogens involved with bloodstream infections (BSI) occurring in Dhaka, Bangladesh between January 2005 to December 2014. It also reveals their antibiotic susceptibility patterns for commonly used antibiotics. We expect our findings to help healthcare professionals to make informed decisions and provide better care for their patients. Also, we hope this study to help researchers and policy makers to prioritize their research options to face future challenges of infectious diseases both at home and abroad.

Additional files

Additional file 1: Table S7. Association of two age groups with distinct bacterial pathogens causing BSI in Dhaka, Bangladesh.

Additional file 2: Table S8. Association of sex with distinct bacterial pathogens causing BSI in Dhaka, Bangladesh.

Additional file 3: Table S1. Percentage of antimicrobial resistance in *Acinetobacter* species strains isolated from blood cultures.

Additional file 4: Table S2. Percentage of antimicrobial resistance in *Pseudomonas* species strains isolated from blood cultures.

Additional file 5: Table S4. Percentage of antimicrobial resistance in *Enterobacter* species strains isolated from blood samples.

Additional file 6: Table S3. Percentage of antimicrobial resistance in *Klebsiella* species strains isolated from blood cultures.

Additional file 7: Table S5. Percentage of antimicrobial resistance in *Streptococcus* species strains isolated from blood cultures.

Additional file 8: Table S6. Percentage of antimicrobial resistance in *Enterococcus faecalis* strains isolated from blood cultures.

Abbreviations

FAN: Fastidious antibiotic neutralization; API: Analytical profile index

Acknowledgement

This research study was funded by core donors which provided unrestricted support to icddr,b for its operations and research. Current donors providing unrestricted support include: Government of the People's Republic of Bangladesh; Global Affairs Canada (GAC); Swedish International Development Cooperation Agency (Sida) and the Department for International Development (UK Aid). We gratefully acknowledge these donors for their support and commitment to icddr,b's research efforts. The funders had no role in study design, data collection and analysis, decision to publish, or preparation of the manuscript. We also thank Dr. Daniel Leung, from University of Utah, for his valuable comments on draft versions of this manuscript.

Funding

This research study was funded by core donors which provide unrestricted support to icddr,b for its operations and research. But the funders had no role in study design, data collection and analysis, decision to publish, or preparation of the manuscript.

Authors' contributions

DA designed the study and reviewed the manuscript for important intellectual content. MAN analyzed the data and wrote the manuscript. ABS took part in data analysis and reviewed the manuscript. FH, NA, TS, MSR performed experimental works. MSBE was responsible for collecting the data. MMR critically revised the manuscript. All the authors read and approved the final manuscript.

Competing interests

The authors declare that they have no competing interests.

Consent for publication

Not applicable.

References

1. Tumbarello M, et al. Costs of bloodstream infections caused by Escherichia coli and influence of extended-spectrum-beta-lactamase production and inadequate initial antibiotic therapy. Antimicrob Agents Chemother. 2010;54(10):4085–91.
2. Kanoksil M, et al. Epidemiology, microbiology and mortality associated with community-acquired bacteremia in northeast Thailand: a multicenter surveillance study. PLoS One. 2013;8(1):e54714.
3. Kollef MH, et al. Epidemiology, microbiology and outcomes of healthcare-associated and community-acquired bacteremia: a multicenter cohort study. J Infect. 2011;62(2):130–5.
4. Reddy EA, Shaw AV, Crump JA. Community-acquired bloodstream infections in Africa: a systematic review and meta-analysis. Lancet Infect Dis. 2010;10(6):417–32.
5. Sogaard M, et al. Temporal changes in the incidence and 30-day mortality associated with bacteremia in hospitalized patients from 1992 through 2006: a population-based cohort study. Clin Infect Dis. 2011;52(1):61–9.
6. Valles J, et al. Evolution over a 15-year period of clinical characteristics and outcomes of critically ill patients with community-acquired bacteremia. Crit Care Med. 2013;41(1):76–83.
7. Valles J, et al. Community-acquired bloodstream infection in critically ill adult patients: impact of shock and inappropriate antibiotic therapy on survival. Chest. 2003;123(5):1615–24.
8. Friedman ND, et al. Health care–associated bloodstream infections in adults: a reason to change the accepted definition of community-acquired infections. Ann Intern Med. 2002;137(10):791–7.
9. Siegman-Igra Y, et al. Reappraisal of community-acquired bacteremia: a proposal of a new classification for the spectrum of acquisition of bacteremia. Clin Infect Dis. 2002;34(11):1431–9.
10. Deen J, et al. Community-acquired bacterial bloodstream infections in

developing countries in south and southeast Asia: a systematic review. Lancet Infect Dis. 2012;12(6):480–7.

11. (CLSI), C.L.S.I. Performance standards for antimicrobial susceptibility testing: twenty second informational supplement ed, CLSI document M100S-S22. Wayne: CLSI; 2012.
12. (CLSI), C.L.S.I. Performance standards for antimicrobial susceptibility testing: 23rd informational supplement, CLSI document M100S-S22. Wayne: CLSI; 2013.
13. (CLSI), C.L.S.I. Performance standards for antimicrobial susceptibility testing: 20th informational supplement, CLSI document M100S-S22. Wayne: CLSI; 2010.
14. (CLSI), C.L.S.I. Performance standards for antimicrobial susceptibility testing: fourteenth informational supplement ed, CLSI document M100-S14. Wayne: CLSI; 2004.
15. Pillar CM, et al. Prevalence of multidrug-resistant, methicillin-resistant staphylococcus aureus in the United States: findings of the stratified analysis of the 2004 to 2005 LEADER surveillance programs. Diagn Microbiol Infect Dis. 2008;60(2):221–4.
16. Cohen AL, et al. Recommendations for metrics for multidrug-resistant organisms in healthcare settings: SHEA/HICPAC Position paper. Infect Control Hosp Epidemiol. 2008;29(10):901–13.
17. Critchley IA, et al. Activity of daptomycin against susceptible and multidrug-resistant gram-positive pathogens collected in the SECURE study (Europe) during 2000–2001. J Antimicrob Chemother. 2003;51(3):639–49.
18. Kallen AJ, et al. Multidrug resistance among gram-negative pathogens that caused healthcare-associated infections reported to the National Healthcare Safety Network, 2006–2008. Infect Control Hosp Epidemiol. 2010;31(5):528–31.
19. O'Fallon E, Gautam S, D'Agata EM. Colonization with multidrug-resistant gram-negative bacteria: prolonged duration and frequent cocolonization. Clin Infect Dis. 2009;48(10):1375–81.
20. Paterson DL, Doi Y. A step closer to extreme drug resistance (XDR) in gram-negative bacilli. Clin Infect Dis. 2007;45(9):1179–81.
21. Falagas ME, Koletsi PK, Bliziotis IA. The diversity of definitions of multidrug-resistant (MDR) and pandrug-resistant (PDR) Acinetobacter baumannii and Pseudomonas aeruginosa. J Med Microbiol. 2006;55(Pt 12):1619–29.
22. Ahmed D, et al. Salmonella enterica serovar typhi strain producing extended-spectrum beta-lactamases in Dhaka, Bangladesh. J Med Microbiol. 2012;61(Pt 7):1032–3.
23. Brooks WA, et al. Bacteremic typhoid fever in children in an urban slum, Bangladesh. Emerg Infect Dis. 2005;11(2):326–9.
24. Naheed A, et al. Burden of typhoid and paratyphoid fever in a densely populated urban community, Dhaka, Bangladesh. Int J Infect Dis. 2010;14 Suppl 3:e93–9.
25. Saha SK, et al. Typhoid fever in Bangladesh: implications for vaccination policy. Pediatr Infect Dis J. 2001;20(5):521–4.
26. Rahman M, Ahmad A, Shoma S. Decline in epidemic of multidrug resistant Salmonella typhi is not associated with increased incidence of antibiotic-susceptible strain in Bangladesh. Epidemiol Infect. 2002;129(1):29–34.
27. Threlfall EJ, Ward LR. Decreased susceptibility to ciprofloxacin in Salmonella enterica serotype typhi, United Kingdom. Emerg Infect Dis. 2001;7(3):448–50.
28. Hassing RJ, et al. Analysis of mechanisms involved in reduced susceptibility to ciprofloxacin in Salmonella enterica serotypes typhi and paratyphi a isolates from travellers to southeast Asia. Int J Antimicrob Agents. 2011;37(3):240–3.
29. Cisneros JM, Rodriguez-Bano J. Nosocomial bacteremia due to Acinetobacter baumannii: epidemiology, clinical features and treatment. Clin Microbiol Infect. 2002;8(11):687–93.
30. Cross A, et al. Nosocomial infections due to Pseudomonas aeruginosa: review of recent trends. Rev Infect Dis. 1983;5 Suppl 5:S837–45.
31. Akram F, et al. Prevalence, clinical features, and outcome of pseudomonas bacteremia in under-five diarrheal children in bangladesh. ISRN Microbiol. 2014;2014:469758.
32. Brauers J, et al. Activities of various beta-lactams and beta-lactam/beta-lactamase inhibitor combinations against Acinetobacter baumannii and Acinetobacter DNA group 3 strains. Clin Microbiol Infect. 2005;11(1):24–30.
33. Fournier PE, Richet H. The epidemiology and control of Acinetobacter baumannii in health care facilities. Clin Infect Dis. 2006;42(5):692–9.
34. Manchanda V, Sanchaita S, Singh N. Multidrug resistant acinetobacter. J Glob Infect Dis. 2010;2(3):291–304.
35. Zavascki AP, et al. Polymyxin B for the treatment of multidrug-resistant pathogens: a critical review. J Antimicrob Chemother. 2007;60(6):1206–15.
36. Talukdar PK, et al. Antimicrobial resistance, virulence factors and genetic diversity of Escherichia coli isolates from household water supply in Dhaka, Bangladesh. PLoS One. 2013;8(4):e61090.
37. Arias CA, Murray BE. The rise of the Enterococcus: beyond vancomycin resistance. Nat Rev Microbiol. 2012;10(4):266–78.
38. Boucher HW, Corey GR. Epidemiology of methicillin-resistant Staphylococcus aureus. Clin Infect Dis. 2008;46 Suppl 5:S344–9.
39. Williams BG, et al. Estimates of world-wide distribution of child deaths from acute respiratory infections. Lancet Infect Dis. 2002;2(1):25–32.
40. Baqui AH, et al. Causes of childhood deaths in Bangladesh: an update. Acta Paediatr. 2001;90(6):682–90.
41. Brooks WA, et al. Effect of weekly zinc supplements on incidence of pneumonia and diarrhoea in children younger than 2 years in an urban, low-income population in Bangladesh: randomised controlled trial. Lancet. 2005;366(9490):999–1004.
42. Farha T, Thomson AH. The burden of pneumonia in children in the developed world. Paediatr Respir Rev. 2005;6(2):76–82.
43. Mamishi S, et al. Penicillin-resistant trend of Streptococcus pneumoniae in Asia: a systematic review. Iran J Microbiol. 2014;6(4):198–210.
44. Brooks WA, et al. Invasive pneumococcal disease burden and implications for vaccine policy in urban Bangladesh. Am J Trop Med Hyg. 2007;77(5):795–801.
45. Klevens RM, et al. Invasive methicillin-resistant Staphylococcus aureus infections in the United States. JAMA. 2007;298(15):1763–71.
46. Chambers HF, Deleo FR. Waves of resistance: Staphylococcus aureus in the antibiotic era. Nat Rev Microbiol. 2009;7(9):629–41.
47. Rasmussen RV, et al. Future challenges and treatment of Staphylococcus aureus bacteremia with emphasis on MRSA. Future Microbiol. 2011;6(1):43–56.

12

Antimicrobials in small-scale urban pig farming in a lower middle-income country – arbitrary use and high resistance levels

G. Ström[1], S. Boqvist[2], A. Albihn[2,3], L.-L. Fernström[2], A. Andersson Djurfeldt[4], S. Sokerya[5], T. Sothyra[6] and U. Magnusson[1*]

Abstract

Background: Administration of antimicrobials to food-producing animals is regarded as a major contributor to the overall emergence of resistance in bacteria worldwide. However, few data are available on global antimicrobial use and resistance (AMR) in livestock, especially from low- and middle-income countries.

Methods: We conducted a structured survey of 91 small-scale pig farms in the urban and peri-urban areas of Phnom Penh, Cambodia, to assess the farmers' knowledge, attitudes and practices related to antimicrobial use in their pig production. Commensal *Escherichia coli* was isolated from three healthy pigs from each farm ($n = 261$) and susceptibility testing was performed against 14 antimicrobials, using broth microdilution. Univariable logistic regression and generalized linear mixed models were used to investigate potential associations between farm characteristics, management factors and resistance to different types of antimicrobials.

Results: We found a widespread and arbitrary use of antimicrobials, often based on the farmer's own judgment. Around 66% of the farmers reported frequently self-adjusting treatment duration and dosage, and 45% had not heard about the term 'antimicrobial resistance'. The antimicrobials most commonly mentioned or kept by the farmers were amoxicillin, tylosin, gentamicin and colistin. Around 37% used a feed concentrate that contained antimicrobials, while antimicrobials for humans were used as a last-line treatment by 10% of the farmers. Commensal *E. coli* exhibited high prevalence of resistance to several antimicrobials considered to be of critical importance for human medicine, including ampicillin, ciprofloxacin and colistin, and multidrug-resistance was found in 79% of the samples. Higher prevalence of resistance was observed on farms that administered prophylactic antimicrobials and on farms that treated the entire group or herd in the event of disease.

Conclusion: The widespread and arbitrary use of antimicrobials in pig farming in Cambodia is highly worrisome. Overall, farmers had a low awareness of the risks and consequences related to antimicrobial use and AMR. The results presented in this study confirm the hypothesis that non-rational use of antimicrobials results in higher prevalence of AMR and highlight the need for professional animal health systems that involve medically rational use of antimicrobials in emerging economies such as Cambodia.

Keywords: Antimicrobial use, Antimicrobial resistance, Pig production, Cambodia

* Correspondence: ulf.magnusson@slu.se
[1]Department of Clinical Sciences, Swedish University of Agricultural Sciences, Uppsala, Sweden
Full list of author information is available at the end of the article

Background

Antimicrobial resistance (AMR) is a major global health concern and our decreased ability within human and veterinary medicine to cure resistant infections will have serious repercussions for future treatment and prevention of infections in humans and for the productivity of livestock [1–3]. The emergence of AMR is believed to be partly caused by the inappropriate use within the livestock sector, where antimicrobials are widely administered to animals for prevention and control of diseases and, more controversially, for growth promotion purposes [4–6]. Although data from several high-income countries indicate extensive antimicrobial use and AMR in livestock in these countries [7, 8], data from most low- and middle-income countries are scarce. Historically, the primary problem in some low- and middle-income countries has been the lack of antimicrobial drugs [9, 10]. Recently, however, the access to antimicrobials has generally increased in urban areas in these countries, with a consequent rise in the inappropriate usage of such drugs in cities and towns [11]. Overall, the use of antimicrobials in animal production is expected to continue to increase globally due to growing demand for animal-source foods, particularly in emerging economies [12]. Facilitated by the ongoing globalization of trade and travel, AMR is rapidly spread throughout the world [13].

Southeast Asia, a region with a high burden of infectious diseases [14] and a dense population of both humans and animals, is considered to be a hotspot for the development of AMR [15]. This partly stems from the expanding pig and poultry sectors [16] and partly from the widespread availability of antimicrobials and an often weak regulatory framework governing their use in human and veterinary medicine. Weak regulations enable inappropriate usage of antimicrobials which, in the livestock sector, often manifests as use without proper diagnosis, poor adherence to dosage and treatment duration, and use of falsified pharmaceuticals, behaviors that may favor AMR emergence [17, 18].

Antimicrobials are presumed to be extensively used in Southeast Asia, but only a few published studies have investigated practices related to antimicrobial usage in the large and expanding pig sector in the region [19–22]. These studies indicate uncontrolled and arbitrary use of antimicrobials with little or no supervision by veterinarians. Concomitantly, other studies have reported high prevalence of AMR in bacteria isolated from pigs and poultry in Southeast Asia, with resistance levels as high as 98% to ampicillin [23], 96% to tetracycline [24], and 97% to gentamicin [25]. Notably, resistance levels have been reported to be higher in pigs than in other species [26, 27].

The present study was undertaken in urban and peri-urban areas of Cambodia, where availability of antimicrobials was assumed to be good and in a country with strong economic growth [28], where regulations governing the use of veterinary antimicrobials are under development, but not yet implemented. The aim was to obtain information on knowledge, attitudes and practices related to antimicrobial use in small-scale pig farming in Phnom Penh, and data on phenotypic AMR in the indicator bacteria *Escherichia coli* isolated from pigs kept by the farming households. This information could assist in the development of strategies for more medically rational use of antimicrobials in the pig sector, not only in Cambodia but also elsewhere in the Global South.

Methods

Study area and study population

This cross-sectional study was conducted in urban and peri-urban areas of Phnom Penh in January and February 2017. Only households keeping pigs under family farm conditions (FAO, 2014) were targeted for the study, and thus larger commercial farms were excluded. Cambodian households have a long tradition of raising animals in their backyards for both subsistence and commercial purposes, with around 80% of the pigs in Cambodia still being raised in backyard systems [29].

In recruitment of farms, a list of pig-keeping households (family farms) in the province of Phnom Penh ($n = 267$) was available from a previous study [30]. In that study, snowball sampling [31] had been used with the ambition to locate all family farms keeping pigs in Phnom Penh. For the present study, all farms on that list were visited and included if they still kept pigs and if the farmers were at home and willing to participate in the study. However, due to failing profitability from pig production, a large proportion of the farms on the list had stopped keeping pigs since the previous study, and thus only 81 farms could be included from the previous study. However, ten farms that had started with pig production since the previous study were found during the fieldwork and were included in the present study.

Study procedure

A semi-structured questionnaire, with questions on farm characteristics, pig husbandry and routines for antimicrobial (i.e. antibacterial) use, was administered to the person responsible for treating sick pigs at the farm. The questionnaire, which took around 20 min to complete, was written in English and interviews were carried out in Khmer with the assistance of the same interpreter throughout the study. The interpreter, an employee at the Centre for Livestock and Agriculture Development (CelAgrid), had extensive knowledge of Cambodian livestock production and was familiar with the different medicines and treatment regimens commonly used in livestock production in Cambodia. In order to determine whether the drugs referred to by respondents contained antimicrobials, probing questions were used together with observations of any medicines, premixes or feed concentrates present at the farm.

The questionnaire is provided as supplementary material [see Additional file 1].

Collection of fecal samples

Fecal samples were collected from three randomly chosen healthy pigs at each farm, using sterile cotton swabs. At two of the 91 farms, no family member was at home when the team arrived for sampling and at some farms only one or two pigs were available for sampling, resulting in a total of 261 samples from 89 farms. Samples were collected either from the rectum or from fresh feces on the ground, if the pig defecated during sample collection. The swabs were placed in sterile plastic tubes containing Amies medium (Amies PS Viscose, Sarstedt), and stored and transported on ice to the National Animal Health and Production Research Institute (NAHPRI) in Phnom Penh within 8 h. Samples were stored at 2–8 °C until analysis, which was performed within 48 h after sampling.

Isolation of *E. coli*

Fecal sampled were cultured on MacConkey agar at 44 °C overnight. Presumptive *E. coli* isolates were subcultured on Tryptone Soya Agar (TSA) and incubated at 37 °C overnight. Selected isolates were tested for production of tryptophanase (indole). One positive isolate was selected from each fecal sample, and bacterial material was transferred to cryogenic vials containing Luria Broth (LB) and 20% glycerol, and stored at – 70 °C before being transported to the Swedish University of Agricultural Sciences (SLU), Uppsala, Sweden.

Antimicrobial susceptibility testing

Susceptibility testing was performed at SLU by broth microdilution, using the growth method for inoculum preparation, according to the standards described by the Clinical and Laboratory Standards Institute [32]. Prior to analysis, all isolates were confirmed as *E. coli* isolates by matrix-assisted laser-desorption/ionization time-of-flight mass spectrometry (MALDI-TOF MS).

Microdilution susceptibility panels (Sensititre™ EUVSEC, Thermo Scientific) were used to determine susceptibility of the bacteria isolates to 14 antimicrobials (ampicillin, azithromycin, cefotaxime, ceftazidime, chloramphenicol, ciprofloxacin, colistin, gentamicin, meropenem, nalidixid acid, sulfamethoxazole, tetracycline, tigecycline, trimethoprim). *Escherichia coli* CCUG 17620 was used as a quality control strain.

The minimum inhibitory concentration (MIC) for each antimicrobial was visually determined and epidemiological cut-off values (ECOFFs), defined by the European Committee on Antimicrobial Susceptibility Testing [33], were used to differentiate between wild-type and non-wild-type strains of the bacteria isolates, henceforth referred to as susceptible and resistant, respectively. Multidrug-resistance (MDR) was defined as isolates resistant to at least three different categories of the antimicrobials tested [34].

Data management and statistical analysis

Data from the questionnaire responses were transcribed into Epi Info™ 7 (CDC, Atlanta, GA) following the interviews, and were exported on to Microsoft Excel 2010 spreadsheets after the fieldwork was finished.

Statistical analyses were conducted in SAS software 9.4 (SAS Institute Inc., Cary, NC). Descriptive statistics were computed to define farm characteristics and to determine knowledge, attitudes and practices among respondents regarding use of antimicrobials. Distributions for continuous variables were tested for normality using the Shapiro-Wilks test. Univariable logistic regression and Chi-square tests were used to examine possible associations between farm size, education level and management factors, such as routines related to antimicrobial use. To investigate associations between farm characteristics, management factors, age group of pigs and the prevalence of resistance to different types of antimicrobials, generalized linear mixed models were used where farm was included as a random effect, to account for clustering. The confounding variable 'age group of pigs' was included in all models as a fixed effect. The statistical significance level was defined as a two-tailed P-value ≤0.05 for all models. For the associations with AMR prevalence, however, all P-values < 0.1 are presented.

Results

Farm characteristics

Among the 91 farms included in the study, 29 farms (32%) also kept cattle and 64 farms (70%) kept poultry, besides keeping pigs. The number of pigs present in at the farm at the time of the visits ranged from 2 to 228 with a median of 20 pigs (5th and 95th percentiles: 7 and 81 pigs). The farm with 228 pigs was a farm that produced piglets to sell on to other producers, which explains its much higher number of pigs compared with the other farms.

Male household heads had in general attained a higher level of education than female household heads ($P < 0.001$). A high level of education was defined as commencing, but not necessarily completing, studies at upper secondary school, which was achieved by 31% of male and 9% of female farmers.

Antimicrobial use

At 60 farms (66%), the male household head was responsible for treating sick animals while the female household head was responsible at 15 farms (16%) and the veterinarian or village animal health worker at nine farms (10%). At the remaining farms (8%), another household member (than the household heads) had the responsibility for treatment. The age of the person responsible for treating sick pigs (not including veterinarians or animal health workers) varied between 20 and 68 years, with a mean of 44 years. At 78 farms (86%) antimicrobials were routinely administered to the pigs to treat an existing disease, as a prophylactic for piglets or sows after farrowing, or as a feed additive commonly included in the feed concentrate. At nine farms (10%), however, it could not be determined with certainty that antimicrobials were used, as the respondent did not remember the names of the drugs used, and no drug packages were present. Nonetheless, all these farmers reported that they received drugs from veterinarians or pharmaceutical companies for treatment. Based on the respondents' descriptions of disease symptoms and treatment regimens, we concluded that these farmers most likely administered antimicrobials to the pigs. Only four farmers (4%) reported that they did not use any antimicrobials, of which three farmers explained that their pigs had not been sick in a long time, while one farmer explained that they had stopped treatment with antimicrobials because their pigs died the last time they received antimicrobial treatment.

At least 70 different brands of antimicrobial drugs were used by the farmers. The antimicrobials most commonly mentioned or kept by the respondents were amoxicillin, tylosin, gentamicin and colistin (Table 1). Most respondents, however, could only name some of the antimicrobials that they used. Furthermore, the majority of piglet-producing farms gave the new-born piglets iron supplements, although only 24 respondents (26%) could specify or show the type of supplement used. Of these, eight farmers (33%) used iron supplements that contained antimicrobials, commonly gentamicin or colistin, in combination with tylosin, streptomycin or spectinomycin.

At least 14 farmers reported to routinely administer antimicrobials to the pigs as a preventive measure (Table 2). However, the antimicrobial content in the feed concentrate is not included in this figure and comprehensive information regarding the contents of the iron supplements administered could not be retrieved. At least 37% of the farms routinely used a concentrate that contained antimicrobials, although the types and concentrations of the antimicrobials were only specified on the concentrates used at three farms. It was commonly the concentrate for younger pigs (as advised by the manufacturer) that contained antimicrobials.

The respondents reported that they commonly received antimicrobials from the veterinarian or village animal health worker. Most veterinarians either operated a pharmaceutical store or were employed by a pharmaceutical company. Respondents described unrestricted access to antimicrobials, and professional prior diagnosis of the animals seemed to be rarely practiced. Many respondents explained that they just went to the store and described the disease symptoms to acquire antimicrobials from the veterinarian. Other respondents claimed that they did not necessarily need veterinary advice, as they could decide which type of antimicrobial and dosage to administer based on previous experiences. In general, treatment based on experience was a common practice among the farmers. On at least 60 farms (66%), the respondent reported frequently deviating from the instructions provided by veterinarians or written on product labels, by adjusting both dosage and duration of treatment based on the severity of the disease and whether the animals recovered quickly or not. Respondents that reported this behavior were also more likely to use human antimicrobials on their pigs ($P = 0.056$). Furthermore, almost half of the respondents (47%) reported that they did not adhere to the withdrawal period stated on drug packaging or prescribed by the veterinarian, and pigs were often sold for slaughter during or directly after antimicrobial treatment. None of the behaviors described above was associated with the level of education of the household head.

Table 1 Antimicrobials most commonly mentioned or kept by the farmers surveyed[a]

Antimicrobial	Number of farms
Amoxicillin[b]	56
Ampicillin[b]	21
Colistin[b]	27
Enrofloxacin[b]	19
Gentamicin[b]	29
Lincomycin	14
Oxytetracycline	17
Penicillin G[b]	15
Spectinomycin	6
Streptomycin[b]	9
Sulfonamides	16
Thiamphenicol	6
Trimethoprim	9
Tylosin[b]	38

[a]This list is not complete, as most farmers could only name a few of the antimicrobials that were used and it does not include potential antimicrobials in the feed concentrate
[b]Antimicrobial considered critically important according to WHO [48]

Knowledge and attitudes about antimicrobials and AMR

Only one respondent (a former animal health worker) explained that he knew what antimicrobials were and their mode of action. For the other respondents, their

Table 2 Practices related to antimicrobial use on the farms that presumably used antimicrobials ($n = 87$)

	Category	*n*	%
How do you administer antimicrobials to the pigs?	Injections when sick	87	100
	In feed/orally when sick	18	21
	In water when sick	1	1
	To sows after farrowing (n=58[a])	5	9
	In feed routinely	8	9
If only some pigs are sick, to which pigs do you administer antimicrobials? ($n = 86$)	Only the sick pigs	65	76
	All pigs[b]	21	24
Do you administer antimicrobials as a prophylaxis?	Yes	14	16
	No	72	83
	Unsure[c]	1	1
Does the feed concentrate contain antimicrobials? (n = 91[d])	Yes	34	37
	No	8	9
	Don't know	42	46
	Don't use concentrates	7	8
Do you sometimes give human medicines that contain antimicrobials to the animals?	Yes	9	10
	No	77	89
	Don't know	1	1
Do you sometimes end treatment prematurely if the animal gets better?	Yes	57	66
	No	30	34
What do you do with antimicrobials that are left (and have expired)? ($n = 84$)	Throw away to pond/environment	36	43
	Bury	20	24
	Burn	3	4
	Take back to veterinarian/animal health worker	8	10
	Throw to the person collecting waste	11	13
	Keep at home	4	5
	Don't know	2	2
Do you have a withdrawal period (according to instructions) between antimicrobial treatment and slaughter/trader collecting animals? ($n = 81$)	Yes	8	10
	No	38	47
	Don't know	1	1
	Never been sick around time of slaughter	32	40
	Other	2	2

[a]Calculated based on number of farms that kept sows
[b]This category does not necessarily includes sows, as some farmers only used traditional medicines to treat sows
[c]Some substance was added to the feed routinely but the respondent did not remember the name
[d]Calculated based on all 91 farms in the study

knowledge was limited to recognizing the names of some antimicrobials they frequently used. In general, all respondents (99%) were of the opinion that antimicrobials were necessary in order to keep their animals healthy (Table 3). All respondents save two considered antimicrobials to be easily accessible. It should be noted that these two respondents stated either that antimicrobials were often sold out when they arrived at the store, or that it was difficult to find 'high quality antimicrobials' from Europe. The latter was mentioned by other respondents too and some expressed concerns that locally produced antimicrobials (commonly imported from Vietnam) were not as efficient as antimicrobials imported from European countries.

Around half of the respondents (55%) stated that they had heard of the term 'antimicrobial resistance'. This was more likely among respondents who had attained a higher level of education (78% vs. 49%; $P = 0.036$; Odds ratio (OR) 3.6; 95% Confidence Interval (CI) 1.1–12.0) and was more often reported by male respondents (74% vs. 39%; $P < 0.001$; OR 4.4; CI 1.8–10.9), and by farms where the respondent was the person responsible for treating sick pigs (65% vs. 41%; $P = 0.021$; OR 2.7; CI 1.6–6.4). Some respondents elaborated on this question and gave examples from their own experience of what they believed to be AMR (Table 4).

Table 3 Knowledge and attitudes about antimicrobials and antimicrobial use among respondents ($n = 91$)

	Category	*n*	%
Is it important to give antimicrobials to animals?	Yes	82	90
	No	4	4
	Don't know	5	5
Are antimicrobials needed to keep animals healthy?	Yes	90	99
	No	0	0
	Don't know	1	1
Will the use of antimicrobials result in better growth of animals? ($n = 90$)	Yes	30	33
	No	58	64
	Don't know	2	2
Do you think it is easy to get access to antimicrobials?	Yes	89	98
	No	2	2
Do you consider antimicrobials to be cheap?	Yes	5	5
	No	55	60
	It's acceptable	29	32
	Don't know	2	2
Do you think giving antimicrobials to animals may result in any negative consequences?	Yes	49	54
	No	3	3
	Don't know	39	43
Have you ever heard of 'antimicrobial resistance'?	Yes	50	55
	No	41	45
Do you feel you have received enough information on how antimicrobials should be used in animals?	Yes	37	41
	No	38	42
	Don't know	16	18

Table 4 Statements by respondents regarding their experiences and reflections on AMR

"When we use too much of one type of antimicrobial and the animal does not recover, it may be because of resistance"
Male, 52 years, higher education
"Sometimes after we use the antimicrobials, the animals get more sick and do not recover"
Female, 36 years, lower education
"If we use only one kind of medicine for a long time and then the animal recovers, the next time it [the medicine] might not work"
Male, 35 years, higher education
"When I use this one [points at antimicrobial] the pigs will no longer recover"
Male, 35 years, lower education

Although many respondents had heard about AMR, when asked to state some possible negative consequences from the use of antimicrobials none mentioned this as a potential problem. Still, respondents expressed some concerns about other possible adverse effects that could arise from antimicrobial use, for example the risk of antimicrobial residues being present in the meat and potential negative effects on the animals when they received too much antimicrobials (Table 5).

Antimicrobial susceptibility in *E. coli*

Escherichia coli bacteria were successfully isolated from all 261 samples, of which 110 were obtained from growers (1–3 months old), 122 were obtained from fatteners (over 3 months old), and 29 were obtained from sows. Overall, bacteria isolates were resistant to a median of five of the 13 antimicrobials tested (no ECOFF was available for azithromycin). Twenty-one isolates (8%) were susceptible to all antimicrobials, whereas 31 isolates (12%) showed resistance to eight or more antimicrobials. Among all isolates tested, resistance levels were as follows: ampicillin (AMP) 75%; cefotaxime (CTX) 1%; ceftazidime (CAZ) 2%; chloramphenicol (CHL) 61%; ciprofloxacin (CIP) 59%; colistin (COL) 20%; gentamicin (GEN) 25%; meropenem (MER) 0%; nalidixic acid (NAL) 19%; sulfamethoxazole (SMX) 71%; tetracycline (TET) 84%; tigecycline (TIG) 1%; and trimethoprim (TMP) 57%. Multidrug-resistance (MDR) was found in 79% of all isolates. Isolates from growers showed higher prevalence of resistance to all antimicrobials compared with isolates from fatteners (Fig. 1), although this difference was only significant for AMP, CHL, COL and SMX, and for MDR. Furthermore, isolates from sows showed significantly higher prevalence of resistance to CIP and NAL, compared with isolates from fatteners. Resistance prevalence and MIC distributions are presented for growers in Table 6, for fatteners in Table 7 and for sows in Table 8.

Table 5 Statements by respondents regarding potential negative effects of antimicrobial use

"If too much medicine, there may be medicine in the meat and it will taste different"
Female, 35 years, lower education
"If too much the pig will grow slower and the cycle will take longer time. Maybe it will affect the consumer if the animal gets too much antimicrobials. The meat will be yellow."
Female, 51 years, lower education
"When a consumer eats an animal that has received a lot of antimicrobials it may have an effect on human health."
Male, 48 years, lower education
"If the people that use the medicine don't know how to use it, the medicine will remain in the meat. [It] may affect the people who eat the meat."
Female, 36 years, lower education

Antimicrobial use, farm characteristics and associations with AMR

The statistical analyses revealed some associations between farm characteristics, practices related to antimicrobial use and the prevalence of resistance to the antimicrobials tested. Age of the person responsible for antimicrobial treatment was positively related to lower prevalence of resistance to CIP ($P = 0.043$) and SMX ($P = 0.021$), and to MDR ($P = 0.029$). Isolates from pigs owned by farmers who had attained a higher level of education showed a higher prevalence of resistance to CIP ($P = 0.007$) and NAL ($P = 0.053$), and to MDR ($P = 0.024$). There was no correlation between age of the farmer and level of education. Higher prevalence of resistance was also found for NAL ($P = 0.031$), TMP ($P = 0.004$) and SMX ($P = 0.023$), and for MDR ($P = 0.089$) in isolates from farms where a veterinarian was responsible for antimicrobial treatment. Furthermore, isolates from farms where antimicrobials were administered preventatively showed higher prevalence of resistance to AMP ($P = 0.081$), CIP ($P = 0.072$), CHL ($P = 0.056$), SMX ($P = 0.028$) and TMP ($P = 0.031$), and farms that often treated the entire group of pigs instead of only the sick individuals had a higher prevalence of resistance to CIP ($P = 0.021$), COL ($P = 0.048$) and NAL ($P = 0.012$). Finally, farms that reported routinely using feed supplements that contained antimicrobials had a higher prevalence of resistance to AMP ($P = 0.070$), CIP ($P = 0.076$), CHL ($P = 0.015$), SMX ($P = 0.031$) and TMP ($P = 0.016$). For farms where it could be concluded that the concentrate included antimicrobials, the prevalence of resistance to CHL ($P = 0.068$) was higher.

Discussion

In the present study, we found that the majority of the participating farms used antimicrobials in their pig

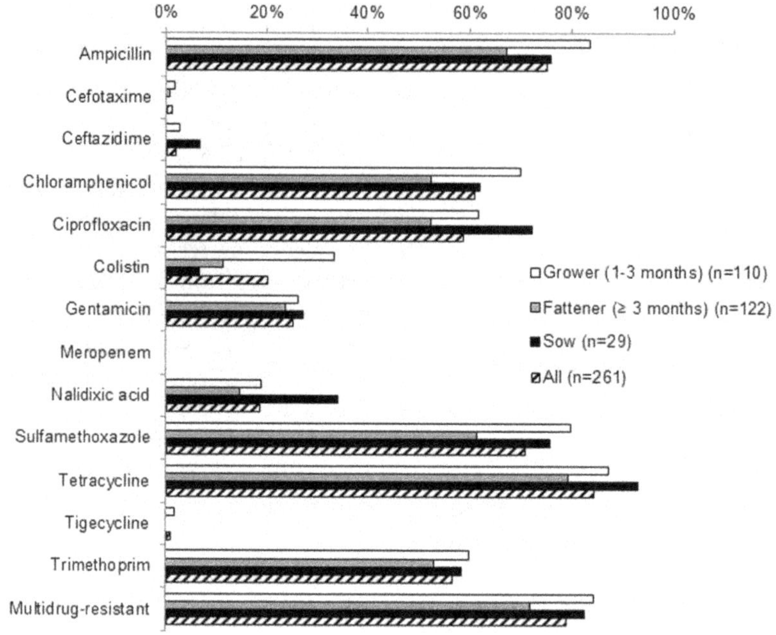

Fig. 1 Prevalence of antimicrobial resistance of commensal *E. coli* isolated from growers, fatteners and sows

production. Overall, knowledge regarding antimicrobial use appeared to be low among the respondents and few reported having received any training in veterinary practices. Antimicrobial use was mainly based on pig-keepers' experiences and on drug sellers' advices according to symptoms described by the owner, rather than being based on professional diagnostics. Similar practices have been reported in other studies conducted in the region [20, 21]. In the present study, we frequently found labels on the veterinary antimicrobials in languages other than Khmer, such as English, Vietnamese or Spanish. Additionally, labelling on concentrate packaging and feed premixes did not always specify the type and concentration of the antimicrobial content. This prevents farmers and retailers from making informed decisions on which drugs to choose and may contribute to inappropriate use of antimicrobials in livestock farming in Cambodia.

In agreement with other studies in Southeast Asia [23, 24, 27] we found a high prevalence of resistance to ampicillin, tetracycline and chloramphenicol, probably

Table 6 Resistance and distribution of Minimum Inhibitory Concentrations (MIC) of antimicrobials for *E. coli* from growers[a] ($n = 110$)

Antimicrobial	Resistance	Distribution (%) of MICs (mg/L)																	
	(%)	0.015	0.03	0.06	0.12	0.25	0.5	1	2	4	8	16	32	64	128	256	512	1024	>1024
Ampicillin	83.6								6.4	8.2	1.8		0.9	2.7	80.8				
Azithromycin[b]	-								0.9	9.1	31.8	44.5	10.9	2.7					
Cefotaxime	1.8					98.2	0.9	0.9											
Ceftazidime	2.7						97.3	1.8	0.9										
Chloramphenicol	70.0										25.5	4.5	3.6	7.3	39.1	20.0			
Ciprofloxacin	61.8	18.2	12.7	7.3		12.7	25.5	8.2	6.4		0.9	8.2							
Colistin	33.6							50.9	15.5	32.7	0.9								
Gentamicin	26.4						5.5	36.4	31.8	2.7	2.7	1.8	1.8	17.3					
Meropenem	0.0		99.1	0.9															
Nalidixic acid	19.0									35.5	29.1	16.4	2.7	0.9		15.5			
Sulfamethoxazole	80.0										3.6	10.0	5.5	0.9					80.0
Tetracycline	87.3								7.3	4.5	0.9		7.3	30.9	49.1				
Tigecycline	1.8					88.2	10.0	0.9			0.9								
Trimethoprim	60.0					4.5	22.7	12.7			0.9			59.1					

White fields represent range of dilutions tested for each antimicrobial. MICs higher than the highest concentration tested are given as the concentration closest above the range. MICs equal to or lower than the lowest concentration tested are underlined. The epidemiological cut-off value (ECOFF) [33] for each antimicrobial is presented as a vertical line

[a]Pigs aged between 1 and 3 months

[b]No ECOFF was available for azithromycin

Table 7 Resistance and distribution of Minimum Inhibitory Concentrations (MIC) of antimicrobials for *E. coli* from fatteners[a] ($n = 122$)

Antimicrobial	Resistance (%)	0.015	0.03	0.06	0.12	0.25	0.5	1	2	4	8	16	32	64	128	256	512	1024	>1024
		Distributions (%) of MICs (mg/L)																	
Ampicillin	67.2								13.1	18.0	1.6			0.8	66.4				
Azithromycin[b]	-								1.6	5.7	36.1	45.9	9.0	0.8	0.8				
Cefotaxime	0.8					99.2				0.8									
Ceftazidime	0.0						100												
Chloramphenicol	52.5										43.4	4.1	9.8	8.2	25.4	9.0			
Ciprofloxacin	52.5	24.6	13.1	9.8	0.8	9.8	24.6	10.7		1.6	0.8	4.1							
Colistin	11.5							81.1	7.4	11.5									
Gentamicin	23.8						8.2	27.0	41.0	11.5			1.6	10.7					
Meropenem	0.0		96.7	3.3															
Nalidixic acid	14.8									41.8	29.5	13.9	6.6		1.6	6.6			
Sulfamethoxazole	61.5										6.6	15.6	14.8	1.6		0.8		0.8	59.8
Tetracycline	79.5								8.2	9.0	3.3		11.5	32.0	36.1				
Tigecycline	0.0					91.8	8.2												
Trimethoprim	53.3					1.6	26.2	17.2	1.6	1.6				51.6					

White fields represent range of dilutions tested for each antimicrobial. MICs higher than the highest concentration tested are given as the concentration closest above the range. MICs equal to or lower than the lowest concentration tested are underlined. The epidemiological cut-off value (ECOFF) [33] for each antimicrobial is presented as a vertical line
[a]Pigs older than 3 months
[b]No ECOFF was available for azithromycin

reflecting a long tradition of use in livestock farming in the region. The high prevalence of resistance to colistin, especially among growers, is a particular concern, as colistin is considered a last-resort antimicrobial for treatment of severe human infections and its use in livestock production may contribute to emerging resistance globally. The high prevalence of resistance detected in this study most likely results from the widespread use of colistin, either for treatment ofdiseases or as a prophylactic for piglets. We also found high prevalence of resistance to the quinolone ciprofloxacin, an antimicrobial not licensed for veterinary use. This is probably explained by cross-resistance with other veterinary quinolones, such as enrofloxacin [35], an antimicrobial commonly used by the farms in the present study. Notably, higher prevalence of AMR was found on farms that reported administering antimicrobials as a prophylactic and on farms that normally treated the entire group or herd in the event of disease. These results support the claim that non-rational use of antimicrobials contributes to increased prevalence of AMR [5].

We found that bacteria isolated from growers (1–3 months) exhibited significantly higher prevalence of resistance to several of the antimicrobials tested, including

Table 8 Resistance and distribution of Minimum Inhibitory Concentrations (MIC) of antimicrobials for E. coli from sows ($n = 29$)

Antimicrobial	Resistance (%)	0.015	0.03	0.06	0.12	0.25	0.5	1	2	4	8	16	32	64	128	256	512	1024	>1024
		Distributions (%) of MICs (mg/L)																	
Ampicillin	75.9								13.8	10.3	3.4				72.4				
Azithromycin[a]	-										37.9	48.3	13.8						
Cefotaxime	0.0					100													
Ceftazidime	6.9						93.1	6.9											
Chloramphenicol	62.1										31.0	6.9	13.8	13.8	17.2	17.2			
Ciprofloxacin	72.4	13.8	10.3	3.4		13.8	34.5	13.8			3.4	6.9							
Colistin	6.9							89.7	3.4	3.4	3.4								
Gentamicin	27.6						6.9	41.4	24.1	20.7				6.9					
Meropenem	0.0		100																
Nalidixic acid	34.5									24.1	20.7	20.7	10.3	6.9	3.4	13.8			
Sulfamethoxazole	75.9											17.2	6.9						75.9
Tetracycline	93.1								6.9				13.8	24.1	55.2				
Tigecycline	0.0					88.2	10.0	0.9			0.9								
Trimethoprim	58.6						34.5	6.9						58.6					

White fields represent range of dilutions tested for each antimicrobial. MICs higher than the highest concentration tested are given as the concentration closest above the range. MICs equal to or lower than the lowest concentration tested are underlined. The epidemiological cut-off value (ECOFF) [33] for each antimicrobial is presented as a vertical line
[a]No ECOFF was available for azithromycin

MDR, than bacteria from fatteners (older than 3 months). Higher prevalence of AMR in younger pigs has been reported in other cross-sectional studies [36, 37]. A longitudinal study by Nguyen et al. [19] presented similar results where the prevalence of resistance to ciprofloxacin and gentamicin, as well as MDR, in *E. coli* declined during the rearing process. The decreasing prevalence of AMR is suggested to be the result of reduced use of antimicrobials during the finishing phase of pig production and may also reflect the potential fitness cost of resistance in bacteria from the intestinal tract [38]. In the present study, however, isolates from sows exhibited significantly higher prevalence of resistance than isolates from fatteners for several of the antimicrobials tested. One explanation might be that sows (and also younger pigs) receive oral antimicrobials to a higher extent than older pigs, as oral administration of antimicrobials has been reported to increase AMR in commensal *E. coli* from pigs [39]. Animal age might thus be an important factor to consider when investigating prevalence of AMR in pigs.

Two thirds of the farmers reported frequently deviating from the instructions provided by veterinarians or those written on drug packaging. Common practices were to stop administering antimicrobials as soon as the animals started to recover, hence not completing the treatment, and to self-adjust the dosage based on the severity of the disease. Poor adherence to recommended instructions may increase the risk of AMR [17, 18] and has been reported to be a common problem in countries with non-prescription access to antimicrobials [40]. A particular concern is the use of human antimicrobials as a last-line treatment and the handling of expired antimicrobials, where almost half of the respondents stated that they commonly dumped the remaining pharmaceuticals in the environment once the expiry date had passed. This implies that discarded antimicrobials may be present locally at high concentrations in the environment, where they may contribute to resistance development [41, 42].

Improper and unregulated use of antimicrobials may pose a risk to public health if antimicrobial residues are present in animal products. Nearly half of the respondents in the present study reported that pigs were commonly sold during or directly after antimicrobial treatment, that is within the prescribed withdrawal time. If withdrawal times are not respected there is a risk of antimicrobial residues remaining in the meat at slaughter [43]. In many low- and middle-income countries, compliance with withdrawal times is not monitored and analysis of animal products is not routinely practiced. Studies in Vietnam, however, have found tetracycline [44] and sulfamethazine [45] residues in 5.5 and 8.8%, respectively, of pork meat sampled at local markets.

The prevalence of resistance to several antimicrobials, including MDR, was lower on farms operated by an older farmer, possibly as a consequence of more experienced farmers having better disease control practices, as previously suggested by Nhung et al. [27]. Notably, farms on which a veterinarian was responsible for antimicrobial treatment had a higher prevalence of resistance to several of the antimicrobials tested, including MDR. This is a concern, as veterinary supervision is a measure often put forward when discussing ways to improve antimicrobial treatment regimens. It is possible that these farmers relied on a veterinarian for treatment as a result of poor knowledge of animal health and veterinary practices, which in turn might result in deficient disease control. However, it is also important to consider the fact that veterinarians in most countries globally (including Cambodia) receive a considerable part of their income from the sale of pharmaceuticals, and therefore may be reluctant to reduce the use of antimicrobials in their practice [46]. It is also possible that these results reflect a need to strengthen veterinary education in Cambodia.

Male respondents more often stated that they had heard about antimicrobial resistance than female respondents. This could be a consequence of men generally attaining a higher level of education than women, or of men most commonly being responsible for treating sick pigs and therefore probably having more discussions with veterinarians. The latter suggestion is reinforced by the fact that previous awareness of antimicrobial resistance was more commonly reported by farms where the respondent was the person responsible for treating sick pigs. Although our aim was to interview the person responsible, this was not possible on all farms. If we had omitted those farms, we would probably have ended up with far fewer farms in our study.

When performing surveys that rely on self-reported practices, there is always the risk of recall bias or of respondents providing answers that they think are 'correct', but which may not correspond to actual practices. In the present study, many of the respondents did not remember the names of the drugs they used and they did not keep any treatment records. Thus we were unable to determine whether higher levels of AMR were the result of higher consumption of certain antimicrobials or to establish any associations between antimicrobial use and explanatory factors, such as farm size or education level.

Conclusions

The emergence of AMR is a truly global issue as it spreads easily between countries, and excessive and inappropriate use of antimicrobials should thus be mitigated everywhere.

In the present study, we found that antimicrobial use in urban and peri-urban pig farming in Cambodia was commonly only based on farmers' experiences or on drug sellers' advices based on descriptions of symptoms, and there was low awareness of the risks and consequences of antimicrobial resistance among the respondents. Commensal *E. coli* from pigs showed high prevalence of AMR to several antimicrobials considered to be of critical importance for human medicine, including ampicillin, ciprofloxacin and colistin, and multidrug-resistance was found in four out of five samples. Higher prevalence of resistance was found on farms that administered antimicrobials as a prophylactic and on farms that treated the entire group or herd in the event of disease. These results confirm the hypothesis that non-rational use of antimicrobials results in higher prevalence of AMR and highlight the need for professional animal health systems that involve medically rational use of antimicrobials in emerging economies such as Cambodia.

Abbreviations
AMP: Ampicillin; AMR: Antimicrobial resistance; CAZ: Ceftazidime; CHL: Chloramphenicol; CIP: Ciprofloxacin; CLSI: Clinical and Laboratory Standards Institute; COL: Colistin; CTX: Cefotaxime; ECOFF: Epidemiological cut-off value; EFSA: European Food Safety Authority; EUCAST: European Committee on Antimicrobial Susceptibility Testing; GEN: Gentamicin; MDR: Multidrug-resistance; MER: Meropenem; MIC: Minimum Inhibitory Concentration; NAHPRI: National Animal Health and Production Research Institute; NAL: Nalidixic acid; Sida: Swedish International Development Cooperation Agency; SLU: Swedish University of Agricultural Sciences; SMX: Sulfamethoxazole; TET: Tetracycline; TIG: Tigecycline; TMP: Trimethoprim; TSA: Tryptone Soya Agar; VR: Swedish Research council; WHO: World Health Organization

Acknowledgements
The authors would like to thank the farmers that participated in the study and Mr. Vor Sina for his assistance with translations and sampling during the fieldwork.

Funding
The study was funded by the Swedish Research Council (VR) (SWE-2012-059).

Authors' contributions
GS, SB, AA, AAD and UM designed the study. SS and TS contributed to the organization and implementation of the study. GS collected the data. GS and LF performed the analyses. GS wrote the paper. All authors read and approved the final manuscript.
All farmers were informed about the purpose of the study and that their participation was voluntary and anonymous. Informed consent was obtained from each participating farmer before the interviews were conducted.

Consent for publication
Not applicable.

Competing interests
The authors declare that they have no competing interest.

Author details
[1]Department of Clinical Sciences, Swedish University of Agricultural Sciences, Uppsala, Sweden. [2]Department of Biomedical Sciences and Veterinary Public Health, Swedish University of Agricultural Sciences, Uppsala, Sweden. [3]Department of Chemistry, Environment and Feed Hygiene, National Veterinary Institute, Uppsala, Sweden. [4]Department of Human Geography, Lund University, Lund, Sweden. [5]Centre for Livestock and Agriculture Development, Phnom Penh, Cambodia. [6]National Animal Health and Production Research Institute, Phnom Penh, Cambodia.

References
1. Ventola CL. The antibiotic resistance crisis: part 1: causes and threats. P T. 2015;40:277–83.
2. WHO. Global action plan on antimicrobial resistance. Switzerland: Geneva; 2015.
3. Adeyi OO, Baris E, Jonas OB, Irwin A, Berthe FCJ, Le Gall FG, Marquez PV, Nikolic IA, Plante CA, Schneidman M, Shriber DE, Thiebaud A. Drug-resistant infections: a threat to our economic future. Washington DC: World Bank. Group. 2017; http://documents.worldbank.org/curated/en/323311493396993758/final-report. Accessed 9 Dec 2017
4. Aarestrup FM. Veterinary drug usage and antimicrobial resistance in bacteria of animal origin. Basic Clin Pharmacol Toxicol. 2005;96:271–81.
5. Marshall BM, Levy SB. Food animals and antimicrobials: impacts on human health. Clin Microbiol Rev. 2011;24:718–33.
6. Tang KT, Caffrey NP, Nóbrega DB, Cork SC, Ronksley PE, Barkema HW, Polachek AJ, Ganshorn H, Sharma N, Kellner JD, Ghali WA. Restricting the use of antibiotics in food-producing animals and its association with antibiotic resistance in food-producing animals and human beings: a systematic review and meta-analysis. Lancet Planet Health. 2017;1:e316-e327.
7. EFSA (European Food Safety Authority), ESDC (European Centre for Disease Prevention and Control). The European Union summary report on antimicrobial resistance in zoonotic and indicator bacteria from humans, animals and food in 2014. EFSA J. 2016;14:207.
8. European Medicines Agency. Sales of veterinary antimicrobial agents in 30 European countries in 2015: Seventh ESVAC Report. 2017. www.ema.europa.eu/ema/index.jsp?curl=pages/regulation/document_listing/document_listing_000302.jsp. Accessed 27 Dec 2017.
9. Planta MB. The role of poverty in antimicrobial resistance. J Am Board Fam Med. 2007;20:533–9.
10. Laxminarayan R, Matsoso P, Pant S, Brower C, Røttingen JA, Klugman K, Davies S. Access to effective antimicrobials: a worldwide challenge. Lancet. 2016;387:168–75.
11. Laxminarayan R, Duse A, Wattal C, Zaidi AK, Wertheim HF, Sumpradit N, Vlieghe E, Hara GL, Gould IM, Goossens H, Greko C, So AD, Bigdeli M, Tomson G, Woodhouse W, Ombaka E, Peralta AQ, Qamar FN, Mir F, Kariuki S, Bhutta ZA, Coates A, Bergström R, Wright GD, Brown ED, Cars O. Antibiotic resistance-the need for global solutions. Lancet Infect Dis. 2013;13:1057–98.
12. Van Boeckel TP, Brower C, Gilbert M, Grenfell BT, Levin SA, Robinson TP, Teillant A, Laxminarayan R. Global trends in antimicrobial use in food animals. Proc Natl Acad Sci U S A. 2015;112:5649–54.
13. Robinson TP, Bu DP, Carrique-mas J, Fevre EM, Gilbert M, Grace D, Hay SI, Jiwakanon J, Kakkar M, Kaiuki S, Laxminarayan R, Lubroth J, Magnusson U, Ngoc PT, van Boeckel TP, MEJ W. Antibiotic resistance is the quintessential one health issue. Trans R Soc Trop Med Hyg. 2016;110:377–80.
14. Coker RJ, Hunter BM, Rudge JW, Liverani M, Hanvoravongchai P. Emerging infectious diseases in southeast Asia: regional challenges to control. Lancet. 2011;377:599–609.
15. Antimicrobial resistance WHO. global report on surveillance. Switzerland: Geneva; 2014.
16. Gilbert M, Conchedda G, Van Boeckel TP, Cinardi G, Linard C, Nicolas G, Thanapongtharm W, D'Aietti L, Wint W, Newman SH, Robinson TP. Income disparities and the global distribution of intensively farmed chicken and pigs. PLoS One. 2015;10:e0133381.
17. Okeke IN, Lamikanra A, Edelman R. Socioeconomic and behavioral factors leading to acquired bacterial resistance to antibiotics in developing countries. Emerg Infect Dis. 1999;5:18–27.
18. Guillemot D, Carbon C, Balkau B, Geslin P, Lecoeur H, Vauzelle-Kervroëdan F, Bouvenot G, Eschwége E. Low dosage and long treatment duration of beta-lactam: risk factors for carriage of penicillin-resistant Streptococcus pneumoniae. JAMA. 1998;279:365–70.

19. Nguyen NT, Nguyen HM, Nguyen CV, Nguyen TV, Nguyen MT, Thai QH, Ho MH, Thwaites G, Ngo HT, Baker S, Carrique-Mas J. Use of Colistin and other critical antimicrobials on pig and chicken farms in southern Vietnam and its association with resistance in commensal Escherichia coli bacteria. Appl Environ Microbiol. 2016;82:3727–35.
20. Dang PK, Saegerman C, Douny C, Ton VD, Bo HX, Binh DV, Ngan HP, Scippo ML. First survey on the use of antibiotics in pig and poultry production in the Red River Delta region of Vietnam. Food. Public Health. 2013;3:247–56.
21. Om C, McLaws ML. Antibiotics: practice and opinions of Cambodian commercial farmers, animal feed retailers and veterinarians. Antimicrob Resist Infect Control. 2016;5:42.
22. Ström G, Halje M, Karlsson D, Jiwakanon J, Pringle M, Fernström LL, Magnusson U. Antimicrobial use and antimicrobial susceptibility in Escherichia coli on small- and medium-scale pig farms in north-eastern Thailand. Antimicrob Resist Infect Control. 2017;6:75.
23. Changkaew K, Intarapuk A, Utrarachkij F, Nakajima C, Suthienkul O, Suzuki Y. Antimicrobial resistance, extended-Spectrum beta-lactamase productivity, and class 1 Integrons in Escherichia coli from healthy swine. J Food Prot. 2015;78:1442–50.
24. Lay KK, Koowattananukul C, Chansong N, Chuanchuen R. Antimicrobial resistance, virulence, and phylogenetic characteristics of Escherichia coli isolates from clinically healthy swine. Foodborne Pathog Dis. 2012;9:992–1001.
25. Nguyen VT, Carrique-Mas J, Ngo TH, Ho HM, Ha TT, Campbell JI, Nguyen TN, Hoang NN, Pham VM, Wagenaar JA, Hardon A, Thai QH, Schultsz C. Prevalence and risk factors for carriage of antimicrobial-resistant Escherichia coli on household and small-scale chicken farms in the Mekong Delta of Vietnam. J Antimicrob Chemother. 2015;70:2144–52.
26. Nhung NT, Cuong NV, Thwaites G, Carrique-Mas J. Antimicrobial usage and antimicrobial resistance in animal production in Southeast Asia: a review. Antibiotics. 2016;5:37.
27. Nhung NT, Cuong NV, Campbell J, Hoa NT, Bryant JE, Truc VN, Kiet BT, Jombart T, Trung NV, Hien VB, Thwaites G, Baker S, Carrique-Mas J. High levels of antimicrobial resistance among escherichia coli isolates from livestock farms and synanthropic rats and shrews in the Mekong Delta of Vietnam. Appl Environ Microbiol. 2015;81:812–20.
28. World Bank. World development indicators. 2017. http://databank.worldbank.org/data/reports.aspx?source=world-development-indicators. Accessed 9 Dec 2017.
29. Sovann S, San S. Pig production in Cambodia. In: Jones R, editor. Priority for research in Southeast Asia and the Pacific to 2010. Canberra: Australian Centre for International Agricultural Research; 2010.
30. Ström G, Andersson Djurfeldt A, Boqvist S, Albihn A, Sokerya S, San S, Davun H, Magnusson U. Urban and peri-urban family-based pig-keeping in Cambodia: characteristics, management and perceived benefits and constraints. PLoS One. 2017;12:e0182247.
31. Faugier J, Sargeant M. Sampling hard to reach populations. J Adv Nurs. 1997;26:790–7.
32. CLSI (Clinical and Laboratory Standards Institute). Performance Standards for Antimicrobial Disk and Dilution Susceptibility Tests for Bacteria Isolated From Animals; Approved Standard - Forth Edition. CLSI document VET01-A4 Clinical and Laboratory Standards Institute. Wayne, Pennsylvania, USA.
33. EUCAST (European Committee on Antimicrobial Susceptibility Testing). MIC distributions and ECOFFs. 2017. http://mic.eucast.org/Eucast2/SearchController/search.jsp?action=performSearch&BeginIndex=0&Micdif=mic&NumberIndex=50&Antib=-1&Specium=162. Accessed 20 Oct 2017.
34. Magiorakos AP, Srinivasan A, Carey RB, Carmeli Y, Falagas ME, Giske CG, Harbarth S, Hindler JF, Kahlmeter G, Olsson-Liljequist B, Paterson DL, Rice LB, Stelling J, Struelens MJ, Vatopoulos A, Weber JT, Monnet DL. Multidrug-resistans, extensively drug-resistant and pandrug-resistant bacteria: an international expert proposal for interim standard definitions for aquired resistance. Clin Microbiol Infect. 2012;18:268–81.
35. Literak I, Reitschmied T, Bujnakova D, Dolejska M, Cizek A, Bardon J, Pokludova L, Alexa P, Halova D, Jamborova I. Broilers as a source of quinolone-resistant and extraintestinal pathogenic Escherichia coli in the Czech Republic. Microb Drug Resist. 2013;19:57–63.
36. Mathew AG, Saxton AM, Upchurch WG, Chattin SE. Multiple antibiotic resistance patterns of Escherichia coli isolates from swine farms. Appl Environ Microbiol. 1999;65:2770–2.
37. Gibbons JF, Boland F, Egan J, Fanning S, Markey BK, Leonard FC. Antimicrobial resistance of Faecal Escherichia coli isolates from pig farms with different durations of in-feed antimicrobial use. Zoonoses Public Health. 2016;63:241–50.
38. Marchant M, Moreno MA. Dynamics and diversity of Escherichia coli in animals and system management of the manure on a commercial farrow-to-finish pig farm. Appl Environ Microbiol. 2013;79:853–9.
39. Burow E, Simoneit C, Tenhagen BA, Käsbohrer A. Oral antimicrobials increase antimicrobial resistance in porcine E. Coli - a systematic review. Prev Vet Med. 2014;113:364–75.
40. Morgan DJ, Okeke IN, Laxminarayan R, Perencevich EN, Weisenberg S. Non-prescription antimicrobial use worldwide: a systematic review. Lancet Infect Dis. 2011;11:692–701.
41. Sarmah AK, Meyer MT, Boxall AB. A global perspective on the use, sales, exposure pathways, occurrence, fate and effects of veterinary antibiotics (VAs) in the environment. Chemosphere. 2006;65:725–59.
42. Larsson DGJ. Antibiotics in the environment. Ups J Med Sci. 2014;119:108–12.
43. Lee MH, Lee HJ, Ryu PD. Public health risks: chemical and antibiotic residues – review. Asian-Australas J Anim Sci. 2001;14:402–13.
44. Duong VM, Paulsen P, Suriyasathaporn W, Smulders FJ, Kyule MN, Baumann MP, Zessin KH, Pham HN. Preliminary analysis of tetracycline residues in marketed pork in Hanoi, Vietnam. Ann N Y Acad Sci. 2006;1081:534–42.
45. Yamaguchi T, Okihashi M, Harada K, Konishi Y, Uchida K, Do MH, Bui HD, Nguyen TD, Nguyen PD, Chau VV, Nguyen HT, Kajimura K, Kumeda Y, Bui CT, Vien MQ, Le NH, Hirata K, YamamotoY. Antibiotic residue monitoring results for pork, chicken, and beef samples in Vietnam in 2012-2013. J Agric Food Chem 2015;63:5141–5145.
46. Wegener HC. Antibiotic resistance - linking human and animal health. In: Institute of Medicin, editor. Improving food safety through a One Health approach: Workshop summary. Washington DC: National Academies Press; 2012.
47. Swedish Code of Statutes. The Act concerning the Ethical Review of Research Involving Humans (2003,460). https://www.riksdagen.se/sv/Dokument-Lagar/Lagar/Svenskforfattningssamling/Lag-2003460-om-etikprovning_sfs-2003-460/ Accessed 30 Nov 2017.
48. WHO. Critically important antimicrobials for human medicine - 5th rev. Switzerland: Geneva; 2017.

13

Antimicrobial use and antimicrobial susceptibility in *Escherichia coli* on small- and medium-scale pig farms in north-eastern Thailand

G. Ström[1], M. Halje[1], D. Karlsson[1], J. Jiwakanon[2], M. Pringle[3], L.-L. Fernström[4] and U. Magnusson[1*]

Abstract

Background: Intensification of livestock production seen in many low- and middle-income countries is often believed to be associated with increased use of antimicrobials, and may hence contribute to the emergence of antimicrobial resistance. The aim of this study was to map antimicrobial use on small- (n = 25) and medium-scale (n = 27) pig farms in north-eastern Thailand, and to compare antimicrobial susceptibility of commensal *Escherichia coli* isolated from sows on these farms.

Methods: Information regarding pig husbandry and antimicrobial treatment regimens was obtained by the use of semi-structured questionnaires. Faecal samples were collected from three healthy sows at each farm, and *Escherichia coli* was cultured and analysed for antimicrobial susceptibility using the broth microdilution method. Multilevel regression models were used to compare antimicrobial susceptibility between isolates from small- and medium-scale farms.

Results: All farms included in the study administered antimicrobials to their sows. Small-scale farmers most commonly (64%) decided themselves when to give antimicrobials and the majority (60%) bought the medicines at the local store or pharmacy, whereas farmers on medium-scale farms always discussed antimicrobial treatment with a veterinarian. Medium-scale farms used a greater diversity of antimicrobials than small-scale farms and did also administer antimicrobials in feed to a higher extent. High levels of antimicrobial resistance to several critically important antimicrobials for human medicine (including ciprofloxacin, streptomycin and ampicillin) were found in isolates from both small- and medium-scale farms. Resistance levels were significantly ($P < 0.05$) higher in isolates from medium-scale farms for several of the antimicrobials tested, as well as the level of multidrug-resistance ($P = 0.026$).

Conclusion: The routines regarding access and administration of antimicrobials differed between the small- and medium-scale farms. Although the level of antimicrobial resistance, as well as multidrug-resistance, was higher in isolates from medium-scale farms, it cannot be concluded if this increase is a consequence of a more abundant use of antimicrobials, or a result of differences in administration routines.

Keywords: Antimicrobial use, Antimicrobial resistance, *E. coli*, Pig production, Farm size, Thailand

* Correspondence: ulf.magnusson@slu.se
[1]Department of Clinical Sciences, Swedish University of Agricultural Sciences, Uppsala, Sweden
Full list of author information is available at the end of the article

Background

The emergence of antimicrobial resistance (AMR) has become a serious global health concern, and imprudent use of antimicrobials has been recognized as a contributing factor in the selection for resistant bacterial populations [1]. Although much of the resistance seen in human medicine originates from inappropriate use in humans [2], antimicrobial use within the livestock sector is believed to contribute to AMR through increased selective pressure and through generating resistance reservoirs [3, 4].

The level of AMR has been shown to be highest in low- and middle-income countries, particularly those in South and Southeast Asia [5]. In Thailand, infections with antimicrobial resistant bacteria in humans have been estimated to be the cause of almost 90,000 hospitalisations and 38,000 mortalities each year [6], and high levels of resistance have been documented in the environment and along the food production chain [7].

As *Escherichia coli* are intestinal commensal bacteria present in both animals and humans, and therefore subjected to a high selection pressure driven by the antimicrobials to which their hosts are exposed, they may serve as a good indicator to monitor the general level of AMR in a human or livestock population [8]. Also, although commensal bacteria are normally harmless, they may constitute a reservoir of resistance genes that may be transmitted to pathogenic bacteria [9].

Today's intensive livestock production often depends on antimicrobials to maintain the health and productivity of the livestock [10]. Antimicrobials are not only used to treat infectious diseases, but are also sometimes used subtherapeutically for growth promotion, a practice associated with a high potential for selection of resistant pathogens [11]. Intensification of livestock production in many low- and middle-income countries, as exemplified by Thailand's pig sector [12, 13], is often believed to be driving an increased use of antimicrobials and thereby also an increased emergence of AMR [10, 14]. Here we explored the validity of that assertion in a country with an expanding pig sector. We therefore investigated antimicrobial use on small- and medium-scale pig farms in north-eastern Thailand, and compared antimicrobial susceptibility of commensal *E. coli* isolated from sows on these farms.

Methods

Study area

This cross-sectional study was conducted on small- and medium-scale pig farms situated near the city Khon Kaen in north-eastern Thailand. In 2013, the country produced more than 16 million pigs for slaughter [12]. Among the 220,000 households that raised pigs, 94% raised less than 50 pigs per year. On the other hand, two large companies owned about 46% of all breeder pigs. Currently, there are about 200 such contractual, company-owned pig farms in the Khon Kaen province and the density of the total number of pigs, as well as small - scale farms (less than 50 heads per farm), are about the averages for the provinces in Thailand [13]. In the last decade, Thailand's pig sector has intensified and farm sizes have increased; a trend that is expected to continue [13].

Study design and data collection

The study was conducted between September and November 2015. Inclusion criteria for small-scale farms were that the farm kept sows for breeding, with a maximum of 20 sows, whereas medium-scale farms were defined as farms with between 100 and 500 sows, a classification relating to previous work in Thailand where such farms have been named "smallholders" and "small large-scale farms", respectively [13]. In order to make a distinct difference in size between the small- and medium-scale farms in the present study, no farms with 21–99 sows were included. From a governmental list of villages with pig farm(s), the heads in randomly selected villages were contacted for checking that there were pig farms at the time of the fieldwork. The villages with positive responses were visited and all farms where the farmers were at home agreed to participate. For the medium-scale farms, that all but one belonged to two companies, the company officers were asked to make a choice of farms to be equally distributed over the province. By this procedure, 25 small-scale and 27 medium-scale farms were included in the study.

A faecal sample was collected, using a rectal swab, from the individual pen of three randomly chosen healthy sows at each farm and added to sterile plastic tubes containing Amies medium. At the small-scale farms, sampling was performed by the authors (MH, DK), and at the medium-scale farms by local veterinary assistants who were thoroughly instructed beforehand how to collect the samples in a correct manner. Sampling was performed at mid-day and samples were transported to Khon Kaen University within 1–6 h and stored at 2-8 °C until analysis, which was performed within 48 h after sampling. Because not all small-scale farms had three healthy sows, only 69 samples were obtained from these farms.

A semi-structured questionnaire, with questions on farm characteristics, pig husbandry and routines for antimicrobial treatment, was administered to the person responsible for the pigs at each farm. The questionnaire was in English and had been pre-tested on pig farms not involved in the subsequent study, after which necessary adjustments were made. Interviews were performed by the authors MH and DK together with a Thai speaking veterinary student at the Khon Kaen University who translated the questions to Thai and the farmer's answers to English. The interviews took about 40 min each.

Antimicrobial susceptibility testing

Each faecal sample was streaked on MacConkey agar and incubated at 44 °C overnight. Suspected *E. coli* isolates were sub-cultured on blood agar, incubated at 37 °C overnight and tested for production of tryptophanase (indole). One indole positive isolate was selected from each faecal sample and further tested for antimicrobial susceptibility.

Susceptibility testing was performed by broth microdilution, using the growth method inoculum preparation, according to the standards described by the Clinical and Laboratory Standards Institute (CLSI) [15]. Microdilution panels (VetMIC GN-mo, National Veterinary Institute, Uppsala, Sweden) were used to determine susceptibility to 13 antimicrobials (ciprofloxacin, nalidixid acid, gentamicin, streptomycin, tetracycline, florfenicol, chloramphenicol, colistin, sulfamethoxazole, trimethoprim, ampicillin, cefotaxime, ceftazidime). *Escherichia. coli* ATCC 25922 was used as quality control strain.

The Minimum Inhibitory Concentration (MIC) for each antimicrobial was recorded and epidemiological cut-off values (ECOFFs), defined by the European Committee on Antimicrobial Susceptibility Testing [16], were used to differentiate between wild-type and non-wild-type isolates. Wild-type and non-wild-type isolates will henceforth be referred to as susceptible and resistant, respectively. Multidrug-resistance was defined as isolates resistant to at least three different categories (i.e. with different mechanisms of action) of the antimicrobials tested [17].

Statistical analyses

Statistical analyses were conducted in SAS software 9.4 (SAS Institute Inc., Cary, NC). Descriptive statistics were computed to define farm characteristics. To investigate associations between management factors, such as use of antimicrobials and veterinary services, and resistance against different types of antimicrobials, univariable logistic regression and Fisher's exact test were used where applicable. Multilevel regression models were used to compare susceptibility patterns between the small- and medium-scale farms. As isolates from the same farm were assumed to be more alike, generalised estimating equations (GEE) were used to account for the effect of clustering within farms. The statistical significance level was defined as a two-tailed P-value <0.05.

Results

Farm characteristics

At the small-scale farms, all privately owned, the number of sows varied from 1 to 19, with a median of 5 sows (25th and 95th percentiles: 3 and 12 sows). Most of these farms (60%) practised a 'farrow-to-finish' system, where pigs were raised from birth to slaughter. The rest of the small-scale farms were either breeding farms (28%), where the piglets were sold to other farmers after weaning, or farms that practised a combination of the two systems (12%).

The medium-scale farms in this study, except for one farm that was privately owned and managed, were contract farms contracted by two different companies. The number of sows ranged from 100 to 400, with a median number of 210 sows (25th and 95th percentiles: 155 and 327 sows). All medium-scale farms were breeding farms, and the privately managed farm also combined this with a 'farrow-to-finish' system.

None of the farms in this study kept their pigs freely roaming; instead the pigs were kept in enclosures, such as concrete pens or metal crates.

Antimicrobial use

All farms in this study administered antimicrobials to their sows, though only 21 of the 25 small-scale farms knew the names of the antimicrobials used. Small-scale farmers most commonly decided themselves when to give antimicrobials and the majority bought the drugs at the local store or pharmacy (Table 1). On all medium-scale farms, the farmer discussed with a veterinarian when to give antimicrobials to the animals, and the contract farms received the antimicrobials through their respective contracting company. The privately managed medium-scale farm received antimicrobials through a pharmaceutical company. Furthermore, antimicrobials were added to the feed on all medium-scale farms, a practice that was performed on only one of the small-scale farms.

The number and types of antimicrobials used differed between small- and medium-scale farms (Table 2). Penicillin and streptomycin were used as injectable drugs on all the medium-scale farms, compared to only 19% of the small-scale farms. Small-scale farms most commonly used amoxicillin (38%) and enrofloxacin (57%) as injectable drugs. For the contract farms, the two contracting companies had

Table 1 Practices related to use and access to antimicrobials on the small- and medium-scale pig farms

	Small-scale % (n = 25)	Medium-scale % (n = 27)
Antimicrobials injected for disease treatment	100 (25)	100 (27)
Antimicrobials added to, or included in, feed[a]	4 (1)	100 (27)
Person who decides on when to give antimicrobials		
Farmer	68 (17)	0 (0)
Veterinarian	32 (8)	100 (27)
Source of antimicrobials		
From veterinarian	32 (8)	0 (0)
From local store/pharmacy	60 (15)	0 (0)
From the contracting company	4 (1)	96 (26)
Other	4 (1)	4 (1)

[a]On regular basis

Table 2 Antimicrobials administered to sows on the small- (n = 21[a]) and medium-scale farms (n = 27)

Antimicrobials	Small-scale[a]																				
Farm no	1	2	3	4	5	6	7	8	9	10	11	12	13	14	15	16	17	18	19	20	21
Injection																					
Penicillin G[b]											•	•				•	•	•			
Streptomycin[b]											•	•				•	•	•			
Amoxicillin[b]				•			•			•		•	•		•			•			•
Oxytetracycline													•								
Cefotaxime[b]																					
Enrofloxacin		•			•	•		•	•			•	•		•	•	•	•		•	
Kanamycin[b]	•	•	•									•							•		
Florfenicol																					
Gentamicin[b]														•							
In feed																					
Amoxicillin[b]		•																			
Colistin[b]																					
Kitasamycin																					
Oxytetracycline		•																			
Sulfonamide		•																			

Antimicrobials	Medium-scale																										
Farm no	26	27	28	29	30	31	32	33	34	35	36	37	38	39	40	41	42	43	44	45	46	47	48	49	50	51	52
Injection																											
Penicillin G[b]	•	•	•	•	•	•	•	•	•	•	•	•	•	•	•	•	•	•	•	•	•	•	•	•	•	•	•
Streptomycin[b]	•	•	•	•	•	•	•	•	•	•	•	•	•	•	•	•	•	•	•	•	•	•	•	•	•	•	•
Amoxicillin[b]																											•
Oxytetracycline																											•
Cefotaxime[b]																											•
Enrofloxacin															•	•	•	•	•	•	•	•	•	•	•	•	
Kanamycin[b]																											
Florfenicol																											
Gentamicin[b]																											
In feed																											
Amoxicillin[b]																											•
Colistin[b]																											•
Kitasamycin	•	•	•	•	•	•	•	•	•	•	•	•	•	•													
Oxytetracycline															•	•	•	•	•	•	•	•	•	•	•	•	
Sulfonamide																											

[a]From four of the small-scale farms, information on which antimicrobials that were used was not obtained and these farms are thus not displayed in the figure
[b]Antimicrobial considered to be critically important for human medicine according to WHO [22]

different regimes regarding treatment with antimicrobials. Both companies provided penicillin and streptomycin as injectable drugs to their contract farms, and one of the companies also provided enrofloxacin. The companies either provided kitasamycin or oxytetracycline as in-feed antimicrobials to their respective farms. On the privately managed medium-scale farm, penicillin, streptomycin, amoxicillin, oxytetracycline and cefotaxime were administered by injection, and amoxicillin and colistin were provided with the feed. Unfortunately, no information regarding the amount of antimicrobials used could be obtained in this study.

Antimicrobial susceptibility

In total, 69 and 81 isolates were obtained from the small- and medium-scale farms, respectively. Around 90% (62/69) of isolates from the small-scale farms showed resistance to at least one category of antimicrobials. The corresponding figure for medium-scale farms was 98% (79/81). The MIC distributions for isolates from the small- and medium-scale farms are presented in Tables 3 and 4, respectively.

For both small- and medium-scale farms, most isolates showed resistance to ampicillin, tetracycline and sulfamethoxazole, ranging from 61% to 86% (for details see Table 5). No isolates showed resistance to colistin, and only a few isolates were resistant to the third generation cephalosporins cefotaxime and ceftazidime. Isolates obtained from medium-scale farms were significantly more likely to be resistant to streptomycin ($P < 0.001$), sulfamethoxazole ($P = 0.006$), trimethoprim ($P < 0.001$) and chloramphenicol ($P = 0.023$), compared to isolates from small-scale farms. Multidrug-resistance was more common ($P = 0.026$) in isolates from medium-scale farms (89%), than in isolates from small-scale farms (74%).

Isolates obtained from farms that used enrofloxacin were more likely to show resistance to ciprofloxacin ($P = 0.02$), but not to nalidixic acid ($P = 0.47$). Moreover, all isolates from medium-scale farms that administered oxytetracycline in the feed were resistant to tetracycline.

Discussion

The overall aim of this study was to investigate possible differences in antimicrobial use in pigs on small- and medium-scale pig farms in Thailand, a country that is experiencing an intensification of the pig sector, like other countries in the region [13]. Furthermore, we compared antimicrobial susceptibility of isolates of *E. coli* from pigs on these farms. This research question stems from the common assertion that farm intensification, in particular in the pig and poultry sectors, is associated with a more abundant use of antimicrobials, and thereby also with higher levels of antimicrobial resistance (AMR) [10, 14].

The levels of AMR presented here are largely similar to those in previous studies on *E. coli* isolated from animals in Southeast Asia, according to a recent review by Nhung et al. [18]. The highest frequencies of resistance in isolates from both small- and medium-scale farms were found against tetracycline, followed by ampicillin. Multidrug-resistance was significantly more commonly observed in isolates from pigs on medium- compared to small-scale farms. These results are in accordance with a study by Love et al. [19], where herd size was reported to be positively associated with higher rates of multidrug-resistance in *E. coli* isolated on pig farms in northern Thailand. Although the medium-scale farms in the present study routinely used a greater diversity of antimicrobials, we do not have any reliable information regarding the amounts of antimicrobials used on the farms. Therefore, no associations between the amounts of administrated antimicrobials and AMR can be determined here.

Penicillin and streptomycin were used on all medium-scale farms, whereas small-scale farms most commonly used enrofloxacin and amoxicillin. Enrofloxacin was also used on almost half of the medium-scale farms. Although this antimicrobial is not used in human medicine, being a quinolone its use in animals selects for resistance to other quinolones that are used for humans. Here we found a positive association between the use of enrofloxacin on the farm and ciprofloxacin resistance in isolates of *E. coli* from the pigs, which indicates the importance of restricting the use of quinolones in animal agriculture. These results are in accordance with studies conducted on pig and chicken farms in Vietnam [20, 21].

Many of the antimicrobials used by the farms in this study are classified by the World Health Organization (WHO) as critically important for human medicine [22], including amoxicillin, cefotaxime and colistin. The recent discovery of the plasmid mediated *mcr-1* gene in bacteria isolated from pigs [23], a gene that confers resistance to colistin and that may be transferred horizontally between bacteria, has emphasised the importance of colistin as a last-resort antimicrobial that should possibly be restricted to human use. Plasmid-mediated colistin resistance has since been detected in almost all regions of the world [24], including in bacteria isolated from Vietnamese pigs [20, 25]. None of the isolates in the present study, however, were resistant to colistin, and it was only used on one of the study farms.

Data presented in this study indicate that medium-scale farms administer antimicrobials to the feed to a higher extent than small-scale farms. Oral administration of antimicrobials is known to increase AMR in *E. coli* from pigs [26]. A possible explanation to the higher use of antimicrobials in feed on the medium-scale farms in this study could be that these farms experience an increased disease pressure that is associated with larger group sizes and

Table 3 Resistance and distributions of Minimum Inhibitory Concentrations (MIC) for *E. coli* isolates from small-scale farms

Antimicrobial	Resistance (%)	≤0.008	0.016	0.03	0.06	0.12	0.25	0.5	1	2	4	8	16	32	64	128	256	512	1024	>1024
		Distributions (%) of MICs (mg/L)																		
Ciprofloxacin	40.5		1.4	18.8	39.1	2.9	5.8	10.1	8.7	13										
Nalidixic acid	20.2									8.7	46.4	20.3	4.3	7.2		2.9	10.1			
Gentamicin	11.4						7.2	36.2	34.8	10.1	4.3		1.4	1.4	4.3					
Streptomycin	37.6									7.2	17.4	21.7	15.9	10.1	1.4	14.5	2.9	8.7		
Tetracycline	75.3								2.9	11.6	7.2	2.9	8.7	30.4	30.4	5.8				
Florfenicol	14.5										5.8	62.3	17.4		14.5					
Chloramphenicol	39.1										20.3	37.7	2.9	21.7	17.4					
Colistin	0							73.9	14.5	11.6										
Sulfamethoxazole	60.8											26.1	10.1	2.9				1.4		59.4
Trimethoprim	42						4.3	36.2	15.9	1.4				42						
Ampicillin	69.6								8.7	20.3	1.4					2.9	66.7			
Cefotaxime	1.4			15.9	66.7	14.5	1.4				1.4									
Ceftazidime	4.3					13	66.7	15.9	2.9			1.4								

White fields denote range of dilutions tested for each substance. MICs higher than the highest concentration tested are given as the concentration closest above the range. MICs equal to or lower than the lowest concentration tested are presented underlined. The ECOFF [16] for each substance is presented as a vertical line

higher densities of animals [27], or simply that these farms were more commercially oriented and therefore pursued better animal performance and higher returns from production. We do not have information whether these antimicrobials were intended to promote growth or to prevent sickness in the animals, therefore these are only speculations. However, Thailand recently, as the first country in the region, banned the inclusion of antimicrobials as growth promotors in animal agriculture [28], which is an important step towards a more prudent use of antimicrobials.

We found a difference between the ways in which small- and medium-scale farms accessed antimicrobials, where the latter always consulted a veterinarian before treating sick animals. This difference, that must be interpreted with caution given the sample size, might however not be resulting from increased farm size, but could merely be a consequence of that the medium-scale farms

Table 4 Resistance and distributions of Minimum Inhibitory Concentrations (MIC) for *E. coli* isolates from medium-scale farms

Antimicrobial	Resistance (%)	≤0.008	0.016	0.03	0.06	0.12	0.25	0.5	1	2	4	8	16	32	64	128	256	512	1024	>1024
		Distributions (%) of MICs (mg/L)																		
Ciprofloxacin	48.1			9.9	42	4.9	4.9	23.5	6.2	8.6										
Nalidixic acid	30.8									14.8	35.8	14.8	3.7	1.2	1.2	4.9	23.5			
Gentamicin	7.4						1.2	29.6	51.9	9.9	3.7		1.2		2.5					
Streptomycin	76.5										3.7	4.9	14.8	27.2	14.8	13.6	8.6	12.3		
Tetracycline	86.3								2.5	3.7	3.7	3.7	12.3	22.2	37	14.8				
Florfenicol	2.4										7.4	38.3	51.9	1.2	1.2					
Chloramphenicol	58										9.9	21.0	11.1	45.7	12.3					
Colistin	0							75.3	19.8	4.9										
Sulfamethoxazole	84											6.2	8.6	1.2						84.0
Trimethoprim	70.4						6.2	18.5	4.9					70.4						
Ampicillin	85.2								4.9	8.6	1.2					2.5	82.7			
Cefotaxime	1.2			7.4	56.8	33.3	1.2				1.2									
Ceftazidime	3.7				1.2	1.2	66.7	27.2	2.5			1.2								

White fields denote range of dilutions tested for each substance. MICs higher than the highest concentration tested are given as the concentration closest above the range. MICs equal to or lower than the lowest concentration tested are presented underlined. The ECOFF [16] for each substance is presented as a vertical line

Table 5 Antimicrobial resistance parameters of *E. coli* isolates from pigs on the small- and medium-scale farms

Antimicrobial	Resistant isolates % (n)		*P*-value	OR (95% CI)[a]
	Small-scale (*n* = 69)	Medium-scale (*n* = 81)		
Ciprofloxacin[†]	41 (28)	48 (39)	0.54	
Nalidixic acid[†]	20 (14)	31 (25)	0.21	
Gentamicin[†]	11 (8)	7 (6)	0.39	
Streptomycin[†]	38 (26)	77 (62)	<0.001	5.4 (2.7-11)
Tetracycline	75 (52)	86 (70)	0.09	2.1 (0.9-4.8)
Florfenicol	14 (10)	2 (2)	0.01	0.1 (0.03-0.7)
Chloramphenicol	39 (27)	58 (47)	0.02	2.2 (1.1-4.1)
Colistin[†]	0 (0)	0 (0)	-	-
Sulfamethoxazole	61 (42)	84 (68)	0.002	3.4 (1.6-7.2)
Trimethoprim	42 (29)	70 (57)	<0.001	3.3 (1.7-6.4)
Ampicillin[†]	70 (48)	85 (69)	0.02	2.5 (1.1-5.6)
Cefotaxime[†]	1 (1)	1 (1)	0.9	
Ceftazidime[†]	4 (3)	4 (3)	0.8	
Multidrug-resistance[b]	74 (51)	89 (72)	0.002	3.7 (1.2-8.8)

[†]Antimicrobial classified as critically important for human medicine according to WHO [22]
[a]For the OR estimates, the small-scale farms were used as reference variable and GEE models were used to account for clustering of isolates within farms
[b]Multidrug-resistance defined as an isolate resistant against at least three different categories of the antimicrobial agents tested

were bound to the routines of the contracting companies, as this was the case for all but one of the medium-scale farms. The two contracting companies, owning about half each of the medium-scale farms in the current study, are very large companies that have operations all over the country, and one may thus assume that the regimes regarding antimicrobial treatment presented here are representative for many medium-scale farms in Thailand.

In this study the emphasis was on antimicrobial use and susceptibility in commensal *E. coli* collected from sows. Sows were sampled as antimicrobial use and resistance in *E. coli* from sows is of epidemiological importance within the herd, as the sow may serve as a reservoir of resistant bacteria and genetic determinants [29]. Whilst the recommendation by the European Food Safety Authority (EFSA) [30] is that samples should be taken from fattener pigs, the approach adopted here was to ensure sufficient number of pigs to sample at each farm, as small-scale farms might not have enough fatteners at the time of visit.

As already mentioned we found a positive association between enrofloxacin use and ciprofloxacin resistance, both being fluoroquinolones used in veterinary and human medicine, respectively. Our analyses also revealed some associations between the use of certain antimicrobials and AMR. Such associations should be interpreted with caution, especially since this study contained relatively few farms and the fact that we could not obtain reliable information from all farms regarding precise treatment regimes, e.g. duration and dosage. Thus, assessing possible associations between the treatment regime and antimicrobial resistance might fall outside the power of this study.

The data from the current study have been interpreted conservatively given the relatively small sample size. Another limitation to take into account when reading the paper is that the selection of farms might not be regarded as entirely random. The antimicrobial activity testing panel used is designed to detect resistance among *E. coli*, therefore there may be resistance in other bacterial species and to other antimicrobials not tested for in this study.

Conclusions

Considerable reservoirs of antimicrobial resistance were observed in *E. coli* from pigs on both small- and medium-scale farms in north-eastern Thailand. Higher rates of resistance, including multidrug-resistance, were observed on medium-scale farms, which could be a consequence of the greater diversity of antimicrobials used on these farms, as well as of the higher extent to which antimicrobials were administered in the feed. Although we found differences in how antimicrobials were accessed and administered between the small- and medium-scale farms, it cannot be concluded whether these differences could be responsible for the higher rate of antimicrobial resistance observed on the medium-scale farms.

Abbreviations

AMR: Antimicrobial resistance; CLSI: Clinical and laboratory standards institute; ECOFF: Epidemiological cut-off value; EFSA: European food safety authority; EUCAST: European Committee on Antimicrobial Susceptibility Testing; GEE: Generalised estimating equations; MIC: Minimum inhibitory concentration; SLU: Swedish University of Agricultural Sciences; WHO: World Health Organization

Acknowledgements
The authors would like to express their gratitude towards the farmers that participated in the study, as well as the veterinary students who assisted during the fieldwork.

Funding
Not applicable.

Authors' contributions
Study design: UM, JK, MP, LF, MH, DK. Data collection and analysis: MH, DK, JK, MP, LF, GS. Manuscript writing: GS, MH, DK, UM. Manuscript review: All authors. All authors read and approved the final manuscript.

Consent for publication
Not applicable.

Competing interests
The authors declare that they have no competing interest.

Author details
[1]Department of Clinical Sciences, Swedish University of Agricultural Sciences, Uppsala, Sweden. [2]Research Group for Preventive Technology in Livestock, Faculty of Veterinary Medicine, Khon Kaen University, Khon Kaen, Thailand. [3]National Veterinary Institute, Uppsala, Sweden. [4]Department of Biomedical Sciences and Veterinary Public Health, Swedish University of Agricultural Sciences, Uppsala, Sweden.

References
1. WHO. Antimicrobial resistance: global report on surveillance 2014. Geneva: World Health Organization; 2014.
2. Aarestrup FM. Veterinary drug usage and antimicrobial resistance in bacteria of animal origin. Basic Clin Pharmacol Toxicol. 2005;96:271–81.
3. Smith DL, Harris AD, Johnson JA, Silbergeld EK, Morris JG Jr. Animal antibiotic use has an early but important impact on the emergence of antibiotic resistance in human commensal bacteria. Proc Natl Acad Sci U S A. 2002;99:6434–9.
4. van den Bogaard AE, Stobberingh EE. Epidemiology of resistance to antibiotics. Links between animals and humans. Int J Antimicrob Agents. 2000;14:327–35.
5. Kang CI, Song JH. Antimicrobial resistance in Asia: current epidemiology and clinical implications. Infect Chemother. 2013;45:22–31.
6. Phumart P, Phodha P, Thamlikitkul P, Riewpaiboon P, Prakongsai P. Health and economic impacts of antimicrobial resistant infections in Thailand: a preliminary study. Journal of Health System Research. 2012;6:352–60.
7. Boonyasiri A, Tangkoskul T, Seenama C, Saiyarin J, Tiengrim S, Thamlikitkul V. Prevalence of antibiotic resistant bacteria in healthy adults, foods, food animals, and the environment in selected areas in Thailand. Pathog Glob Health. 2014;108:235–45.
8. EFSA (European Food Safety Authority) and ECDC (European Centre for Disease Prevention and Control). EU Summary Report on antimicrobial resistance in zoonotic and indicator bacteria from humans, animals and food in 2013. EFSA J. 2015; doi:10.2903/j.efsa.2015.4036.
9. Marshall BM, Ochieng DJ, Levy SB. Commensals: underappreciated reservoir of antibiotic resistance. Microbe. 2009;4:231–8.
10. Robinson TP, Bu DP, Carrique-Mas J, Fevre EM, Gilbert M, Grace D, Hay SI, Jiwakanon J, Kakkar M, Kariuki S, Laxminarayan R, Lubroth J, Magnusson U, Thi Ngoc P, Van Boeckel TP, Woolhouse MEJ. Antibiotic resistance: mitigation opportunities in livestock sector development. Animal. 2017;11:1–3.
11. Hughes P, Heritage J. Antibiotic Growth-Promoters in Food Animals. Assessing Quality and Safety of Animal Feeds. FAO Animal Production and Health Papers Series No 160. Rome: Food and Agriculture Organization of the United Nations; 2004. pp. 129–152.
12. Tantasuparuk W, Kunavongkrit A. Pig production in Thailand. In: Country report. 2014; 2014.
13. Thanapongtharm W, Linard C, Chinson P, Kasemsuwan S, Visser M, Gaughan AE, Epprech M, Robinson TP, Gilbert M. Spatial analysis and characteristics of pig farming in Thailand. BMC Vet Res. 2016;12:218.
14. Van Boeckel TP, Brower C, Gilbert M, Grenfell BT, Levin SA, Robinson TP, Teillant A, Laxminarayan R. Global trends in antimicrobial use in food animals. Proc Natl Acad Sci U S A. 2015;112:5649–54.
15. CLSI (Clinical and Laboratory Standards Institute. Performance standards for antimicrobial disk and dilution susceptibility tests for bacteria isolated from animals; approved standard. In: CLSI document VET01-A4. Forth ed. Wayne, Pennsylvania, USA: Clinical and Laboratory Standards Institute.
16. EUCAST (European Committee on Antimicrobial Susceptibility Testing). MIC distributions and ECOFFs. 2016. http://mic.eucast.org/Eucast2/SearchController/search.jsp?action=performSearch&BeginIndex=0&Micdif=mic&NumberIndex=50&Antib=–1&Specium=162. Accessed 28 Dec 2016.
17. Magiorakos AP, Srinivasan A, Carey RB, Carmeli Y, Falagas ME, Giske CG, Harbarth S, Hindler JF, Kahlmeter G, Olsson-Liljequist B, Paterson DL, Rice LB, Stelling J, Struelens MJ, Vatopoulos A, Weber JT, Monnet DL. Multidrug-resistans, extensively drug-resistant and pandrug-resistant bacteria: an international expert proposal for interim standard definitions for aquired resistance. Clin Microbiol Infect. 2012;18:268–81.
18. Nhung NT, Cuong NV, Thwaites G, Carrique-Mas J. Antimicrobial usage and antimicrobial resistance in animal production in Southeast Asia: a review. Antibiotics. 2016;5:37.
19. Love DC, Tharavichitkul P, Arjkumpa O, Imanishi M, Hinjoy S, Nelson K, Nachman KE. Antimicrobial use and multidrug-resistant salmonella spp., *Escherichia coli*, and Enterococcus faecalis in swine from northern Thailand. Thai J Vet Med. 2015;45:43–53.
20. Nguyen NT, Nguyen HM, Nguyen CV, Nguyen TV, Nguyen MT, Thai QH, Ho MH, Thwaites G, Ngo HT, Baker S, Carrique-Mas J. Use of Colistin and other critical antimicrobials on pig and chicken farms in southern Vietnam and its association with resistance in Commensal *Escherichia coli* bacteria. Appl Environ Microbiol. 2016;82:3727–35.
21. Nguyen VT, Carrique-Mas J, Ngo TH, Ho HM, Ha TT, Campbell JI, Nguyen TN, Hoang NN, Pham VM, Wagenaar JA, Hardon A, Thai QH, Schultsz C. Prevalence and risk factors for carriage of antimicrobial-resistant *Escherichia coli* on household and small-scale chicken farms in the Mekong Delta of Vietnam. J Antimicrob Chemother. 2015;70:2144–52.
22. WHO. Critically important antimicrobials for human medicine – 3rd revision. Geneva: World Health Organization; 2012.
23. Liu YY, Wang Y, Walsh TR, Yi LX, Zhang R, Spencer J, Doi Y, Tian G, Dong B, Huang X, Yu LF, Gu D, Ren H, Chen X, Lv L, He D, Zhou H, Liang Z, Liu JH, Shen J. Emergence of plasmid-mediated colistin resistance mechanism MCR-1 in animals and human beings in China: a microbiological and molecular biological study. Lancet Infect Dis. 2016;16:161–8.
24. Baron S, Hadjadj L, Rolain JM, Olaitan AO. Molecular mechanisms of polymixine resistance: knows and unknowns. Int J Antimicrob Agents. 2016;48:583–91.
25. Malhotra-Kumar S, Xavier BB, Das AJ, Lammens C, Hoang HTT, Pham NT, Goossens H. Colistin-resistant *Escherichia coli* harbouring mcr-1 isolated from food animals in Hanoi, Vietnam. Lancet Infect Dis. 2016;16:286–7.
26. Burow E, Simoneit C, Tenhagen BA, Kasbohrer A. Oral antimicrobials increase antimicrobial resistance in porcine *E. coli* - a systematic review. Prev Vet Med. 2014;113:364–75.
27. Maes D, Deluyker H, Verdonck M, Castryck F, Miry C, Vrijes B, de Kruif A. Herd factors associated with the seroprevalences of four major respiratory pathogens in slaughter pigs from farrow-to-finish pig herds. Vet Res. 2000;31:313–27.
28. Thamlikitkul V, Rattanaumpawan P, Boonyasiri A, Pumsuwan V, Judaeng T, Tiengrim S, Paveenkittiporn W, Rojanasthien S, Jaroenpoj S, Issaracharnvanich S. Thailand antimicrobial resistance containment and prevention program. J Glob Antimicrob Resist. 2015;3:290–4.
29. Callens B, Faes C, Maes D, Catry B, Boyen F, Francoys D, de Jong E, Haesebrouck F, Dewulf J. Presence of antimicrobial resistance and antimicrobial use in sows are risk factors for antimicrobial resistance in their offspring. Microb Drug Resist. 2015;21:50–8.
30. EFSA (European Food Safety Authority). Manual for reporting on antimicrobial resistance within the framework of directive 2003/99/EC and decision 2013/652/EU for information deriving from the year 2015. In: EFSA supporting publication 2016:EN-990; 2016. p. 35.
31. Central Ethical Review Board, Sweden, 2017. http://www.epn.se/en/start/the-organisation/ Accessed July 2 2017.

14

Genetic markers associated with resistance to beta-lactam and quinolone antimicrobials in non-typhoidal *Salmonella* isolates from humans and animals in central Ethiopia

Tadesse Eguale[1*], Josephine Birungi[2], Daniel Asrat[3], Moses N. Njahira[4], Joyce Njuguna[2], Wondwossen A. Gebreyes[5], John S. Gunn[6], Appolinaire Djikeng[2] and Ephrem Engidawork[7]

Abstract

Background: Beta-lactam and quinolone antimicrobials are commonly used for treatment of infections caused by non-typhoidal *Salmonella* (NTS) and other pathogens. Resistance to these classes of antimicrobials has increased significantly in the recent years. However, little is known on the genetic basis of resistance to these drugs in *Salmonella* isolates from Ethiopia.

Methods: *Salmonella* isolates with reduced susceptibility to beta-lactams ($n = 43$) were tested for genes encoding for beta-lactamase enzymes, and those resistant to quinolones ($n = 29$) for mutations in the quinolone resistance determining region (QRDR) as well as plasmid mediated quinolone resistance (PMQR) genes using PCR and sequencing.

Results: Beta-lactamase genes (*bla*) were detected in 34 (79.1%) of the isolates. The dominant *bla* gene was *bla*TEM, recovered from 33 (76.7%) of the isolates, majority being TEM-1 (24, 72.7%) followed by TEM-57, (10, 30.3%). The *bla*OXA-10 and *bla*CTX-M-15 were detected only in a single *S.* Concord human isolate. Double substitutions in *gyr*A (Ser83-Phe + Asp87-Gly) as well as *par*C (Thr57-Ser + Ser80-Ile) subunits of the quinolone resistance determining region (QRDR) were detected in all *S.* Kentucky isolates with high level resistance to both nalidixic acid and ciprofloxacin. Single amino acid substitutions, Ser83-Phe ($n = 4$) and Ser83-Tyr ($n = 1$) were also detected in the *gyr*A gene. An isolate of *S.* Miami susceptible to nalidixic acid but intermediately resistant to ciprofloxacin had Thr57-Ser and an additional novel mutation (Tyr83-Phe) in the *par*C gene. Plasmid mediated quinolone resistance (PMQR) genes investigated were not detected in any of the isolates. In some isolates with decreased susceptibility to ciprofloxacin and/or nalidixic acid, no mutations in QRDR or PMQR genes were detected. Over half of the quinolone resistant isolates in the current study 17 (58.6%) were also resistant to at least one of the beta-lactam antimicrobials.

Conclusion: Acquisition of *bla*TEM was the principal beta-lactamase resistance mechanism and mutations within QRDR of *gyr*A and *par*C were the primary mechanism for resistance to quinolones. Further study on extended spectrum beta-lactamase and quinolone resistance mechanisms in other gram negative pathogens is recommended.

Keywords: Non-typhoidal *Salmonella*, Antimicrobial resistance, Mechanisms of resistance, Beta-lactamase, Quinolone, Fluoroquinolone, Human strains, Animal strains, Ethiopia

* Correspondence: tadesse.eguale@aau.edu.et
[1]Aklilu Lemma Institute of Pathobiology, Addis Ababa University, P.O. Box 1176, Addis Ababa, Ethiopia
Full list of author information is available at the end of the article

Background

Salmonellosis in humans is caused by several serovars belonging to *Salmonella enterica* subspecies enterica. Infection by *Salmonella* causes two forms of diseases; typhoid fever, a febrile illness caused by a few host specific serovars such as *Salmonella enterica* subspecies enterica serovar Typhi (*S.* Typhi,) and *S.* Paratyphi A, while the majority of *Salmonella* serovars cause non-typhoidal salmonellosis characterized by self limiting gastoentritis and occasional invasive salmonellosis in immunocompromised, young and elderly patients. Infection with non-typhoidal *Salmonella* (NTS) serovars is one of the leading causes of foodborne illnesses worldwide [1]. NTS infection is commonly associated with consumption of contaminated food of animal origin such as poultry products, beef and pork as well as contact with infected animals [2–4].

Antimicrobial treatment is usually not recommended due to the self-limiting nature of the disease. However, in cases of invasive complicated salmonellosis, treatment with beta-lactam antimicrobials such as ampicillin, ceftriaxone and quinolone drugs are employed as lifesaving agents [5]. Resistance to beta-lactam antimicrobials and quinolones has increased dramatically in NTS isolates from humans as well as food animals worldwide [6–9]. The common mechanism of resistance to beta-lactam antimicrobials is due to production of beta-lactamase enzymes with variable level of activity against different generations of beta-lactam antimicrobials. In addition to the first generation beta-lactamases: *bla*TEM1, *bla*SHV1, several extended spectrum *bla*TEM and *bla*SHV variants, other extended spectrum beta-lactamase enzymes such as *bla*CTX-M, *bla*CMY, *bla*OXA and AmpC have been reported in *Salmonella* serotypes from different parts of the world [10–13].

Resistance to quinolone drugs is primarily mediated by mutations in Quinolone Resistance Determining Region (QRDR) of *gyr*A and *par*C genes in *Salmonella* and other Gram-negative organisms. Specifically, high level resistance to ciprofloxacin is frequently attributed to double mutations in the *gyr*A gene and single or double mutation in the *par*C gene [14]. In addition to chromosomal mutations, other mechanisms such as activation of efflux pumps (multidrug efflux pump and quinolone specific plasmid mediated efflux pump encoded by *qep* genes), *qnr* (plasmid-mediated quinolone resistance), porins, and quinolone-modifying enzyme (*aac(6')-Ib-cr*) have been associated with decreased susceptibility to quinolones [14]. Of particular concern is the occurrence, within the last few years in different parts of the world, of plasmid-mediated quinolone resistance encoded by several *qnr* genes. These genes encode for pentapeptide proteins that protect bacterial topoisomerases from the effect of quinolones. They do not induce high level resistance but their presence leads to mutation in the QRDR [15]. However, recent report from Senegal indicated the presence of *qnrB1* together with the quinolone modifying enzyme *aac(6')-Ib-cr* in *Salmonella* associated with high level resistance to ciprofloxacin even in the absence of mutations in the QRDR [16]. These resistance determinants have been observed in various gram negative organisms including *Salmonella* [16, 17]. In recent years, the rate of resistance to ciprofloxacin has increased considerably in both clinical and food isolates of *Salmonella* [6, 18, 19].

In Ethiopia, reports revealed resistance to beta-lactam antimicrobials and quinolones in *Salmonella* isolates from human patients and food of animal origin [20, 21]. However, little data is available on the genetic basis of the observed phenotypic drug resistance. Multidrug resistant *S.* Concord isolates obtained from children adopted from Ethiopia in different European countries and USA were reported to harbor *bla*CTX-M-15, *bla*TEM1, *bla*SHV-12 genes encoding for resistance to third generation cephalosporins, *qnrA* and *qnrB* encoding for reduced susceptibility to fluoroquinolones [22, 23]. The aim of this study was to investigate the genetic markers associated with resistance to beta-lactam and quinolone antimicrobials among NTS isolates collected from humans and animals in central Ethiopia.

Methods

Bacterial isolates

Non-typhoidal *Salmonella* strains investigated in the current study were isolated from feces of food animals (cattle $n = 50$, poultry $n = 26$, swine $n = 8$) in Addis Ababa and surrounding districts of Oromia region namely: Ada, Barake, Sebeta and Sululta. In addition, *Salmonella* isolates obtained from stool of temporally and spatially related diarrheic human patients from primary health centers and Tikur Anbessa Specialized Hospital in Addis Ababa ($n = 68$) were also included. All human and animal isolates were collected from 2013 to 2014.

Antimicrobial susceptibility testing, serotyping and phage typing

Susceptibility of each isolate to beta-lactam and quinolone antimicrobials was determined using disk diffusion method according to the guidelines of the Clinical and Laboratory Standards Institute (CLSI). The interpretation of the categories of susceptible, intermediate or resistant was also based on the CLSI guidelines [24]. For purposes of analysis, all readings classified as intermediate were considered resistant unless otherwise mentioned. *Escherichia coli* ATCC 25922 was used as a quality control. *Salmonella* isolates were serotyped and phage-typed at the Public Health Agency of Canada, World Organization for Animal Health

(OIÉ), Reference Laboratory for Salmonellosis, Guelph, Ontario, Canada as described previously [25].

Bacterial DNA extraction

Isolates were grown on Luria Bertani (LB) agar (37 °C, over night). A single colony was inoculated to 5 ml of LB broth and grown in a shaking incubator at 37 °C for 16–18 h. Genomic DNA was then extracted using the QIAGEN genomic DNA extraction kit (QIAGEN, USA) according to the manufacturer's recommendation.

Detection and characterization of beta-lactamase enzymes

A total of 43 isolates, 12 from humans and 31 from animals, with reduced susceptibility to one or more of beta-lactam antimicrobials (ampicillin, amoxicillin + clavulanic acid, cephalothin, ceftriaxone) were tested for genes encoding for beta-lactamase enzymes. PCR and DNA sequencing were performed for the detection and characterization of beta-lactamase (*bla*) genes with oligonucleotide primers previously described for *bla*TEM, *bla*SHV, *bla*PER, *bla*PSE, *bla*OXA1, *bla*OXA4, *bla*OXA10, *bla*CMY, and *bla*CTX-M genes (Table 1). The PCR conditions for all reactions involved an initial denaturation for 3 min at 95 °C followed by 30 cycles of (95 °C for 30 s, specific annealing temperature for 1 min, and extension at 72 °C for 30 s) followed by a final extension at 72 °C for 5 min. Specific annealing temperature for each PCR reaction is shown in Table 1. Group specific primers were used to characterize *bla*CTX-M enzymes [26]. The PCR amplicons were purified using QIAGEN PCR purification kit (QIAGEN, USA) and sequenced with forward and reverse primers at Sequencing, Genotyping, Oligosynthesis and Proteomics (Segolip) unit of Biosciences eastern and central Africa (BecA). All amplicon sequences were assembled and translated to

Table 1 List of primers used for detection and characterization of beta-lactamases

Gene/target	Primer	Sequence 5'-3'	Amplicon size	AT °C	Ref	Remark
BLA_{Tem} Gene	TEM-F1	ATGAGTATTCAACATTTCCG	862-bp	55	[34]	
	TEM-R1	GACAGTTACCAATGCTTAATCA				
	blaTEM-F2	TAA CCA TGAGTGATAACACT			[34]	sequencing
	blaTEM-R2	CCGATCGTT GTCAGAAGTAA				
BLA_{SHV} gene	Bla SHV-F1	CTTTACTCGCCTTTATCG	827-bp	56	[34]	
	Bla SHV-R1	TCCCGC AGATAAATCACCA				
	blaSHV-F2	ACTGCCTTTTTG CGCCAGAT			[34]	sequencing
	blaSHV-R2	CAGTTCCGTTTCCCAGCGGT				
Bla OXA-1	OXA-1-F	ATGAAAAACACAATACATATCAAC	755-bp	48	[13]	
	OXA-1-R	TTTCCTGTAAGTGCGGACAC				
Bla OXA −4	OXA-4-F	TCAACAGATATCTCTACTGGT	216 bp	54	[13]	
	OXA-4-R	TTTATCCCATTTGAATATG				
Bla OXA-10	OXa 10-F	TCAACAAATCGCCAGAGAAG	277 bp	57	[13]	
	Oxa-10-R	TCCCACACCAGAAAAACCA				
bla PER	Per1-F	AATTTGGGCTTAGGGCAGAA	925 bp	55	[50]	
	Per1-R	ATGAATGTCATTATAAAAGC				
blaPSE	blaPSE-F	TGCTTCGCAACTATGACTAC			[42]	
	blaPSE-R	AGCCTGTGTTTGAGCTAGAT				
blaCYM	blaCMY2-F	TGGCCGTTGCCGTTATCTAC	868	57	[9]	
	blaCMY2-R	CCCGTTTATGCACCCATGA				
CTX-M group I	CTXM1-F3	GACGATGTCACTGGCTGAGC	499	55	[38]	
	CTXM1-R2	AGCCGCCGACGCTAATACA				
CTX-M group II	TOHO1-2 F	GCGACCTGGTTAACTACAATCC	351	55	[38]	
	TOHO1-1R	CGGTAGTATTGCCCTTAAGCC				
CTX-M group III	CTXM825F	CGCTTT GCCATGTGCAGCACC	307	55	[38]	
	CTXM825R	GCT CAGTACGATCGAGCC				
CTX-M group IV	CTXM914F	GCTGGAGAAAAGCAGCGGAG	474	62	[38]	
	CTXM914R	GTAAGCTGACGCAACGTCTG				

amino acid sequences using CLC Main Work Bench (Inqaba Biotechnical Industries, (Pty) Ltd, Denmark) and compared with protein sequences in the Genbank database. Classification of *bla*TEM enzymes was based on beta-lactamase classification database (https://www.lahey.org/studies/temtable.asp).

Investigation of quinolone resistance mechanism

Isolates with reduced susceptibility to nalidixic acid and/or ciprofloxacin ($n = 29$), three human isolates and 26 animal isolates were examined for the presence of known quinolone resistance determinants. Quinolone resistance determining region (QRDR): *gyr*A, *gyr*B, *par*C and *par*E genes were amplified using PCR. PCR was also used to examine for various plasmid mediated quinolone resistance genes: *qnr*A, *qnr*B, *qnr*D, *qnr*S, *qep*A, and *aac(6′)-Ib-cr* as described previously (Table 2). Similar PCR conditions described previously were used and annealing temperature for each primer set is presented in Table 2. PCR ampilicons were purified using QIAGEN PCR purification kit and sequenced as previously described. Presence of mutation in the QRDR was examined by translating nucleotide sequences into proteins and aligning against reference sequence of *S.* Typhimurium strain LT2 on NCBI database (Accession Number AE006468).

Results

Resistance to beta-lactam antimicrobials and beta-lactamase genes in *Salmonella* isolates from animals and humans

Of the 20 different serotypes investigated in the current study, resistance to at least one beta-lactam antimicrobial was detected in nine serotypes and the *bla* gene was detected only in isolates belonging to six serotypes. Of the 43 isolates resistant to one or more beta-lactam antimicrobials (ampicillin, amoxicillin + clavulanic acid, cephalothin, ceftriaxone), *bla* genes were detected in 34/43 (79.1%) of the isolates. The dominant *bla* gene responsible for resistance to beta-lactam antimicrobials in the majority of *Salmonella* isolates, 33 (76.7%) was found to be variants of *bla*TEM gene. Most of these were TEM-1 type, 24 (72.7%) followed by TEM-57, 10 (30.3%). Both phenotypic resistance to beta-lactam antimicrobials and detection of *bla* genes was more common in isolates obtained from poultry compared to isolates from other sources (Table 3). In one of the human isolates of *S.* Concord, two *bla* genes (*bla*OXA-10 and *bla*CTX-M-15) were detected. Both of these genes

Table 2 List of primers used for detection of quinolone resistance mechanism

Gene	Primer name	Primer sequence (5′ to 3′)	Product size	AT in °C	References
gyrA	GyrAFP	AAATCTGCCCGTGTCGTTGGT	344 bp	58	[16]
	GyrARP	GCCATACCTACTGCGATACC			
gyrB	GyrB FP	GAATACCTGCTGGAAAACCCAT	446 bp	57	[16]
	GyrB RP	CGGATGTGCGAGCCGTCGACGTCCGC			
parC	ParC FP	AAGCCGGTACAGCGCCGCATC	395 bp	57	[16]
	ParC RP	GTGGTGCCGTTCAGCAGG			
ParE	ParE FP	TCTCTTCCGATGAAGTGCTG	240 bp	55	[12]
	ParE RP	ATACGGTATAGCGGCGGTAG			
qnrA	qnrA FP	ATTTCTCACGCCAGGATTTG	516 bp	53	[43]
	qnrA RP	GATCGGCAAAGGTTAGGTCA			
qnrB	qnrB FP	GATCGTGAAAGCCAGAAAGG	469 bp	53	[43]
	qnrB RP	ACGATGCCTGGTAGTTGTCC			
aac(6′)-Ib	aac(6′)-Ib FP	TTGCGATGCTCTATGAGTGGCTA	482-bp	55	[36]
	aac(6′)-Ib-RP	CTCGAATGCCTGGCGTGTTT			
	aac(6′)-Ib-cr-seq	CGTCACTCCATACATTGCAA (for sequencing of aac(6′)-Ib-cr			
qepA	QepA FP	CGTGTTGCTGGAGTTCTTC	403 bp	59	[7]
	QepA RP	CTGCAGGTACTGCGTCATG			
QnrD	QnrD FP	CGAGATCAATTTACGGGGAATA	565 bp	53	[8]
	QnrD RP	AACAAGCTGAAGCGCCTG			
QnrS	QnrS FP	ACGACATTCGTCAACTGCAA	417 bp	53	[43]
	QnrS RP	TAAATTGGCACCCTGTAGGC			

FP forward primer, *RP* Reverse primer

Table 3 Occurrence of *bla* genes in *Salmonella* isolates from different sources with reduced susceptibility to beta-lactam antimicrobials

Source	Total no. of isolates	[a]Resistant to ≥ one of beta-lactams (%)	*bla* genes detected[b]			Not detected	No.(%) positive for bla genes
			blaTEM	*blaOXA10*	*blaCTX-M*		
Cattle	50	16(32)	12	-	-	4	8(75)
Poultry	26	13(50)	12	-		1	12(92.3)
Swine	8	2(25)	1	-	-	1	1(50)
Human	68	12(17.7)	9	1	1	2	[c]10(83.3)
Total	152	43(28.3)	34	1	1	8	34(79.1)

[a]Ampicillin, Cephalothin, Cefoxitin, Ceftriaxone, amoxicillin and clavulanic acid
[b]Though all isolates were screened for *bla*SHV, *bla*OXA1, *bla*OXA4, *bla*PER, *bla*PSE and *bla*CMY2, none of them were positive for these genes
[c]*blaOXA10* and *blaCTX-M-15* were detected in a single isolate

encode for enzymes capable of extended spectrum beta-lactamase activity. This isolate was resistant to the third generation cephalosporin, ceftriaxone in addition to ampicillin, and cephalothin. In eight (18.6%) of the isolates, none of the tested *bla* genes were detected (Table 3).

Among the dominant serotypes, 66.7, 92.3, 50 and 100% of *S.* Typhimurium, *S.* Saintpaul, *S.* Virchow and *S.* Kentucky were positive for variants of the *bla*TEM gene, respectively. All of the 10 *S.* Kentucky isolates collected from cattle, poultry and humans were resistant to ampicillin, cephalothin and amoxicillin + clauvlanic acid and were all positive for *bla*TEM-1 gene (Table 4).

Interestingly, all 10 *bla*TEM-57 were recovered from *S.* Saintpaul isolated from poultry, while those *S.* Saintpaul strains obtained from cattle and human were all TEM-1 type. Despite a change in amino-acid sequences, there was no distinct difference in phenotypic antimicrobial susceptibility pattern to beta-lactam antimicrobials among isolates carrying *bla*TEM-57 and *bla*TEM-1 enzymes.

Among eight isolates in which none of the tested *bla* genes were detected, most of them were susceptible to the major beta-lactams and were at the margin of susceptibility and intermediate; *S.* Dublin ($n = 2$) and *S.* Typhimurium ($n = 2$) only to cephalothin and *S.* Haifa to ampicillin ($n = 1$) On the other hand, three *S.* Virchow isolates and one *S.* V:ROUGH-O;-:- were completely resistant to ampicillin and cephalothin.

Mechanism of resistance to quinolone antimicrobials

Out of the 29 *Salmonella* isolates with reduced sensitivity to quinolones, high level resistance to both nalidixic acid and ciprofloxacin was observed in only 10 *S.* Kentucky isolates (34.5%) (Table 5). All of these *S.* Kentucky isolates had double mutations in *gyr*A (Ser83-Phe + Asp87-Gly) and *par*C (Thr57-Ser + Ser80-Ile) genes. Single mutation in *gyr*A (Ser83-Phe) was observed in four isolates (*S.* Livingstone var.14+ (2), *S.* Virchow (1), *S.* I:6;7,14:-:I,w (1). All these isolates were resistant to nalidixic acid and intermediately resistant to ciprofloxacin. A single amino acid substitution in *gyr*A (Ser83-Tyr) was detected in one *S.* Haifa from poultry with an R-phenotype [resistant to nalidixic acid and intermediately resistant to ciprofloxacin]. Overall, double and single substitutions in *gyr*A were detected in 15 (51.7%) of the isolates. Double substitution in *par*C (Thr57-Ser + Tyr83-Phe) was detected in one *S.* Miami isolated from swine. This strain was sensitive to nalidixic acid and intermediately resistant to ciprofloxacin. The Tyr83-Phe is a novel mutation. A strain of *S.* Agona with only single substitution at Thr57-Ser was intermediately resistant to nalidixic acid but sensitive to ciprofloxacin. Double substitution in the *gyr*B gene (Val423-Gly + Asp459-His) was detected in two isolates; *S.* Mikawasima and *S.* Braenderup, the latter having additional substitution in *par*C gene (Thr57-Ser) associated with intermediate susceptibility to both nalidixic acid and ciprofloxacin, whereas the former with intermediate susceptibility only to naldixic acid. A strain of serotype V: rough-O;-:- that was susceptible to nalidixic acid but intermediately resistant to ciprofloxacin had single substitution of Ser463-Ala on *gyr*B gene. Over half of the quinolone resistant isolates in the current study 17 (58.6%) were also resistant to at least one of the beta-lactam antimicrobials (Table 5) and all *S.* Kentucky isolates resistant to nalidixic acid and ciprofloxacin were also shown to be MDR to several antimicrobials in our previous works [27, 28]. No mutation was detected in *par*E gene in any of the isolates examined in the current study. Nine isolates with reduced sensitivity to nalidixic acid and or ciprofloxacin had no mutation in any of the QRDR (Table 5).

Plasmid mediated quinolone resistance

None of the tested plasmid mediated quinolone resistance genes were detected in the isolates examined in the current study. Seven isolates belonging to serotypes Saintpaul, Typhimurium, Aberdeen, Virchow and Haifa were susceptible to nalidixic acid but had shown reduced sensitivity to ciprofloxacin according to CLSI (2013) cutoff points, with zone of inhibition ranging from 25 to 28 mm. There appears to be other resistance mechanisms responsible for the observed decreased sensitivity.

Table 4 Beta-lactam resistance profile among different *Salmonella* serotypes from various hosts, occurrence of betalactamses genes and *bla*-types based on amino acid sequences

Serotype	Total	Host (No.)	No. resistant to Beta-lactam(%)	Beta-lactam R-profile		*bla* positive(%)	*bla* type
				Intermediate	Resistant		
Aberdeen	1	C	-	-	-	-	-
Agona	1	C	-	-	-	-	-
Braenderup	3	C(2), H(1)	-	-	-	-	-
Concord	1	H	1(100)	Fox	AmpAmcCroCf	1(100)	OXA-10 and blaCTX-M-15
Dublin	3	C	2(66.7)	Cf	-	-	-
Enteritidis	2	H	-	-	-	-	-
Haifa	4	C(3), P(1)	1P(25)	Amp	-	-	-
Heidelberg	1	S	1(100)	Amc	AmpCf	1(100)	TEM-1
I:6;7,14:-:l,w	1	C	1(100)	-	AmpAmcCf	1(100)	TEM-1
I: Rough-O:l:1,2	1	S	-	-	-	-	-
Kentucky	10	C(6),	6(100)	-	AmpAmcCf	6(100)	TEM-1
		P(2)	2(100)	-	AmpAmcCf	2(100)	TEM-1
		H(2)	2(100)	Fox	AmpAmcCf	2(100)	TEM-1
				Amc	AmpCf		
Kottbus	8	C(1), H(7)	-	-	-	-	-
Livingstone var.14+	2	C(1), S(1)	-	-	-	-	-
Miami	5	H(3), S(2)	-	-	-	-	-
Mikawasima	2	C(2)	-	-	-	-	
Newport	2	H(2)	-	-	-	-	-
Saintpaul	33	P(20)	10(50)	AmcCf	Amp	4(100)	TEM-57
				-	AmpAmcCf	4(100)	TEM-57
				Amc	AmpCf	2(100)	TEM-57
		C(10)	2(20)	Amc	AmpCf	2(100)	TEM-1
		S(2)	-	-	-	-	-
		H(1)	1(100)	Amc	AmpCf	1	TEM-1
Typhimurium	42	C(12)	2(16.7)	-	AmpAmcCf	2(100)	TEM-1
		P(3)	-	-	-	-	-
		S(1)	1(100)				
		H(26)	6(64.5)			5(83.3)	TEM-1
				Cf	-	-	-
				Amc	AmpCf	2(100)	TEM-1
				Amp	-	1(100)	TEM-1
				-	AmpAmcCf	2(100)	TEM-1
Virchow	28	C(6)	3(50)	Amc	AmpCf	1(33.3)	TEM-1
		H(22)	1(4.6)	-	AmpAmcCf	1(100)	TEM-1
V:ROUGH-O;-;-	1	H(1)	1	-	AmpCf	-	-

C Cattle, *H* Human, *P* poultry, *S* swine, – = not detected, *Amp* ampicillin, *Amc* amoxicillin and clavulanic acid, *Cf* cephalothin, *Cro* ceftriaxone

Discussion

Detection of a high resistance rate to beta-lactam antimicrobials (50%) and the presence of *bla* genes in isolates from poultry could be due to the fact that drugs like ampicillin and amoxicillin are frequently employed in poultry farms in Ethiopia leading to selection pressure. The dominant beta-lactamase genes detected in the current study were variants of *bla*TEM with the majority being *bla*TEM-1, which is concordant with the observed spectrum of resistance to only ampicillin and

Table 5 Susceptibility of isolates to quinolone drugs and mutation in QRDR

	Serotype	Zone of inhibition mm (susceptibility category)		R-pattern betalactams[a]	Mutation in QRDR		
		Na	Cip		*gyrA*	*gyrB*	*parC*
Cattle	Aberdeen	19[S]	27[I]	-	-	-	-
Cattle	Virchow	20[S]	25[I]	-	-	-	-
Cattle	Typhimurium PT 3	21[S]	25[I]	**AmpAmcCf**	-	-	-
Cattle	Typhimurium PT 4	22[S]	27[I]	**AmpAmcCf**	-	-	-
Cattle	Haifa	21[S]	25[I]	-	-	-	-
Poultry	Saintpaul	20[S]	31[S]	*AmcCf*	-	-	-
Cattle	Saintpaul	17[I]	25[I]	**AmpAmcCCf**	-	-	-
Cattle	Saintpaul	21[S]	27[I]	-	-	-	-
Poultry	Saintpaul	20[S]	27[I]	-	-	-	-
Human	V:ROUGH-O;-:-	22[S]	28[I]	**AmpCf**	-	Ser463Ala	-
Cattle	Mikawasima	20[S]	25[I]	-	-	Val423Gly + Asp459His	-
Cattle	Agona	17[I]	31[S]	-	-	-	Thr57Ser
Cattle	Braenderup	17[I]	25[I]	-	-	Val423Gly + Asp459His	Thr57Ser
Swine	Miami	22[S]	27[I]	-	-	-	Thr57Ser + Tyr83Phe
Poultry	Haifa	0[R]	25[I]	-	Ser83Tyr	-	-
Cattle	Virchow	0[R]	26(I)	**Amp***Amc***Cf**	Ser83Phe	-	-
Cattle	Livingstone var.14+	0[R]	24(I)	-	Ser83Phe	-	-
Cattle	I:6;7,14:-:l,w	7[R]	30(I)	**AmpAmcCf**	Ser83Phe	-	-
Swine	Livingstone var.14+	0[R]	20[I]	-	Ser83Phe	-	-
Cattle	Kentucky	0[R]	14[R]	**AmpAmcCf**	Ser83Phe + Asp87Gly	-	Thr57Ser + Ser80Ile
Cattle	Kentucky	0[R]	12[R]	**AmpCf***Amc*	Ser83Phe + Asp87Gly	-	Thr57Ser + Ser80Ile
Cattle	Kentucky	0[R]	11[R]	**AmpCf***Amc*	Ser83Phe + Asp87Gly	-	Thr57Ser + Ser80Ile
Cattle	Kentucky	0[R]	9[R]	**AmpAmcCf**	Ser83Phe + Asp87Gly	-	Thr57Ser + Ser80Ile
Cattle	Kentucky	0[R]	12[R]	**AmpCf***Amc*	Ser83Phe + Asp87Gly	-	Thr57Ser + Ser80Ile
Cattle	Kentucky	0[R]	10[R]	**AmpAmcCf**	Ser83Phe + Asp87Gly	-	Thr57Ser + Ser80Ile
Human	Kentucky	0[R]	8[R]	**AmpAmcCf***Fox*	Ser83Phe + Asp87Gly	-	Thr57Ser + Ser80Ile
Human	Kentucky	0[R]	10[R]	**AmpCf***Amc*	Ser83Phe + Asp87Gly	-	Thr57Ser + Ser80Ile
Poultry	Kentucky	0[R]	9[R]	**AmpAmcCf**	Ser83Phe + Asp87Gly	-	Thr57Ser + Ser80Ile
Poultry	Kentucky	0[R]	11[R]	**AmpAmcCf**	Ser83Phe + Asp87Gly	-	Thr57Ser + Ser80Ile

PT Phagetype, *Amp* Ampicillin, *Amc* Amoxicillin and clavulanic acid, Cf Cephalothin, *Cip* Ciprofloxacin, *Na-* Nalidixic acid, *S* susceptible, *I* intermediately resistant, *R* resistant
[a]Resistance status, isolates were fully resistant to antimicrobials written in Bold and intermediately resistant to those written in italics

first generation cephalosporin in most of the isolates. In Africa, *bla*TEM-1 has been reported from *Salmonella* isolated from poultry in Egypt [29], from children adopted from Mali [30], and *S.* Enteritidies in Senegal [31].

All *S.* Saintpaul isolated from poultry in the current study carried *bla*TEM-57, while those from cattle and human carried *bla*TEM-1. This is probably due to mutation of a *bla*TEM gene in a strain of *S.* Saintpaul in one of the poultry farms and clonal spread of strain carrying this mutant gene to farms in the area. All poultry *S.* Saintpaul were isolated from farms in the Adaa district. Compared to TEM-1, TEM-57 has a substitution of Gly to Asp at position 92 of amino acid sequence, which was first reported from *Proteus mirabilis* [32] and later on from *E. coli* in China [33]. To our knowledge, this is the first report of detection of *bla*TEM-57 in *Salmonella*. Fortunately, this mutation was not associated with extended spectrum activity against second and third generation cephalosporins.

One of the human isolates, *S.* Concord, resistant to ampicillin, cephalothin, cefoxitin and ceftriaxone was shown to produce *bla*CTX-M-15 and *bla*OXA-10. Previous studies have also reported *bla*CTX-M-15 in *S.* Concord isolated from children adopted from Ethiopia to different European countries and USA [34, 35]. In fact, a separate study also showed that *bla*CTX-M-15 isolated from

S. Concord from Ethiopia was chromosomally encoded [35]. Nevertheless, the previous studies also showed production of *bla*SHV-12 in most of the *S.* Concord from Ethiopia, but OXA-10 was not reported. This is presumably due to loss of a plasmid encoding for SHV-12 and acquisition of OXA-10 in a new isolate from Ethiopia. During the last few years, CTX-M-15 and other related CTX-M enzymes have been widely reported from various *Enterobacteriaceae* including *Salmonella* in different African countries from both hospital and community settings [16, 36–39]. Oxacilinases including OXA-10 have also been commonly isolated from different enterobacteriaceae including *Salmonella* [40].

The possible reason for the absence of *bla* genes in a few isolates with reduced susceptibility in the current study despite testing for most of the known *bla* reported in *Salmonella* could be due to poor sensitivity of phenotypic resistance detection methods. In two *S.* Typhimurium and two *S.* Dublin intermediately resistant only to cephalothin and one *S.* Haifa intermediately resistant to ampicillin, the reading was at the margin of intermediate and susceptible. However, all the three *S.* Virchow were fully resistant to ampicillin and cephalothin and intermediately resistant to amoxicillin + clauvlanic acid. For these isolates, other resistance mechanisms not investigated in this study such as alterations in the beta-lactam targets (PBPs) [41], absence or down-regulation of the production of outer membrane porins [42], over expression of efflux pumps [43] and different *amp*C betalactamases [44] might be responsible for the observed reduction in susceptibility. In general, the rate of occurrence of extended spectrum beta-lactamases in *Salmonella* isolates in the current study is low. This could be due to the fact that most of the human isolates were obtained from primary health care centers and use of 2nd and 3rd generation cephalosporins is not a common practice in veterinary medicine [28, 45]. The single MDR *S.* Concord in the current study was isolated from hospitalized 1 year old child.

Amino acid substitutions at codon 83 and 87 of *gyr*A gene have been associated with high level fluoroquinolone resistance [46–49] whereas resistance to only nalidixic acid is associated with single or double mutation in *par*C gene in *Salmonella* and other Gram-negative pathogens [14, 50]. Detection of two amino acid substitutions in the *gyr*A gene at codon 83 and 87 and the *par*C gene at codon 57 and 80 in all *S.* Kentucky isolates with high level resistance to both nalidixic acid and ciprofloxacin obtained from humans and animals suggests the possibility of clonal spread of *S.* Kentucky strain in the human and animal population in the study area. Similar mutations in *gyr*A and *par*C genes were reported from *S.* Kentucky from French travelers returning from north east and eastern Africa [51]. Studies of *S.* Kentucky ST198 from different countries have also shown a similar substitution in *gyr*A at codon 83 (Ser83-Phe) for all isolates and substitution of aspartate at codon 87 with asparagine, tyrosine or glycine residues. *S.* Kentucky isolates in the current study also belonged to ST198 suggesting the clonal relatedness of our isolates to the internationally spreading clone of *S.* Kentucky (unpublished data). However, only single substitution in the *par*C gene at codon 80 (Ser80-Ile) was reported previously and none of them had substitution at codon 57 of *par*C gene [52]. Additional substitution at codon 57 of the *par*C gene in the Ethiopian isolates might have occurred separately. Contrary to these local and global spread of MDR fluoroquinolone resistant *S.* Kentucky, a previous study on *S.* Typhimurium showed that mutation based fluoroquinolone resistance is associated with fitness cost and resistant strains are less invasive [53]. This suggests that this internationally dispersed clone of *S.* Kentucky has unique mechanisms. Furthermore, we have previously shown that *S.* Kentucky strains from Ethiopia has strong biofilm forming ability which is one of the important traits for persistence of the organism in the host or the environment [54] that might have contributed to its dissemination.

Four of the *Salmonella* isolates resistant to nalidixic acid and intermediately resistant to ciprofloxacin had only a single substitution in the *gyr*A, Ser83-Phe, whereas one isolate *S.* Haifa from poultry had a Ser83-Tyr substitution. Previous studies have also shown that a single mutation in *gyr*A results only in resistance to nalidixic acid and not to ciprofloxacin [47, 53]. Although isolates with a single mutation in *par*C gene resulted only with reduced susceptibility to nalidixic acid, an *S.* Miami isolate with no mutation in *gyr*A gene but double substitution in *par*C gene: (Thr57-Ser) and a novel substitution (Tyr83-Phe) was fully susceptible to nalidixic acid and intermediately resistant to ciprofloxacin. This suggests that the novel mutation at codon 83 of *par*C gene might accentuate the activity of nalidixic acid and attenuate the activity of ciprofloxacin.

The observation of double substitution in *gyrB* gene (Val423-Gly + Asp459-His) associated with intermediate susceptibility only to nalidixic acid shows a minor contribution of mutation in *gyr*B compared to *gyr*A for development of resistance to quinolones. Interestingly, nine isolates with reduced sensitivity to ciprofloxacin and some to nalidixic acid had no mutation in QRDR. We have also not detected PMQR genes in any of the isolates. Other resistance mechanisms not tested in this study such as multidrug efflux pumps, other PMQR mechanisms recently described in *Salmonella* such as oqxAB efflux pump [19], and altered outer membrane porins might be involved [14].

Conclusion

Co-occurrence of beta-lactamases with ciprofloxacin resistant determinants in large proportion of isolates is a major threat. Occurrence of MDR *S.* Kentucky with high level fluoroquinolone resistance mediated by double mutations in *gyr*A and *par*C genes in cattle, poultry, and human in the study area suggests clonal spread of this strain and the need for strict pathogen control strategies to hamper further spread of this pathogen. As the majority of the isolates in this study were from healthy animals at the farm level and human patients from primary health care centers, the data presented here may not represent the national status. Further studies on extended spectrum beta-lactamase and fluoroquinolone resistance mechanisms in *Salmonella* and other gram negative pathogens in hospital and community settings is recommended.

Abbreviations

bla: Betalactamase gene; CLSI: Clinical and Laboratory Standards Institute; MDR: Multi-drug resistance; NTS: Non-typhoidal *Salmonella*; PMQR: Plasmid mediated quinolone resistance; QRDR: Quinolone resistance determining region

Acknowledgments

We are grateful to Dr Roger Johnson, Linda Cole, Shaun Kernaghan, Ketna Mistry, Ann Perets and Betty Wilkie of the Public Health Agency of Canada, National Microbiology Laboratory at Guelph for serotyping and phagetyping of the *Salmonella* isolates. Technical assistance of Mr. Nega Nigusie and Mr Haile Alemayehu during sample collection and laboratory isolation is highly appreciated.

Funding

This study was supported by the BecA-ILRI Hub through the Africa Biosciences Challenge Fund (ABCF) program. The ABCF Program is funded by the Australian Department for Foreign Affairs and Trade (DFAT) through the BecA-CSIRO partnership; the Syngenta Foundation for Sustainable Agriculture (SFSA); the Bill & Melinda Gates Foundation (BMGF); the UK Department for International Development (DFID) and; the Swedish International Development Cooperation Agency (Sida). It was also supported by The National Institutes of Health (NIH) Fogarty International Center (grant 043TW008650) to W.A.G./J.S.G.

Authors' contributions

TE, EE, WG, JSG and DA JB and AD, participated in conception of the study and review of the draft manuscript. TE was involved in sample collection laboratory investigation and preparation of the draft manuscript. MN and JN participated in laboratory work. All authors read and approved the final manuscript.

Competing interests

The authors declare that they have no competing interests.

Consent for publication

Not applicable.

Author details

[1]Aklilu Lemma Institute of Pathobiology, Addis Ababa University, P.O. Box 1176, Addis Ababa, Ethiopia. [2]Biosciences Eastern and Central Africa-International Livestock Research Institute (BecA-ILRI) Hub, P O Box 30709, Nairobi, Kenya. [3]Department of Microbiology, Immunology & Parasitology, School of Medicine, College of Health Sciences, Addis Ababa University, Churchill Avenue, P.O. Box 9086, Addis Ababa, Ethiopia. [4]ICIPE-African Insect Science for Food and Health, P.O. Box 30772-00100, Nairobi, Kenya. [5]Department of Veterinary Preventive Medicine, The Ohio State University, 1920 Coffey Rd., Columbus, OH 43210, USA. [6]Department of Microbial Infection and Immunity, Center for Microbial Interface Biology, The Ohio State University, Biomedical Research Tower, 460 West 12th, Columbus, OH 432101214, USA. [7]Department of Pharmacology and Clinical Pharmacy, School of Pharmacy, College of Health Sciences, Addis Ababa University, Churchill Avenue, P.O. Box 1176, Addis Ababa, Ethiopia.

References

1. Majowicz SE, Musto J, Scallan E, Angulo FJ, Kirk M, O'Brien SJ, Jones TF, Fazil A, Hoekstra RM, Studies ICoEDBoI. The global burden of nontyphoidal Salmonella gastroenteritis. Clin Infect Dis. 2010;50(6):882–9.
2. DE Knegt LV, Pires SM, Hald T. Attributing foodborne salmonellosis in humans to animal reservoirs in the European Union using a multi-country stochastic model. Epidemiol Infect. 2015;143(6):1175–86.
3. Jansen A, Frank C, Stark K. Pork and pork products as a source for human salmonellosis in Germany. Berl Munch Tierarztl Wochenschr. 2007;120(7–8):340–6.
4. Braden CR. Salmonella enterica serotype Enteritidis and eggs: a national epidemic in the United States. Clin Infect Dis. 2006;43(4):512–7.
5. Hohmann EL. Nontyphoidal salmonellosis. Clin Infect Dis. 2001;32(2):263–9.
6. Wong MH, Yan M, Chan EW, Biao K, Chen S. Emergence of clinical Salmonella enterica serovar Typhimurium isolates with concurrent resistance to ciprofloxacin, ceftriaxone, and azithromycin. Antimicrob Agents Chemother. 2014;58(7):3752–6.
7. Wadula J, von Gottberg A, Kilner D, de Jong G, Cohen C, Khoosal M, Keddy K, Crewe-Brown H. Nosocomial outbreak of extended-spectrum beta-lactamase-producing Salmonella isangi in pediatric wards. Pediatr Infect Dis J. 2006;25(9): 843–4.
8. Kruger T, Szabo D, Keddy KH, Deeley K, Marsh JW, Hujer AM, Bonomo RA, Paterson DL. Infections with nontyphoidal Salmonella species producing TEM-63 or a novel TEM enzyme, TEM-131, in South Africa. Antimicrob Agents Chemother. 2004;48(11):4263–70.
9. Olesen I, Hasman H, Aarestrup FM. Prevalence of beta-lactamases among ampicillin-resistant Escherichia coli and Salmonella isolated from food animals in Denmark. Microb Drug Resist. 2004;10(4):334–40.
10. Carattoli A. Animal reservoirs for extended spectrum beta-lactamase producers. Clin Microbiol Infect. 2008;14 Suppl 1:117–23.
11. Seiffert SN, Perreten V, Johannes S, Droz S, Bodmer T, Endimiani A. OXA-48 carbapenemase-producing Salmonella enterica serovar Kentucky isolate of sequence type 198 in a patient transferred from Libya to Switzerland. Antimicrob Agents Chemother. 2014;58(4):2446–9.
12. Li XZ, Mehrotra M, Ghimire S, Adewoye L. beta-Lactam resistance and beta-lactamases in bacteria of animal origin. Vet Microbiol. 2007;121(3–4):197–214.
13. Whichard JM, Gay K, Stevenson JE, Joyce KJ, Cooper KL, Omondi M, Medalla F, Jacoby GA, Barrett TJ. Human Salmonella and concurrent decreased susceptibility to quinolones and extended-spectrum cephalosporins. Emerg Infect Dis. 2007;13(11):1681–8.
14. Redgrave LS, Sutton SB, Webber MA, Piddock LJ. Fluoroquinolone resistance: mechanisms, impact on bacteria, and role in evolutionary success. Trends Microbiol. 2014;22(8):438–45.
15. Robicsek A, Jacoby GA, Hooper DC. The worldwide emergence of plasmid-mediated quinolone resistance. Lancet Infect Dis. 2006;6(10):629–40.
16. Harrois D, Breurec S, Seck A, Delaune A, Le Hello S, Pardos de la Gandara M, Sontag L, Perrier-Gros-Claude JD, Sire JM, Garin B, et al. Prevalence and characterization of extended-spectrum beta-lactamase-producing clinical Salmonella enterica isolates in Dakar, Senegal, from 1999 to 2009. Clin Microbiol Infect. 2014;20(2):O109–16.
17. Jacoby GA, Strahilevitz J, Hooper DC. Plasmid-mediated quinolone resistance. Microbiol Spectr. 2014; 2(2). doi: 10.1128/microbiolspec. PLAS-0006-2013.
18. Raveendran R, Wattal C, Sharma A, Oberoi JK, Prasad KJ, Datta S. High level ciprofloxacin resistance in Salmonella enterica isolated from blood. Indian J Med Microbiol. 2008;26(1):50–3.
19. Lin D, Chen K, Wai-Chi Chan E, Chen S. Increasing prevalence of ciprofloxacin-resistant food-borne Salmonella strains harboring multiple PMQR elements but not target gene mutations. Sci Rep. 2015;5:14754.
20. Beyene G, Nair S, Asrat D, Mengistu Y, Engers H, Wain J. Multidrug resistant Salmonella Concord is a major cause of salmonellosis in children in Ethiopia. J Infect Dev Ctries. 2011;5(1):23–33.
21. Zewdu E, Cornelius P. Antimicrobial resistance pattern of Salmonella serotypes isolated from food items and personnel in Addis Ababa, Ethiopia. Trop Anim Health Prod. 2009;41(2):241–9.
22. Kalender H, Sen S, Hasman H, Hendriksen RS, Aarestrup FM. Antimicrobial susceptibilities, phage types, and molecular characterization of Salmonella

enterica serovar Enteritidis from chickens and chicken meat in Turkey. Foodborne Pathog Dis. 2009;6(3):265–71.
23. Hendriksen RS, Mikoleit M, Kornschober C, Rickert RL, Duyne SV, Kjelso C, Hasman H, Cormican M, Mevius D, Threlfall J, et al. Emergence of multidrug-resistant salmonella concord infections in Europe and the United States in children adopted from Ethiopia, 2003–2007. Pediatr Infect Dis J. 2009;28(9):814–8.
24. CLSI. Performance Standards for Antimicrobial Susceptibility Testing; Twenty-Third Informational SupplementM100-S23. In., vol. 33; 2013.
25. Grimont P, Weill F-X. Antigenic formulas of Salmonella Serotypes. 9th ed. WHO Collaborating Centre for Reference and Research on Salmonella: France; 2007.
26. Pitout JD, Hossain A, Hanson ND. Phenotypic and molecular detection of CTX-M-beta-lactamases produced by Escherichia coli and Klebsiella spp. J Clin Microbiol. 2004;42(12):5715–21.
27. Eguale T, Gebreyes WA, Asrat D, Alemayehu H, Gunn JS, Engidawork E. Non-typhoidal Salmonella serotypes, antimicrobial resistance and co-infection with parasites among patients with diarrhea and other gastrointestinal complaints in Addis Ababa, Ethiopia. BMC Infect Dis. 2015;15:497.
28. Eguale T, Engidawork E, Gebreyes AW, Asrat D, Alemayehu H, Medhin G, Johnson RP, Gunn JS. Fecal prevalence, serotype distribution and antimicrobial resistance of Salmonellae in dairy cattle in central Ethiopia. BMC Microbiol. 2016;16(1):1–11.
29. Ahmed AM, Shimamoto T. Genetic analysis of multiple antimicrobial resistance in Salmonella isolated from diseased broilers in Egypt. Microbiol Immunol. 2012;56(4):254–61.
30. Boisrame-Gastrin S, Tande D, Munck MR, Gouriou S, Nordmann P, Naas T. Salmonella carriage in adopted children from Mali: 2001–08. J Antimicrob Chemother. 2011;66(10):2271–6.
31. Sow AG, Wane AA, Diallo MH, Boye CS, Aidara-Kane A. Genotypic characterization of antibiotic-resistant Salmonella enteritidis isolates in Dakar, Senegal. J Infect Dev Ctries. 2007;1(3):284–8.
32. Bonnet R, De Champs C, Sirot D, Chanal C, Labia R, Sirot J. Diversity of TEM mutants in Proteus mirabilis. Antimicrob Agents Chemother. 1999;43(11):2671–7.
33. Yuan L, Liu JH, Hu GZ, Pan YS, Liu ZM, Mo J, Wei YJ. Molecular characterization of extended-spectrum beta-lactamase-producing Escherichia coli isolates from chickens in Henan Province, China. J Med Microbiol. 2009;58(Pt 11):1449–53.
34. Hendriksen RS, Kjelso C, Torpdahl M, Ethelberg S, Molbak K, Aarestrup FM. Upsurge of infections caused by Salmonella Concord among Ethiopian adoptees in Denmark, 2009. Euro Surveill. 2010;15(23). Available online: http://www.eurosurveillance.org/ViewArticle.aspx?ArticleId=19587.
35. Fabre L, Delaune A, Espie E, Nygard K, Pardos M, Polomack L, Guesnier F, Galimand M, Lassen J, Weill FX. Chromosomal integration of the extended-spectrum beta-lactamase gene blaCTX-M-15 in Salmonella enterica serotype Concord isolates from internationally adopted children. Antimicrob Agents Chemother. 2009;53(5):1808–16.
36. Fam N, Leflon-Guibout V, Fouad S, Aboul-Fadl L, Marcon E, Desouky D, El-Defrawy I, Abou-Aitta A, Klena J, Nicolas-Chanoine MH. CTX-M-15-producing Escherichia coli clinical isolates in Cairo (Egypt), including isolates of clonal complex ST10 and clones ST131, ST73, and ST405 in both community and hospital settings. Microb Drug Resist. 2011;17(1):67–73.
37. Rafai C, Frank T, Manirakiza A, Gaudeuille A, Mbecko JR, Nghario L, Serdouma E, Tekpa B, Garin B, Breurec S. Dissemination of IncF-type plasmids in multiresistant CTX-M-15-producing Enterobacteriaceae isolates from surgical-site infections in Bangui, Central African Republic. BMC Microbiol. 2015;15:15.
38. Kiiru J, Kariuki S, Goddeeris BM, Butaye P. Analysis of beta-lactamase phenotypes and carriage of selected beta-lactamase genes among Escherichia coli strains obtained from Kenyan patients during an 18-year period. BMC Microbiol. 2012;12:155.
39. Usha G, Chunderika M, Prashini M, Willem SA, Yusuf ES. Characterization of extended-spectrum beta-lactamases in Salmonella spp. at a tertiary hospital in Durban, South Africa. Diagn Microbiol Infect Dis. 2008;62(1):86–91.
40. Hendriksen RS, Joensen KG, Lukwesa-Musyani C, Kalondaa A, Leekitcharoenphon P, Nakazwe R, Aarestrup FM, Hasman H, Mwansa JC. Extremely drug-resistant Salmonella enterica serovar Senftenberg infections in patients in Zambia. J Clin Microbiol. 2013;51(1):284–6.
41. Sun S, Selmer M, Andersson DI. Resistance to beta-lactam antibiotics conferred by point mutations in penicillin-binding proteins PBP3, PBP4 and PBP6 in Salmonella enterica. PLoS One. 2014;9(5), e97202.
42. Delcour AH. Outer membrane permeability and antibiotic resistance. Biochim Biophys Acta. 2009;1794(5):808–16.
43. Piddock LJ. Multidrug-resistance efflux pumps - not just for resistance. Nat Rev Microbiol. 2006;4(8):629–36.
44. Jacoby GA. AmpC beta-lactamases. Clin Microbiol Rev. 2009;22(1):161–82. Table of Contents.
45. Beyene T, Endalamaw D, Tolossa Y, Feyisa A. Evaluation of rational use of veterinary drugs especially antimicrobials and anthelmintics in Bishoftu, Central Ethiopia. BMC Res Notes. 2015;8:482.
46. Baucheron S, Chaslus-Dancla E, Cloeckaert A, Chiu CH, Butaye P. High-level resistance to fluoroquinolones linked to mutations in gyrA, parC, and parE in Salmonella enterica serovar Schwarzengrund isolates from humans in Taiwan. Antimicrob Agents Chemother. 2005;49(2):862–3.
47. Zurfluh K, Abgottspon H, Hachler H, Nuesch-Inderbinen M, Stephan R. Quinolone resistance mechanisms among extended-spectrum beta-lactamase (ESBL) producing Escherichia coli isolated from rivers and lakes in Switzerland. PLoS One. 2014;9(4), e95864.
48. Eaves DJ, Randall L, Gray DT, Buckley A, Woodward MJ, White AP, Piddock LJ. Prevalence of mutations within the quinolone resistance-determining region of gyrA, gyrB, parC, and parE and association with antibiotic resistance in quinolone-resistant Salmonella enterica. Antimicrob Agents Chemother. 2004; 48(10):4012–5.
49. Lin CC, Chen TH, Wang YC, Chang CC, Hsuan SL, Chang YC, Yeh KS. Analysis of ciprofloxacin-resistant Salmonella strains from swine, chicken, and their carcasses in Taiwan and detection of parC resistance mutations by a mismatch amplification mutation assay PCR. J Food Prot. 2009;72(1):14–20.
50. Hsueh PR, Teng LJ, Tseng SP, Chang CF, Wan JH, Yan JJ, Lee CM, Chuang YC, Huang WK, Yang D, et al. Ciprofloxacin-resistant Salmonella enterica Typhimurium and Choleraesuis from pigs to humans, Taiwan. Emerg Infect Dis. 2004;10(1):60–8.
51. Weill FX, Bertrand S, Guesnier F, Baucheron S, Cloeckaert A, Grimont PA. Ciprofloxacin-resistant Salmonella Kentucky in travelers. Emerg Infect Dis. 2006;12(10):1611–2.
52. Le Hello S, Hendriksen RS, Doublet B, Fisher I, Nielsen EM, Whichard JM, Bouchrif B, Fashae K, Granier SA, Jourdan-Da Silva N, et al. International spread of an epidemic population of Salmonella enterica serotype Kentucky ST198 resistant to ciprofloxacin. J Infect Dis. 2011;204(5):675–84.
53. Fabrega A, du Merle L, Le Bouguenec C, Jimenez de Anta MT, Vila J. Repression of invasion genes and decreased invasion in a high-level fluoroquinolone-resistant Salmonella typhimurium mutant. PLoS One. 2009; 4(11), e8029.
54. Eguale T, Marshall J, Molla B, Bhatiya A, Gebreyes WA, Engidawork E, Asrat D, Gunn JS. Association of multicellular behaviour and drug resistance in Salmonella enterica serovars isolated from animals and humans in Ethiopia. J Appl Microbiol. 2014;117(4):961–71.

15

Retrospective report of antimicrobial susceptibility observed in bacterial pathogens isolated from ocular samples at Mount Sinai Hospital, 2010 to 2015

Marko Oydanich[1*], Tanis C. Dingle[2], Camille L. Hamula[2], Claudia Ghisa[1] and Penny Asbell[1]

Abstract

Background: Antimicrobial resistance has emerged as a major threat to global public health. Thus, the surveillance of changes in antimicrobial resistance in local and global settings is a paramount necessity. While many studies have tracked antimicrobial resistance, only a small percentage surveyed ocular isolates. The purpose of this study was to report the in vitro susceptibility of bacterial pathogens isolated from ocular samples in New York, NY from 2010 to 2015.

Methods: A retrospective review of ocular isolates was conducted. All organisms were collected by 25 separate inpatient wards and outpatient clinics, and were analyzed by the clinical microbiology laboratory at Mount Sinai Hospital. Clinical Laboratory and Standards Institute (CLSI) guidelines were followed for susceptibility testing and breakpoint interpretations.

Results: A total of 549 bacterial organisms were isolated from 1664 cultures (33%) during the 6-year study period. Of these, 358 isolates (65.2%) underwent susceptibility testing. 182 (50.8%) isolates were Gram-positive. The most common Gram-positive bacterium was *Staphylococcus aureus* (62.1%). Methicillin-resistance decreased in *S. aureus* isolates (31.3% in 2010, 14.1% in 2015) but was without significant change ($p = 0.25$). When analyzing all *S. aureus* isolates recovered during the study period, there were significantly more methicillin-resistant *S. aureus* (MRSA) isolates resistant to fluoroquinolones ($p < 0.0001$), erythromycin ($p < 0.0001$), and trimethoprim/sulfamethoxazole (TMP/SMZ; $p < 0.05$). Overall, *Streptococcus pneumoniae* isolates showed reduced susceptibility to erythromycin, but were otherwise susceptible to the other antimicrobials tested. *Haemophilus influenzae* (26.1%) and *Pseudomonas aeruginosa* (23.9%) were the most common Gram-negative bacteria isolated. Resistance to ampicillin and TMP/SMZ was observed in several of the *H. influenzae* isolates. *P. aeruginosa* isolates did not show high resistance overall, however, it was noted that isolates resistant to meropenem were also resistant to other antimicrobials ($p < 0.01$).

Conclusion: Overall, antimicrobial resistance was infrequent for the Gram-negative and Gram-positive bacteria analyzed. While the MRSA isolates demonstrated increased resistance to multiple antimicrobial classes, this is expected for this pathogen. Due to the continued use of broad-spectrum oral and systemic antimicrobials to treat ocular infections, findings of this study and other surveillance studies specific to ocular isolates should be used as resources in effective decision making in the treatment of ocular disease.

Keywords: Antimicrobial, Multi-drug resistance, Ocular isolates, Susceptibility, New York

* Correspondence: marko.oydanich@mssm.edu
[1]Department of Ophthalmology, Icahn School of Medicine at Mount Sinai, New York, NY, USA
Full list of author information is available at the end of the article

Background

Antimicrobial resistance is an issue that has been impacting medicine for many years. Whether in primary care or specialized care settings, antimicrobial resistance has been on the rise and has affected the way healthcare providers treat bacterial infections. Particularly in ophthalmic settings, physicians tend to treat ocular infections by prescribing empiric antibiotics because they often do not have data from culture analysis. As a result, there is a lack of awareness of fluctuating trends in antimicrobial resistance of many common pathogens [1–4]. This is an important concern, especially due to the fact that many ocular pathogens, if shown to possess multi-drug resistance (MDR), i.e. non-susceptibility to at least one agent in three or more antimicrobial classes [5], can be difficult to treat, which increases the chances of severe ocular damage and vision loss [3, 6, 7].

Generally, broad-spectrum antibiotics are used to treat many ocular infections, including microbial keratitis, conjunctivitis, and endophthalmitis; however, the pathogenic organisms that cause these conditions have shown increased resistance to antibiotics over the past decade. For example, *Staphylococcus* species and *Pseudomonas aeruginosa* have demonstrated resistance to fluoroquinolones, macrolides, and β-lactams [2, 3, 6, 8]. *Haemophilus influenzae*, a common Gram-negative bacterium, has also shown increased resistance to trimethoprim [9–12].

There have been a few nationwide surveillance studies, such as Ocular TRUST and ARMOR, which have tracked resistance patterns in many common ocular pathogens [9, 13]. However, given the growing importance of this issue, there is also a need for smaller, regional studies to obtain local data. Many such single-center studies have been surveying and tracking antimicrobial resistance in order to establish effective treatment methods against ocular infections on a local level [6, 14–19]. The goal of this retrospective study was to determine resistance patterns in ocular pathogens isolated and analyzed by the Mount Sinai Hospital clinical microbiology laboratory in New York, NY and contribute our findings to the growing knowledge base regarding antimicrobial resistance of ocular pathogens. In turn, these findings can also help influence intelligent and effective antibiotic use in the New York City metropolitan area, with the potential to help develop informed treatment protocols against common ocular pathogens.

Methods

A retrospective, consecutive data review study was conducted. The study was approved by the institutional review board of Mount Sinai Hospital and the tenets of the Declaration of Helsinki were followed.

Collection of ocular isolates

A total of 1664 ocular cultures were performed from over 25 separate inpatient wards and outpatient clinics over a 6-year period (January 2010 to December 2015). The clinical microbiology laboratory at Mount Sinai Hospital performed all cultures and antimicrobial susceptibility testing for these facilities. For the purposes of this review, only specimens that tested positive for a bacterial organism were included in the study. Fungal isolates were not analyzed.

Eye culture workup and organism identification

Eye culture specimens (swabs of various ocular anatomic sites, corneal scrapings, and vitreous/aqueous fluids) were either directly plated to agar at the time of collection or sent to the clinical microbiology laboratory for plating. The routine culture media used for eye cultures included blood agar, chocolate agar, and CDC anaerobe 5% sheep blood agar. Providers collecting specimens at the bedside would also frequently add a thioglycollate broth during collection. All media was incubated aerobically in a 5% CO_2 environment or under anaerobic conditions at 35–37 °C per laboratory standard operating protocols. Positive cultures were determined by the laboratory's standard operating protocol. For specimens that were directly plated (isolated from corneal scrapings or vitreous fluids), the organism had to be localized to the area of the plate where the specimen was planted. For those specimens collected with a swab, the organism had to be localized in the first quadrant (first streak area) of the plate. If growth was observed in the 2nd, 3rd, or 4th area, consultation with the microbiology director typically resulted in the organism being labeled as a contaminant.

Significant ocular pathogens were primarily identified using routine biochemical testing and the VITEK-2 instrument (bioMérieux, Inc., Durham, NC). If the VITEK-2 result failed, alternate identification systems used by the laboratory included API strips (bioMérieux, Inc., Durham, NC) and the rapID identification system (Remel, Lenexa, KS).

Susceptibility testing

All susceptibility testing was performed in the Mount Sinai Hospital clinical microbiology laboratory. A total of 358 isolates underwent susceptibility testing from a total of 549 isolated bacterial isolates. Only significant ocular pathogens as defined by the laboratory standard operating protocol underwent susceptibility testing. Organisms identified that were believed to be contaminants or normal flora (i.e. Coagulase-negative *Staphylococcus* and *Corynebacterium* species) were excluded from analysis since susceptibility testing was not performed. This included 152 coagulase-negative *Staphylococcus* (CoNS) isolates that were collected during the 6-year period. Providers always had the opportunity to call the laboratory and request susceptibility testing on these isolates if they deemed them significant. The panel of antimicrobials tested was determined by the microbiology director and antimicrobial stewardship based on the institution's antibiotic formulary. The primary susceptibility testing method used in the laboratory during the study was VITEK-2 (bioMérieux, Inc., Durham, NC), which was performed per manufacturer's recommendations. *Streptococcus* species, infrequently isolated, and fastidious organisms were tested by E-test (bioMérieux Inc., Durham, NC) per manufacturer's recommendations. Interpretations (susceptible, intermediate, susceptible dose-dependent, or resistant) were determined using Clinical Laboratories and Standards Institute (CLSI) guidelines (M100 [20] or M45 [21] documents) relevant to the year the organism was tested.

Data organization & inclusion procedures

All data was collected from the Laboratory Information System used by the Mount Sinai Hospital clinical microbiology laboratory. The data was imported into a Microsoft Excel spreadsheet file and all important patient identifiers were properly and securely discarded in accordance with IRB guidelines. The data imported included date of collection, age of patient, ward, collection site, organism isolated and MIC values against a variety of antibiotics. Only isolates that underwent susceptibility testing were included in this study. Susceptibility profiles are shown for microbial species that were tested at least 30 times during the study period with the exception of MRSA ($n = 28$), though not all antimicrobials were tested against each isolate. MIC_{50} and MIC_{90} values were also calculated.

Statistical analysis

Statistical analysis was conducted using the program Prism (software version 7.0a; GraphPad software). A Fisher's exact test was used to study the prevalence of methicillin-resistance amongst all *Staphylococcus aureus* isolates during the study period as well as to compare differences in resistance between methicillin-resistant *Staphylococcus aureus* (MRSA) and methicillin-susceptible *Staphylococcus aureus* (MSSA) isolates. Comparisons amongst *S. aureus* and age of infection were conducted using a Chi-Squared test. Statistical significance was defined as $p < 0.05$.

Results

Of a total of 1664 cultures performed during the study period, 549 bacterial organisms were isolated. Of these, 358 ocular pathogens (65.2%) underwent susceptibility testing, which included 113 *S. aureus*, 30 *S. pneumoniae*, 42 *P. aeruginosa*, & 46 *H. influenzae* isolates (Table 1). Of the 358 isolates, 41 (11.5%), 30 (8.4%), 11 (3.1%), 17 (4.7%), and 3 (0.8%) samples were isolated from the conjunctiva, cornea, eyelid, contact lens, and vitreous fluid respectively. The remaining 256 (71.5%) samples were collected from unspecified ocular sites. Gram-positive bacteria accounted for 50.8% of the total isolates. *S. aureus* was the most common Gram-positive bacterium [113 of 182 (62.1%)] while *H. influenzae* was the most common Gram-negative bacterium [46 of 176 (26.1%)]. Comparison by patient age, in years, (Table 2) shows that the amount of Gram-positive organisms (*S. aureus*, coagulase-negative *Staphylococcus* (CoNS), and *S. pneumoniae* isolates) was higher in the elderly group (>65 years) than in any other group and increased in an age-dependent manner. MRSA infections were statistically more likely to occur in the two oldest age groups, i.e. >40 years, when compared to the younger age groups ($p < 0.05$). Gram-negative organisms, with the exception of *H. influenzae*, were more prevalent in the middle-aged groups, i.e. 18–64 years. Interestingly, *H. influenzae* isolates were more prevalent in the youngest and oldest age groups, presenting a bimodal distribution.

Staphylococcus aureus

MRSA

Over the 6-year period that was evaluated, the prevalence of methicillin-resistant *S. aureus* showed a decreasing yet statistically insignificant trend (Fig. 1), with 31.30% resistance in 2010 compared to 14.30% resistance in isolates collected in 2015 ($p = .25$).

A total of 28 cultures tested positive for methicillin-resistant *S. aureus* (Table 3a). MRSA isolates exhibited high resistance against erythromycin (89.29%), clindamycin (35.7%), levofloxacin (50%), and ciprofloxacin (80%) and high susceptibility to the remainder of the antimicrobials tested. No MRSA isolates showed resistance to vancomycin, daptomycin or linezolid.

MSSA

A total of 85 cultures tested positive for methicillin-susceptible *S. aureus* (Table 3a). MSSA isolates exhibited high susceptibility to the majority of antimicrobials tested with the exception of clindamycin (34.12%) and erythromycin (44.05%). No isolates were found to be resistant to vancomycin, daptomycin, gentamicin, or linezolid. Unlike MRSA, MSSA isolates were highly susceptible to levofloxacin and ciprofloxacin.

Resistance in MRSA and MSSA was also compared (Fig. 2). As expected, the resistance observed against ciprofloxacin ($p < 0.0001$), erythromycin ($p < 0.0001$), levofloxacin ($p < 0.0001$), and TMP/SMZ ($p < 0.05$) was significantly higher for the MRSA isolates compared to the MSSA isolates. This increased resistance is also seen in the MIC_{50}/MIC_{90} values, in which MRSA had equal or higher MIC_{50}/MIC_{90} values than MSSA in response to ciprofloxacin, erythromycin, levofloxacin, and TMP/SMZ.

Table 1 Ocular Isolates Collected & Analyzed at Mount Sinai Hospital (2010–2015)

Gram-Positive Organisms	No.	%Gram-Positive	%Total	Gram-Negative Organisms	No.	%Gram-Negative	%Total
Staphylococcus aureus				**Non-Fermenting Gram-Negative Bacilli**			
MSSA	85	46.70%	23.74%	***Pseudomonas aeruginosa***	42	23.86%	11.73%
MRSA	28	15.38%	7.82%	*Stenotrophomonas maltophilia*	7	3.98%	1.96%
CoNS				*Achromobacter xylosoxidans*	6	3.41%	1.68%
Staphylococcus epidermidis	13	7.14%	3.63%	*Moraxella catarrhalis*	4	2.27%	1.12%
Staphylococcus haemolyticus	2	1.10%	0.56%	*Acinetobacter baumannii*	3	1.70%	0.84%
Staphylococcus warneri	2	1.10%	0.56%	*Pseudomonas luteola*	1	0.57%	0.28%
Staphylococcus capitis	1	0.55%	0.28%	*Pseudomonas putida*	1	0.57%	0.28%
Unspecified CoNS	2	1.10%	0.56%	*Pseudomonas (Flavimonas) oryzihabitans*	1	0.57%	0.28%
Other				*Unspecified Acinetobacter spp.*	1	0.57%	0.28%
Streptococcus pneumoniae	30	16.48%	8.38%	*Moraxella lacunata*	1	0.57%	0.28%
Corynebacterium pseudodiphthericum	3	1.65%	0.84%	*Unspecified Moraxella spp.*	1	0.57%	0.28%
Streptococcus pyogenes (Group A)	2	1.10%	0.56%	*Achromobacter (Alcaligenes) denitrificans*	1	0.57%	0.28%
Streptococcus intermedius	2	1.10%	0.56%	*Chryseobacterium indologenes*	1	0.57%	0.28%
Unspecified Corynebacterium spp.	2	1.10%	0.56%	*Elizabethkingia meningoseptica*	1	0.57%	0.28%
Bacillus cereus	2	1.10%	0.56%	**Enterobacteriaceae**			
Streptococcus anginosus	1	0.55%	0.28%	*Serratia marcescens*	18	10.23%	5.03%
Streptococcus mitis	1	0.55%	0.28%	*Escherichia coli*	10	5.68%	2.79%
Enterococcus faecium	1	0.55%	0.28%	*Klebsiella oxytoca*	7	3.98%	1.96%
Enterococcus faecalis	1	0.55%	0.28%	*Klebsiella pneumoniae*	5	2.84%	1.40%
Corynebacterium (CDC Group G)	1	0.55%	0.28%	*Enterobacter cloacae*	2	1.14%	0.56%
Gemella morbillorum	1	0.55%	0.28%	*Citrobacter koseri*	2	1.14%	0.56%
Unspecified Bacillus spp.	1	0.55%	0.28%	*Pantoea agglomerans*	2	1.14%	0.56%
Aerococcus viridans	1	0.55%	0.28%	*Raoultella ornithinolytica*	1	0.57%	0.28%
				Citrobacter freundii	1	0.57%	0.28%
				Providencia rettgeri	1	0.57%	0.28%
				Morganella morganii	1	0.57%	0.28%
				Proteus mirabilis	1	0.57%	0.28%
				Other			
				Haemophilus influenzae	46	26.14%	12.85%
				Haemophilus parainfluenzae	2	1.14%	0.56%
				Aggregatibacter aphrophilus	2	1.14%	0.56%
				Eikenella corrodens	2	1.14%	0.56%
				Neisseria meningitidis	1	0.57%	0.28%
				Pasteurella multocida	1	0.57%	0.28%

Bolded organisms are commonly observed bacterial pathogens
Bolded and underlined terms represent important classes of microorganisms
Abbreviation: MSSA methicillin-susceptible *S. aureus*, *MRSA* methicillin-resistant *S. aureus*, *CoNS* coagulase-negative *Staphylococcus*, *spp.* species

Streptococcus pneumoniae

A total of 30 cultures tested positive for *S. pneumoniae* (Table 3b). Overall, *S. pneumoniae* isolates exhibited relatively low resistance to all of the antimicrobials tested against them. This is further supported by the low MIC_{50} and MIC_{90} values for these antimicrobials. Only erythromycin showed moderate resistance, in which five of the isolates (16.67%) were resistant, as well as a large MIC range from .016 to 32 ug/ml. Vancomycin, clindamycin, and levofloxacin remained effective against *S. pneumoniae*, with each antimicrobial generating over 93% susceptibility.

Pseudomonas aeruginosa

A total of 42 cultures tested positive for *P. aeruginosa* (Table 4a). The majority of antimicrobials were greater

Table 2 Frequency of ocular pathogens by age group

Microorganism	Age Distribution (years)				
	≤2	3–17	18–39	40–64	≥65
	N (%)	*N* (%)	*N* (%)	*N* (%)	*N* (%)
MSSA	14 (16.5%)	8 (9.4%)	15 (18.8%)	18 (21.2%)	30 (35.3%)
MRSA	2 (7.1%)	2 (7.1%)	2 (7.1%)	11 (39.3%)	11 (39.3%)
CoNS	2 (10.0%)	1 (5.0%)	1 (5.0%)	6 (30.0%)	10 (50.0%)
Streptococcus pneumoniae	5 (16.7%)	2 (6.7%)	2 (6.7%)	12 (40.0%)	9 (30.0%)
Pseudomonas aeruginosa	1 (2.4%)	3 (7.1%)	12 (28.6%)	17 (40.5%)	9 (21.4%)
Haemophilus influenzae	14 (30.4%)	5 (10.9%)	3 (6.5%)	12 (26.1%)	12 (26.1%)
Klebsiella spp.	4 (33.3%)	0 (0%)	3 (25%)	2 (16.7%)	3 (25%)
Serratia marcescens	1 (5.6%)	1 (5.6%)	8 (44.4%)	6 (33.3%)	2 (11.1%)

Abbreviations: MSSA = methicillin-susceptible *Staphylococcus aureus, MRSA* = methicillin-resistant *Staphylococcus aureus, CoNS* = coagulase-negative *Staphylococcus, spp* = species

than 90% effective against *P. aeruginosa* with the exception of both meropenem and piperacillin/tazobactam (11.91 and 12.20% resistance respectively). The five isolates that were resistant to meropenem were more likely to be resistant to other classes of antimicrobials ($p = 0.008$), including aminoglycosides and fluoroquinolones.

Haemophilus influenzae

A total of 46 cultures tested positive for *H. influenzae* (Table 4b). The vast majority of isolates were susceptible to most of the antimicrobials tested with the exception of TMP/SMZ and ampicillin, both of which showed high MIC_{90} values. All isolates were tested against TMP/SMZ, with 17 (37%) isolates showing resistance. Of the 33 isolates tested against ampicillin, 10 (30.30%) were resistant.

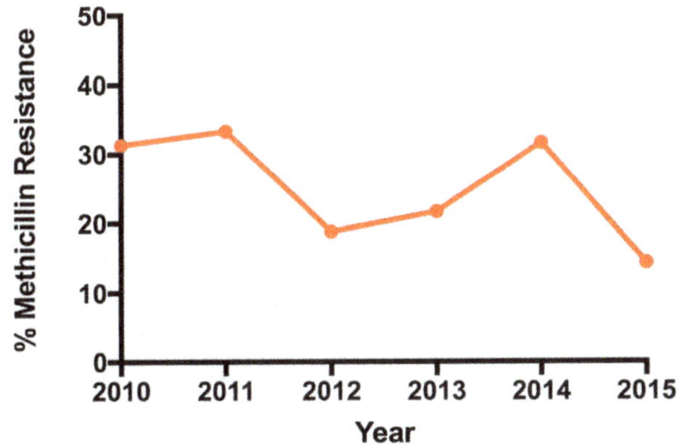

Fig. 1 Prevalence of MRSA from 2010–2015. An overall decreasing trend in MRSA prevalence is observed from 2010–2015. However, the trend is not statistically significant ($p = 0.25$).

Discussion

In this retrospective review, 358 microorganisms were analyzed by a single-center institution over a 6-year study period. A wide variety of Gram-positive and Gram-negative organisms were collected including CoNS, *S. marcescens, K. oxytoca,* and *E. coli,* as well as more common bacterial pathogens such as *S. aureus, S. pneumoniae, H. influenzae,* and *P. aeruginosa.* In this study the number of Gram-negative organisms (49.2%) was nearly equal to the number of Gram-positive organisms (50.8%). While other single-center studies have found a much higher proportion of Gram-positive organisms in collected samples [1, 7, 18, 22–24], this study exhibited a nearly equivalent Gram-positive to Gram-negative ratio. This difference is likely due to the clinical microbiology laboratory protocols that did not require susceptibility testing of CoNS until mid-2015 from eye sources due to the likelihood of these isolates being contaminants. Specifically, there were an additional 152 CoNS isolates, the majority isolated from conjunctival swabs, which did not undergo susceptibility testing. If these isolates had undergone susceptibility testing, the distribution between Gram-positive and Gram-negative bacteria would change considerably (65.5 and 34.5% respectively) and be more in line with previously published studies.

This study also showed an uneven distribution of ocular isolates among age groups. Gram-positive organisms were most common in the elderly, while Gram-negative organisms, except *H. influenzae,* were most common in the middle age ranges. *H. influenzae* isolates had a bimodal distribution, being more common in the youngest and oldest age groups. Additionally MRSA was statistically more likely ($p < 0.05$) to be found in the two oldest age groups (40–64 years and >65 years) when compared to the younger age groups suggesting a higher possibility of MRSA infection with increasing

Table 3 Susceptibility profiles for selected Gram-positive species, *S. aureus* (a) and *S. pneumoniae* (b)

3a: Susceptibility Profile for 113 S. *aureus* isolates

Antimicrobial		MIC (ug/mL)			Interpretation N (%)		
	Organism	Range	MIC_{50}	MIC_{90}	Susceptible	Intermediate	Resistant
Clindamycin	MRSA	0.25 – ≥8	0.25	≥8	18 (64.3)	0 (0)	10 (35.7)
	MSSA	≤0.12 – ≥8	0.25	<0.5	56 (65.9)	0 (0)	29 (34.1)
Ciprofloxacin*	MRSA	≤0.5 – ≥8	≥8	≥8	5 (20)	0 (0)	20 (80)
	MSSA	≤0.5 – ≥8	≤0.5	≤0.5	74 (91.4)	1 (1.2)	6 (7.4)
Daptomycin	MRSA	0.25 – 1	0.5	1	28 (100)	0 (0)	0 (0)
	MSSA	≤0.12 – 1	0.25	0.5	85 (100)	0 (0)	0 (0)
Erythromycin	MRSA	≤0.25 – ≥8	≥8	≥8	3 (10.7)	0 (0)	25 (89.3)
	MSSA	≤0.25 – ≥8	0.5	≥8	47 (56)	0 (0)	37 (44)
Gentamicin	MRSA	≤0.5 – ≥16	≤0.5	8	24 (85.7)	2 (7.1)	2 (7.1)
	MSSA	≤0.5 – 4	≤0.5	≤0.5	85 (100)	0 (0)	0 (0)
Levofloxacin	MRSA	0.25 – ≥8	4	≥8	6 (21.4)	8 (28.6)	14 (50)
	MSSA	≤0.12 – ≥8	0.25	2	80 (94.1)	2 (2.4)	3 (3.5)
Linezolid	MRSA	2 – 4	2	2	28 (100)	0 (0)	0 (0)
	MSSA	1 – 4	2	2	85 (100)	0 (0)	0 (0)
Trimethoprim/Sulfamethoxazole	MRSA	≤0.5 – ≥16	≤0.5	8	25 (89.3)	0 (0)	3 (10.7)
	MSSA	≤0.5 – ≥16	0.5	0.5	84 (98.8)	0 (0)	1 (1.2)
Tetracycline*	MRSA	≤1 – ≥16	≤1	4	22 (91.7)	0 (0)	2 (8.3)
	MSSA	≤1 – ≥16	≤1	4	48 (94.1)	0 (0)	3 (5.9)
Vancomycin	MRSA	≤0.5 – 2	1	2	28 (100)	0 (0)	0 (0)
	MSSA	≤0.5 – 2	1	1	37 (100)	0 (0)	0 (0)

3b: Susceptibility Profile for 30 S. *pneumoniae* isolates

Antimicrobial	MIC (ug/mL)			Interpretation N (%)		
	Range	MIC_{50}	MIC_{90}	Susceptible	Intermediate	Resistant
Ceftriaxone (non-meningitis)#	.004 – 0.5	0.032	0.25	23 (100)	0 (0)	0 (0)
Clindamycin#	.032 – 1	0.125	0.25	27(93.2)	1 (3.4)	1 (3.4)
Erythromycin	.016 – 32	0.25	2	22 (73.3)	3 (10)	5 (16.7)
Levofloxacin	0.25 – 4	1	1	29 (96.7)	0 (0)	1 (3.3)
Penicillin (non-meningitis)#	.008 – 2	0.032	0.5	25 (100)	0 (0)	0 (0)
Vancomycin	.25 – 2	0.5	1	29 (96.7)	0 (0)	1 (3.3)

*Antimicrobials that were not tested against all 28 MRSA isolates
#Antimicrobials that were not tested against 30 or more *S. pneumoniae* isolates
Abbreviations: MSSA = methicillin-susceptible *Staphylococcus aureus, MRSA* = methicillin-resistant *Staphylococcus aureus, MIC* = minimum inhibitory concentration (at 50% and 90%)

age. While the link between age and risk of infection remains unclear, it may be due to the underdeveloped immune system common in infants and children as well as the depressed immune function observed in the elderly, making the risk of microbial infection in these groups higher [25].

Several drugs are used to treat ocular infections, each with a different mechanism of action. Despite this, many of the pathogens observed in this study are adapting in ways that lead to increased resistance to several classes of antibiotics. Fluoroquinolones, which are a class of drugs often used as first-line treatment for ocular infections, have generally been successful, especially as newer generations have been introduced [1, 22]. However, just like other antimicrobial classes, the systemic use of these fluoroquinolones as first-line broad-spectrum antibiotics tends to lead to increases in resistance due to selective pressure [4, 15, 16, 19]. In this study, 50 and 80% of MRSA isolates showed resistance to levofloxacin and ciprofloxacin respectively, while 3.53 and 7.41% of

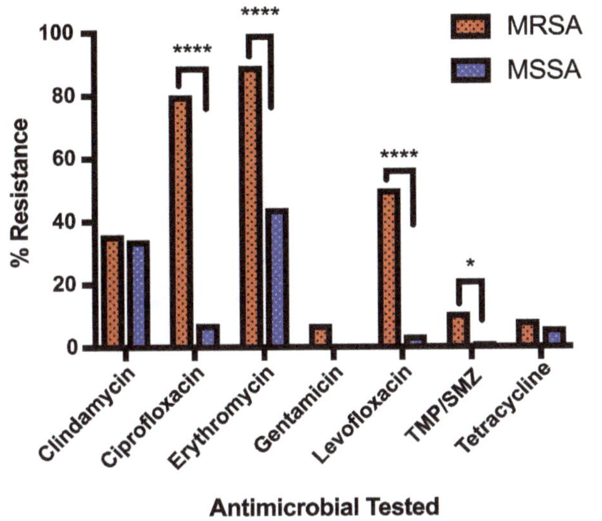

Fig. 2 Antimicrobial Resistance Observed in MRSA & MSSA Isolates. Significant differences in antimicrobial resistance between MRSA & MSSA isolates were observed for ciprofloxacin, erythromycin, levofloxacin, and TMP/SMZ. Note: Daptomycin, vancomycin, and linezolid are not included because no resistance was shown for either MRSA or MSSA isolates. Abbreviations: MSSA = methicillin-susceptible *Staphylococcus aureus;* MRSA = methicillin-resistant *Staphylococcus aureus;* TMP/SMZ = trimethoprim/sulfamethoxazole; **** = ($p < .0001$); * = ($p < .05$)

MSSA isolates showed resistance to levofloxacin and ciprofloxacin, respectively.

Multi-drug resistance (MDR) was observed in many of the MRSA isolates collected in this study ($n = 12$; 42.9%). When compared to MSSA isolates, MRSA isolates have shown statistically significant increases in MDR when compared to MSSA isolates, making them resilient pathogens. However, even with this increased resistance, *S. aureus* isolates have shown limited to no resistance to vancomycin, daptomycin or linezolid, making these treatments reliably effective in bacterial populations that have already shown high resistance to fluoroquinolones, aminoglycosides, and macrolides.

Fluctuating trends in the prevalence of MRSA strains have been reported. Some studies have presented increasing trends in MRSA over extended periods of time [23, 24], while others, including those presented by the CDC, state a decline in MRSA prevalence [26–28]. This study shows a non-statistically significant, decreasing trend over the 6-year study period suggesting that MRSA prevalence has not fluctuated drastically over the last several years. While it is unclear why MRSA prevalence has remained relatively stable in our review, it may result from successful infection control strategies in both hospitals and surrounding communities, or perhaps the cyclical replacement of dominant, infective MRSA strains by MSSA strains over time [27].

In contrast to MRSA, resistance among *S. pneumoniae* and *P. aeruginosa* isolates was low against the antimicrobials tested while resistance among *H. influenzae* isolates was evident primarily against ampicillin and TMP/SMZ. Overall these three organisms did not show alarming resistance to the antimicrobials tested and are consistent with other antimicrobial surveillance studies that have been conducted recently [1, 7, 13, 19].

Several factors are important in the development of antimicrobial resistance in ocular isolates. Overuse of antibiotics is one of the main causes [16]. Other causes include use of an antibiotic when it is not warranted, as in the case of a viral infection, or improper use, such as stopping a course of antibiotics early or using them prophylactically [17]. Since most ocular infections are often resolved through topical application rather than through systemic use, the inherent pharmacokinetic differences between the two must be taken into account when evaluating antimicrobial resistance [29, 30]. Given the high risk of permanent vision loss with eye infection, such as corneal ulcers and endopthalmitis, topical antibiotics tend to be at higher concentrations and are often used as prophylaxis despite limited evidence on their efficacy. The role that topical antibiotics play in antimicrobial resistance is still ambiguous due to the lack of research in this specific area as well as the lack of standardized ocular tissue-specific breakpoints. With the lack of these breakpoints to qualify resistance, CLSI breakpoints have been agreed upon by many researchers as useful indicators of resistance in topical antibiotics and even with the differences mentioned, similar resistance trends are observed in both topical and systemic antibiotic use [31, 32]. Additionally, since systemic antibiotics are still used to treat chronic ocular infections, in such usage, CLSI breakpoints are appropriate. In fact, systemic use of antibiotics may be the key cause of resistance in all isolates, regardless of the source of infection [33, 34]. However, the uncertainty of the role of topical antibiotics is still apparent and therefore requires further attention in order to fully delineate their role.

Limitations of this study include the retrospective nature of this study, which predetermined our sample size, ultimately limiting our analysis of all possible antimicrobial resistance trends. Because there was no standardized protocol for collection of isolates, inevitably there was a large variation in the culturing procedure among physicians. This lack of uniformity may have affected organism recovery in culture. Additionally, the antimicrobial panel underwent small fluctuations from year to year leading to slightly inconsistent susceptibility testing and excluded testing on more recently introduced fluoroquinolones, such as gatifloxacin.

Table 4 Susceptibility profiles of selected Gram-negative species, *P. aeruginosa* (a) and *H. influenzae* (b)

4a: Susceptibility Profile for 42 *P. aeruginosa* isolates

Antimicrobial	MIC (ug/mL)			Interpretation N (%)		
	Range	MIC_{50}	MIC_{90}	Susceptible	Intermediate	Resistant
Amikacin	≤2 – <16	≤2	16	42 (100)	0 (0)	0 (0)
Ceftazidime	≤1 – 8	4	8	42 (100)	0 (0)	0 (0)
Ciprofloxacin	≤0.25 – ≥4	≤0.25	1	41 (97.6)	0 (0)	1 (2.4)
Cefepime	≤1 – 8	2	<8	42 (100)	0 (0)	0 (0)
Gentamicin	≤1 – ≥16	≤1	4	41 (97.6)	0 (0)	1 (2.4)
Imipenem	≤1 – ≥16	2	4	38 (90.5)	1 (2.4)	3 (7.1)
Levofloxacin	≤0.12 – ≥8	1	2	41 (97.6)	0 (0)	1 (2.4)
Meropenem	0.125 – >32	1	8	35 (83.3)	2 (4.8)	5 (11.9)
Piperacillin/Tazobactam	≤4 – ≥128	8	≥128	36 (87.8)	0 (0)	5 (12.2)
Tobramycin*	≤1 – <4	≤1	<4	18 (100)	0 (0)	0 (0)

4b: Susceptibility Profile for 46 *H. influenzae* isolates

Antimicrobial	MIC (ug/mL)			Interpretation N (%)		
	Range	MIC_{50}	MIC_{90}	Susceptible	Intermediate	Resistant
Ampicillin	0.25 – >256	0.5	>256	22 (66.7)	1 (3)	10 (30.3)
Amoxicillin/Clavulanate	0.5 – 8	1	4	41 (95.3)	0 (0)	2 (4.7)
Ceftriaxone	.004 – 32	0.016	0.125	42 (97.7)	0 (0)	1 (2.3)
Ciprofloxacin*	.008 – 1	0.032	0.5	27 (100)	0 (0)	0 (0)
Levofloxacin	.008 – 2	0.064	0.5	30 (100)	0 (0)	0 (0)
Trimethoprim/Sulfamethoxazole	0.032 – >32	0.5	>32	23 (50)	6 (13)	17 (36.9)

*Antimicrobials that that weren't tested against 30 or more *P. aeruginosa* and *H. influenzae* isolates
Abbreviation: MIC = minimum inhibitory concentration (50 and 90%)

Conclusion

This 6-year retrospective study reported the numbers of common ocular bacterial isolates and their susceptibility profiles. The study demonstrated a relatively even ratio of Gram-negative to Gram-positive organisms and a variable distribution amongst age groups, depending on the organism. This study also found increased resistance to other drugs among MRSA strains when compared to MSSA strains, as well as moderately low resistance in Gram-negative organisms. Future studies should include a panel of commonly used antimicrobials for ocular infections, including more recently introduced fluoroquinolones. To prevent further progression of resistance, findings of this study and other surveillance data on ocular isolates should be used as resources in effective decision making in the treatment of ocular disease and infection.

Abbreviations

ARMOR: Antibiotic Resistant Monitoring in Ocular Microorganisms; CDC: Center for Disease Control; CLSI: Clinical Laboratory & Standards Institute; CoNS: Coagulase-Negative *Staphylococcus*; MRSA: Methicillin-resistant *S. aureus*; MSSA: Methicillin-Susceptible *S. aureus*; TMP/SMZ: Trimethoprim-Sulfamethoxazole; TRUST: Tracking Resistance in U.S. Today

Acknowledgements

The authors would like to acknowledge the kind and invaluable assistance of the Pathology Department of the Icahn School of Medicine at Mount Sinai, as well as Dhiraj Patel, a student at Stuyvesant High School, New York, NY.

Funding

No funding was obtained from any sources in order to conduct this study.

Authors' contributions

MO, TD, CH, & PA were responsible for the study design. MO and TD collected and analyzed the data incorporated into this review. CG contributed to the drafting of the manuscript. All authors have read and approved the final manuscript.

Competing interests

The authors declare that they have no competing interests.

Consent for Publication

Not applicable.

Author details

[1]Department of Ophthalmology, Icahn School of Medicine at Mount Sinai, New York, NY, USA. [2]Department of Pathology, Icahn School of Medicine at Mount Sinai, New York, NY 10029, USA.

References

1. Sand D, et al. Microbial keratitis in los angeles: the doheny eye institute and the los angeles county hospital experience. Ophthalmology. 2015;122(5): 918–24.
2. Vazirani J, Wurity S, Ali MH. Multidrug-resistant pseudomonas aeruginosa keratitis: risk factors, clinical characteristics, and outcomes. Ophthalmology. 2015;122(10):2110–4.
3. Oldenburg CE, et al. Emerging moxifloxacin resistance in Pseudomonas aeruginosa keratitis isolates in South India. Ophthalmic Epidemiol. 2013; 20(3):155–8.
4. Paul-Satyaseela M, et al. Characterization of antibiotic resistance profiles of ocular enterobacteriaceae isolates. Eur J Microbiol Immunol (Bp). 2016;6(1):40–8.
5. Magiorakos AP, et al. Multidrug-resistant, extensively drug-resistant and pandrug-resistant bacteria: an international expert proposal for interim standard definitions for acquired resistance. Clin Microbiol Infection. 2012;18(3):268–81.
6. Fernandes M, et al. Extensively and pan-drug resistant Pseudomonas aeruginosa keratitis: clinical features, risk factors, and outcome. Graefes Arch Clin Exp Ophthalmol. 2016;254(2):315–22.
7. Muluye D, et al. Types and drug susceptibility patterns of bacterial isolates from eye discharge samples at Gondar university hospital, northwest Ethiopia. BMC Res Notes. 2014;7:292.
8. Haas W, et al. Monitoring antibiotic resistance in ocular microorganisms: results from the antibiotic resistance monitoring in ocular micRorganisms (ARMOR) 2009 surveillance study. Am J Ophthalmol. 2011;152(4):567–74. e3.
9. Asbell PA, et al. Ocular TRUST: nationwide antimicrobial susceptibility patterns in ocular isolates. Am J Ophthalmol. 2008;145(6):951–8.
10. Thornsberry C, et al. Regional trends in antimicrobial resistance among clinical isolates of streptococcus pneumoniae, haemophilus influenzae, and moraxella catarrhalis in the united states: results from the TRUST surveillance program, 1999–2000. Clin Infect Dis. 2002;34 Suppl 1:S4–S16.
11. Karlowsky JA, et al. Susceptibility to fluoroquinolones among commonly isolated gram-negative bacilli in 2000: TRUST and TSN data for the united states. Tracking resistance in the united states today. The surveillance network. Int J Antimicrob Agents. 2002;19(1):21–31.
12. Sahm DF, et al. Tracking resistance among bacterial respiratory tract pathogens: summary of findings of the TRUST surveillance initiative, 2001–2005. Postgrad Med. 2008;120(3 Suppl 1):8–15.
13. Asbell PA, et al. Antibiotic resistance among ocular pathogens in the united states: five-year results from the antibiotic resistance monitoring in ocular microorganisms (ARMOR) surveillance study. JAMA Ophthalmol. 2015; 133(12):1445–54.
14. McDonald M, Blondeau JM. Emerging antibiotic resistance in ocular infections and the role of fluoroquinolones. J Cataract Refract Surg. 2010; 36(9):1588–498.
15. Gentile RC, et al. Microbiological spectrum and antibiotic sensitivity in endophthalmitis: a 25-years review. Ophthalmology. 2014;121(8):1634–42.
16. Blanco AR, et al. Susceptibility of methicillin-resistant Staphylococci clinical isolates to netilmicin and other antibiotics commonly used in ophthalmic therapy. Curr Eye Res. 2013;38(8):811–6.
17. Willcox MD. Review of resistance of ocular isolates of Pseudomonas aeruginosa and staphylococci from keratitis to ciprofloxacin, gentamicin and cephalosporins. Clin Exp Optom. 2011;94(2):161–8.
18. Ong SJ, et al. Staphylococcus aureus keratitis: a review of hospital cases. PLoS One. 2013;8(11):e80119.
19. Al-Dhaheri HS, et al. Ocular pathogens and antibiotic sensitivity in bacterial keratitis isolates at king khaled Eye specialist hospital, 2011 to 2014. Cornea. 2016;35(6):789–94.
20. Clinical Laboratory and Standards Institute. Performance standards for antimicrobial susceptibility testing, in M100. 2010–2016.
21. Clinical Laboratory Standards Institute. Methods for antimicrobial dilution and disk susceptibility testing of infrequently isolated fastidious bacteria, M45 S2. 2nd ed. 2011.
22. Mantadakis E, et al. Antimicrobial susceptibility of Gram-positive cocci isolated from patients with conjunctivitis and keratitis in Crete, Greece. J Microbiol Immunol Infect. 2013;46(1):41–7.
23. Asbell PA, et al. Increasing prevalence of methicillin resistance in serious ocular infections caused by Staphylococcus aureus in the United States: 2000 to 2005. J Cataract Refract Surg. 2008;34(5):814–8.
24. Adebayo A, et al. Shifting trends in in vitro antibiotic susceptibilities for common bacterial conjunctival isolates in the last decade at the New York Eye and Ear Infirmary. Graefes Arch Clin Exp Ophthalmol. 2011;249(1):111–9.
25. Kale SS, Namita A, Sachin Y. The epidemiology of aging, Aging, infection, and immunity. Netherlands: Springer; 2012.
26. Chuang CC, et al. Staphylococcus aureus ocular infection: methicillin-resistance, clinical features, and antibiotic susceptibilities. PLoS One. 2012; 8(8):e42437.
27. Rolain JM, et al. Worldwide decrease in methicillin-resistant Staphylococcus aureus: do we understand something? Clin Microbiol Infect. 2015;21(6):515–7.
28. Centers for Disease Control and Prevention. Antibiotic resistance threats in the United States, 2013. Atlanta: CDC; 2013.
29. Bertino Jr JS. Impact of antibiotic resistance in the management of ocular infections: the role of current and future antibiotics. Clin Ophthalmol. 2009; 3:507–21.
30. Sharma S. Antibiotic resistance in ocular bacterial pathogens. Indian J Med Microbiol. 2011;29(3):218–22.
31. Parmar P, et al. Comparison of topical gatifloxacin 0.3% and ciprofloxacin 0. 3% for the treatment of bacterial keratitis. Am J Ophthalmol. 2006;141(2): 282–6.
32. Kaliamurthy J, et al. Comparison of in vitro susceptibilities of ocular bacterial isolates to gatifloxacin and other topical antibiotics. Ophthalmic Res. 2005; 37(3):117–22.
33. Ray KJ, et al. Fluoroquinolone treatment and susceptibility of isolates from bacterial keratitis. JAMA Ophthalmol. 2013;131(3):310–3.
34. Rameshkumar G, et al. Prevalence and antibacterial resistance patterns of extended-spectrum beta-lactamase producing Gram-negative bacteria isolated from ocular infections. Indian J Ophthalmol. 2016;64(4):303–11.

16

Estimating the burden of antimicrobial resistance

Nichola R. Naylor[1*], Rifat Atun[3,1], Nina Zhu[1], Kavian Kulasabanathan[2], Sachin Silva[3], Anuja Chatterjee[1], Gwenan M. Knight[1] and Julie V. Robotham[4,1]

Abstract

Background: Accurate estimates of the burden of antimicrobial resistance (AMR) are needed to establish the magnitude of this global threat in terms of both health and cost, and to paramaterise cost-effectiveness evaluations of interventions aiming to tackle the problem. This review aimed to establish the alternative methodologies used in estimating AMR burden in order to appraise the current evidence base.

Methods: MEDLINE, EMBASE, Scopus, EconLit, PubMed and grey literature were searched. English language studies evaluating the impact of AMR (from any microbe) on patient, payer/provider and economic burden published between January 2013 and December 2015 were included. Independent screening of title/abstracts followed by full texts was performed using pre-specified criteria. A study quality score (from zero to one) was derived using Newcastle-Ottawa and Philips checklists. Extracted study data were used to compare study method and resulting burden estimate, according to perspective. Monetary costs were converted into 2013 USD.

Results: Out of 5187 unique retrievals, 214 studies were included. One hundred eighty-seven studies estimated patient health, 75 studies estimated payer/provider and 11 studies estimated economic burden. 64% of included studies were single centre. The majority of studies estimating patient or provider/payer burden used regression techniques. 48% of studies estimating mortality burden found a significant impact from resistance, excess healthcare system costs ranged from non-significance to $1 billion per year, whilst economic burden ranged from $21,832 per case to over $3 trillion in GDP loss. Median quality scores (interquartile range) for patient, payer/provider and economic burden studies were 0.67 (0.56-0.67), 0.56 (0.46-0.67) and 0.53 (0.44-0.60) respectively.

Conclusions: This study highlights what methodological assumptions and biases can occur dependent on chosen outcome and perspective. Currently, there is considerable variability in burden estimates, which can lead in-turn to inaccurate intervention evaluations and poor policy/investment decisions. Future research should utilise the recommendations presented in this review.

Keywords: Antimicrobial resistance, Antibiotic resistance, Burden, Cost

Background

Antimicrobial resistance (AMR) is a cause for global concern due to the current and potential impact on global population health, costs to healthcare systems and Gross Domestic Product (GDP), mainly through reduced treatment options [1]. Recent reports suggest that absolute numbers of infections due to resistant microbes are increasing globally [2–4]. Estimates of the potential economic burden of AMR from recent reports, such as 'The Review on Antimicrobial Resistance' [1], are being utilised by policy makers to push AMR up the political agenda [5]. However, more precise estimates of AMR burden are needed to inform policy through health economic models evaluating interventions attempting to prevent, treat or stop the spread of resistant infections [6, 7].

In order to establish burden, the perspective being taken should be defined. The patient perspective refers to

* Correspondence: n.naylor@imperial.ac.uk
[1]National Institute for Health Research Health Protection Research Unit in Healthcare Associated Infection and Antimicrobial Resistance at Imperial College, Hammersmith Campus, London W12 0NN, UK
Full list of author information is available at the end of the article

associated mortality and morbidity (including clinical outcomes), while the payer perspective can include attributable costs to the payers of healthcare including insurers or national payers [6]. The provider perspective estimates the burden to certain providers of healthcare, such as hospitals and primary care practices [6]. In cases where there is national/governmental provision and payment of healthcare services, the provider and payer perspectives may align to be the same, such as in the case of the National Health Service and the Department of Health in England [6]. The economic (or societal) perspective generally includes the potential impact on the labour force through lost productivity [8, 9], but can also include the burden on carers and patient out-of-pocket expenses [10, 11]. AMR may also create burden through secondary effects, referred to in this review as secondary burden. Secondary patient burden, and onward effects to healthcare system or society, occurs when procedures that utilise antimicrobials to reduce the risk of post-intervention adverse events (such as surgical procedures utilising prophylactic antibiotics) are performed less frequently due to AMR increasing the risk of adverse events [12].

The different perspectives of burden produce varying outcome measures. For example, from a patient perspective an excess mortality figure may be determined [13], whilst looking from a payer or provider perspective could produce an excess cost of hospital treatment in monetary terms [14], and economic burden could refer to excess GDP losses for a country [15]. Obtaining estimates for these different outcomes, may require different methodologies, ranging from case-control studies with regression analyses to complex mathematical and economic models [16, 17].

Past descriptive review articles have discussed the methods of estimating the burden of AMR [9, 18, 19]. However, since an update in 2012 of a previous systematic review [8, 20], there has been no formal systematic assessment of the methods used in AMR burden estimation, or the variation in resulting outcomes. The 2012 update concluded economic evidence was lacking, and that over the 21 studies included there were large variations in the estimates of AMR burden [8]. However, there been no formal quality assessment of recent AMR burden evidence across the stated perspectives, which is needed when discussing study methodology and its limitations. Given the growing media coverage of and policy interest in AMR over recent years [21, 22], there has been a corresponding marked increase in the published evidence on AMR impact. As such, this review aimed to capture and assess this recent portion of the literature, by reviewing the evidence published since the review in 2012 by Smith and Coast [8]. This review aimed to capture both the burden in the sense of the incremental impact of resistance (in addition to infection) and the burden of resistant infections among all of the population. Therefore this systematic review aimed to address the following research questions in regards to the human population, with no limitation on microbe of interest; (i) what perspectives and resulting methodologies have been used to estimate AMR burden in the recent published literature? (ii) Do AMR burden estimates differ by perspective and methodology? (iii) What is the quality of this recent evidence on the burden of AMR?

Methods

This Systematic review is in line with PRISMA guidance, is registered with PROSPERO (registration number PROSPERO CRD42016037510) and has a previously published protocol [23–25].

Search strategy and eligibility criteria

Studies which aimed to quantify the burden of AMR (in humans) published since the Smith and Coast review in 2012 [8] were of interest, and as such, the search was limited from January 2013 – December 2015. Ovid 'Medline & EMBASE,' Scopus and EconLit were searched utilising a search string, which employed combinations of the following terms; excess, associated, attributable, burden, morbidity, mortality, cost, economic, clinical, global, impact, outcome, burden, antibiotic, antimicrobial, multi-drug, microbial-drug, resistan*, gram-positive, gram-negative, susceptib*,nonsusceptib*, enterococc*, Escherichia, streptococc*, staphylococc*, klebsiealla, pseudomonas, neisseria, chlamydia, clostridi*, mycobacteri*. In deviation to the published protocol [25], an additional search of PubMed was conducted for literature published within the stated time period, whereby titles were searched using the following string; "(((((mortality[Title]) OR cost[Title]) OR length of stay[Title]) OR productivity[Title]) AND resistant[Title]) AND infection*[Title]" [26]. The following websites were also searched for grey literature: Public Health England, Public Health Wales, Health Protection Scotland, NHS Health Scotland, Department of Health (UK), Health Protection Agency, National Institute for Health and Care Excellence, Centers for Disease Control and Prevention, World Health Organisation, European Commission for Public Health, Review on Antimicrobial Resistance.

The modified PICO inclusion/exclusion criteria (Table 1) were utilised to screen title/abstracts and subsequently full-texts [27].

Data extraction and quality assessment

Data were extracted from each study into a Data Extraction Table using Microsoft Excel. The following variables were collected as part of this process; study identifier, perspective, infection of interest (exposure, non-exposure, case and control definitions), outcome, country setting, study population, study design, data setting, epidemiological scope, method, sample size, (resistance-related) result, stated limitations and quality (risk of bias).

Table 1 Inclusion/Exclusion Criteria Applied [25]

Criteria	Inclusion	Exclusion
Population	Humans	Animals only
	All ages	Plants only
	All sexes	
	Infection with antimicrobial resistant organism (or similar such as Extended Spectrum Beta-lactamase producing organisms). This includes future predictions of related infected populations, such as in the case of a "post-antibiotic" era	
Outcomes	Associated health burden, including mortality and morbidity	Health-Related Quality of Life only
	Associated healthcare cost burden, including resource use and opportunity cost	Molecular biology only
	Economic burden, including loss of productivity	Epidemiology only
	Burden from not being able to use antibiotics in ways previously or currently used in healthcare, including reduced surgery or chemotherapy	Outcomes associated with the evaluation of an intervention only
Study design	Case–control studies	Editorials
	Cohort studies	Letters
	Cross–sectional studies	Case series reports
	Longitudinal studies	Conference reports
	Randomised controlled trials	Evaluations of interventions
	Modelling studies	Reviews
	Economic Evaluations	

To establish what perspectives and resulting methodologies have been used in establishing AMR burden, study perspectives were grouped into either patient, healthcare system (representing payer and/or provider perspectives) or economic/societal burden. Studies estimating the secondary effects of AMR can do so by estimating the potential impact on health (such as excess deaths), healthcare system or economic burden (excess cost), so could be marked under each of these perspectives. Study methodologies were grouped into the following categories; regression analysis (parametric regression models), survival analysis (this included semi-parametric Cox proportional hazard models and non-parametric time to event analysis), matching, multistate models (including decision trees), economic models (including total factor or computable general equilibrium models), stepwise calculations (for example synthesising evidence from the literature and applying simple calculations to arrive at an estimate), significance tests and other (if none of the former categories applied).

The outcome of particular interest for patient burden was mortality, using odds ratio (OR) and hazard ratio (HR) measures. In this review, length of stay (LoS), alongside monetary cost, was recorded as a healthcare system burden outcome, as it has been shown that for healthcare associated infections LoS is a major contributing factor to hospital costs [28]. For economic burden, monetary cost was considered the main outcome of interest, however reporting of productivity, GDP and other such economic measures were also recorded. Impact significance was defined by p values (less than 0.05) and 95% confidence intervals (CIs), where appropriate.

Risk of bias within individual studies was assessed using the Newcastle-Ottawa scales for cohort and case-control studies [29]. For this review a case-control study was defined when outcomes of interest (such death) were used to select the case and control groups, whereas cohort studies selected cases based on exposure to resistance [30]. The Newcastle-Ottawa checklists include four domains of quality and eight possible stars [29]. The Philips checklist was used for modelling studies, which includes three domains of quality and 57 possible stars [31]. A quality score was derived as the proportion of applicable checklist stars achieved (zero and one representing no checklist items achieved and all checklist items achieved respectively), please see Additional file 1: Tables S1, S2 and S3 for the full checklists utilised.

Risk of bias across the evidence was presented using the median and interquartile ranges of the quality score by perspective. This was a deviation in methodology from the published protocol, which proposed evaluating sign and significance of results [25], and was chosen as any other summary figures would be flawed due to the high heterogeneity in infection of interest and outcome [32].

Data analysis

Due to study heterogeneity no meta-analyses were performed. Monetary costs found were converted into 2013 United States dollars (USD) by inflating the cost to 2013 original-currency estimates using annual inflation rates [33, 34], then converting this into USD utilising 2013 average exchange rates [35].

Descriptive statistics (such as proportions of papers and average quality scores), tables and graphs to collate and present ORs, HRs, LoS and monetary cost were executed in Microsoft Excel and R version 3.3.2 using packages 'plyr', 'metafor' and 'ggplot2' [36–38].

Results

A total of 5187 unique titles and abstracts were retrieved over the specified search period. Applying the selection process resulted in a total of 214 studies being included in the final review (Fig. 1). One hundred eighty-seven studies included a patient burden measure, 75 a

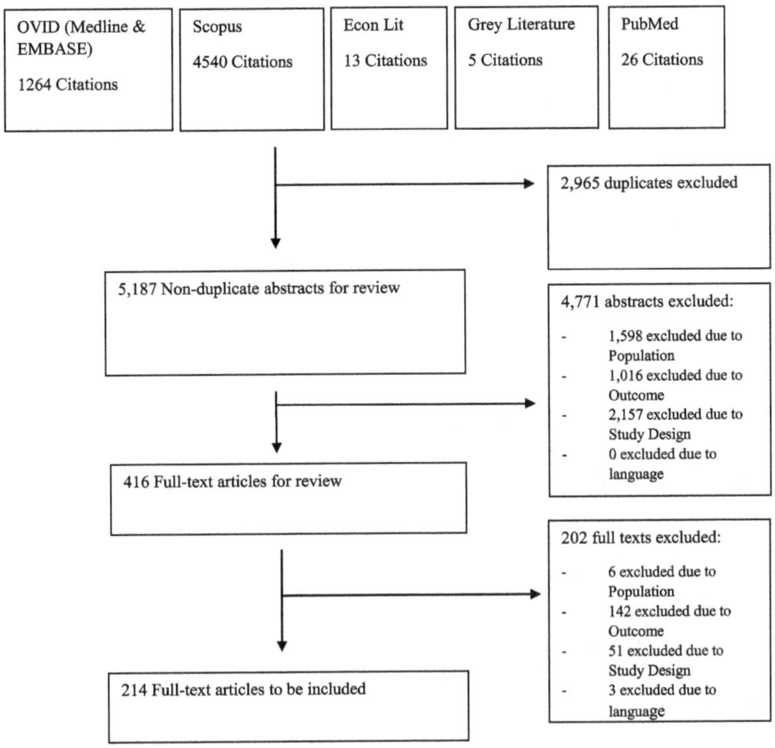

Fig. 1 PRISMA Diagram of Article Retrieval & Inclusion

healthcare system burden measure, and only 11 studies included an economic burden measure (Table 2). The most individually studied genus was *Staphylococcus* (23%, 50/214), followed by *Klebsiella* (9%, 19/214) and *Acinetobacter* (8%, 18/214) respectively. The countries which individually produced the highest number of studies were the USA (19%, 40/214), followed by South Korea (7%, 15/214) and Spain (6%, 13/214). 64% of studies (138/214) used data from just one centre. The majority of studies (89%, 190/214) did not specify the epidemiological scope in estimating AMR burden, for example by stating whether relevant included infections were due to endemic- or outbreak-related microbes. See Additional file 1: Table S4 for individual study details.

Estimating the patient burden of AMR

For estimating the patient burden of AMR, regression analyses and significance tests were the most utilised methods (Table 2). 95% (177/187) of studies estimating patient burden calculated mortality burden, with the remaining 5% (10/187) focusing on morbidity burden. Of those estimating a mortality burden, 48% (85/177) of studies found that AMR had a significant impact on mortality. Studies which aimed to estimate the impact of resistance on morbidity mainly focused on

Table 2 Perspectives & Methods used to Estimate the Burden of Antimicrobial Resistance

	Patient % (*n* = 187)	Healthcare System % (*n* = 75)	Economic % (*n* = 11)
Regression Analysis	44.9%	34.7%	9.1%
Survival Analysis	20.9%	9.3%	0.0%
Matching	4.8%	10.7%	9.1%
Multistate model	2.1%	6.7%	27.3%
Economic Model	0.0%	0.0%	18.2%
Significance Tests	26.2%	32.0%	0.0%
Stepwise calculation	1.1%	6.7%	27.3%
Qualitative	0.0%	0.0%	9.1%

Note that some studies included more than one burden perspective per study (for example a study reporting impact on mortality and costs would appear in multiple perspective categories)

clinical outcomes such as clinical failure, time to stability, recurring infections or development of secondary infections [39–47].

The majority of studies that utilised standard regression techniques to estimate ORs of a mortality event found resistance to be associated with higher mortality (Fig. 2a and Fig. 2b). Focusing on those which directly compared resistant and susceptible infections explicitly, 50% (7/14) and 47% (9/19) of the studies for Gram-positive and Gram-negative exposures, respectively, had 95% confidence intervals which crossed this OR = 1 threshold. This suggests non-statistical significance of such results. Across Gram-positive and Gram-negative infections, this occurred in 4/15 studies investigating resistant cases against "non-exposed" controls and in 2/8 studies investigating the burden of additional resistance mechanisms on already resistant infections (for example the impact of vancomycin resistance on Methicillin resistant *Staphylococcus aureus* (MRSA) patients).

Comparing Figs. 2 and 3 would suggest there is no clear consensus from either method (parametric regression or Cox proportional hazards regression) as to whether there is a significant impact of bacterial resistance mechanisms on mortality outcomes, though it should be noted that different measures of mortality have been used across these studies (see Additional file 1: Table S4). 32% (8/25) of these studies estimating mortality-related hazard ratios, did so in relation to in-hospital mortality. Such analysis may not accurately estimate the impact of exposure (versus non-exposure) on outcome, due to the failure of the non-informative censoring assumption, as the cause of being discharged may be related to the likelihood of experiencing death. As the infection type, resistance type and outcomes are different across the aforementioned studies a rigorous comparison cannot be made.

Only one study estimated the potential patient burden of AMR via secondary effects (secondary patient burden), by evaluating the impact on mortality (excess deaths) of reduced prophylactic antibiotic efficacy in the United States [12]. Utilising an evidence synthesis and stepwise calculation approach, this study estimated that a 30% reduction in the efficacy of antibiotic prophylaxis for certain surgical and chemotherapeutic procedures would result in 6300 infection-related deaths annually [12].

Estimating the healthcare system burden of AMR

For estimating the healthcare system burden (which incorporates the payer and provider perspectives) of AMR, regression analyses and significance tests were the most utilised methods. Seventy-five studies estimated healthcare system burden, 64 of these estimated LoS burden due to AMR and 31 estimated monetary cost (with some studies estimating both). The majority of studies evaluating LoS (69%, 44/64) found that resistance had a statistically significant impact, however 39% (17/44) of these utilised significance testing against descriptive statistics (such as median length of stay). Thirteen studies estimated excess LoS due to resistant infections (Fig. 4), with 3 studies using a multistate modelling methodology to estimate LoS. Multistate models attempt to adjust for time dependency bias [48–50], however this bias has also been adjusted for in other ways, such as shifting forward the index date from the date of hospital admission to the first day of the second calendar month of the patient's stay [51]. The majority of excess LoS estimates were for Gram-positive bacteria, with only two estimates for a Gram-negative bacteria (Fig. 4). Excess LoS was estimated at 12.8 days for MRSA bloodstream infections [95% CI 6.2 - 26.1 days] [48] in Australia, 11.5 [95% CI: 7.9-15] days for MRSA in Switzerland [49] and 11.43 [95% CI; 10.44 – 12.43] days for MRSA in American Veterans, utilising time dependency adjusted methods described above [50]. These are similar to those computed by regression but much higher than that estimated by stepwise calculations (Fig. 4), though all are from different populations.

A variety of methods have been used to calculate healthcare system monetary costs, with no clear majority of one method seen (Table 3). After conversion to 2013 USD for comparing excess/attributable costs, for Extended-Spectrum beta-Lactamase (ESBL) in bloodstream infections, a matching study found no significant impact on healthcare system costs [52], whilst a multistate model found an associated $10,154 loss per case [49]. For MRSA estimates ranged from non-significance [53] to $28,553 per case [51] (across different populations for different infections, Table 3).

Estimating the economic burden of AMR

From the economic perspective stepwise calculations, multistate modelling and economic models were commonly used (Table 2). Only a small number of studies were found in this perspective category, with 11 studies assessing the burden to the economy resulting from AMR. Eight of these reported an estimate for the monetary impact of resistance (Table 4). In addition, two studies found investigated the potential psycho-social impact of having multi-drug resistant Tuberculosis, concluding that many patients in the qualitative study felt that multi-drug resistant Tuberculosis increased stigma and social isolation [54], and increased the odds of incurring catastrophic costs (in which [OR = 1.61 (95% CI = 0.98–2.64), $p < 0.06$]) [43]. A report from 'The Review on Antimicrobial Resistance' did mention the secondary effects of AMR from the economic perspective, however did not attempt to quantify an exact figure for this, instead stating that some proportion of the 120 trillion USD gained from caesareans, joint operations, chemotherapy and organ transplants could be lost [1].

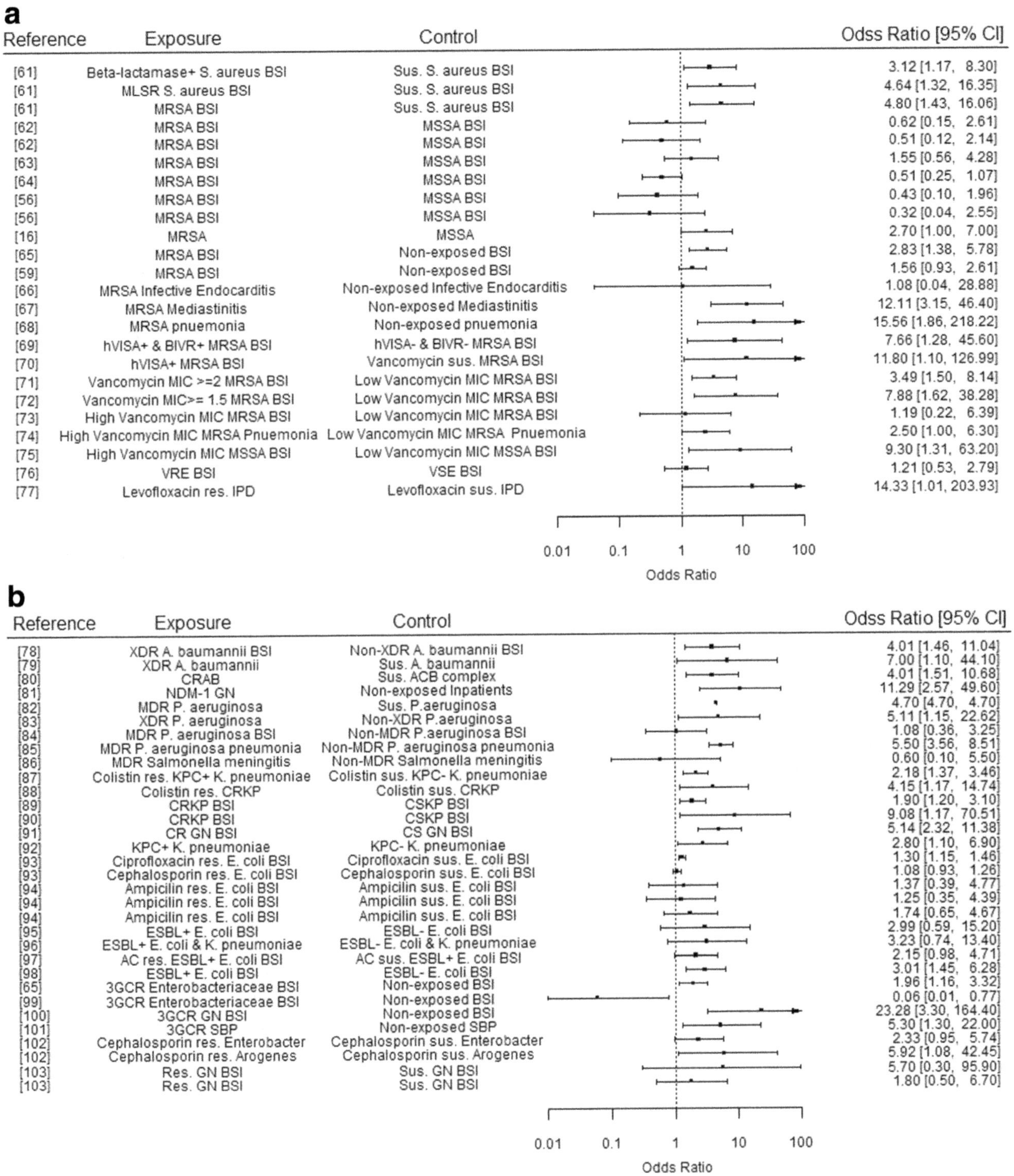

Fig. 2 Odds ratios of Mortality Outcomes for Resistant Infections. Results presented are from studies utilising regression techniques, where 1.0 represents the point at which exposure does not affect the odds of the outcome occurring. The box point represents the reported OR value, with horizontal lines representing the reported 95% Confidence Interval. Results have not been adjusted or adapted to represent sample size, and are presented grouped by genera. **a** Gram-positive Bacteria. **b** Gram-negative Bacteria. [16, 56, 59, 61–103]

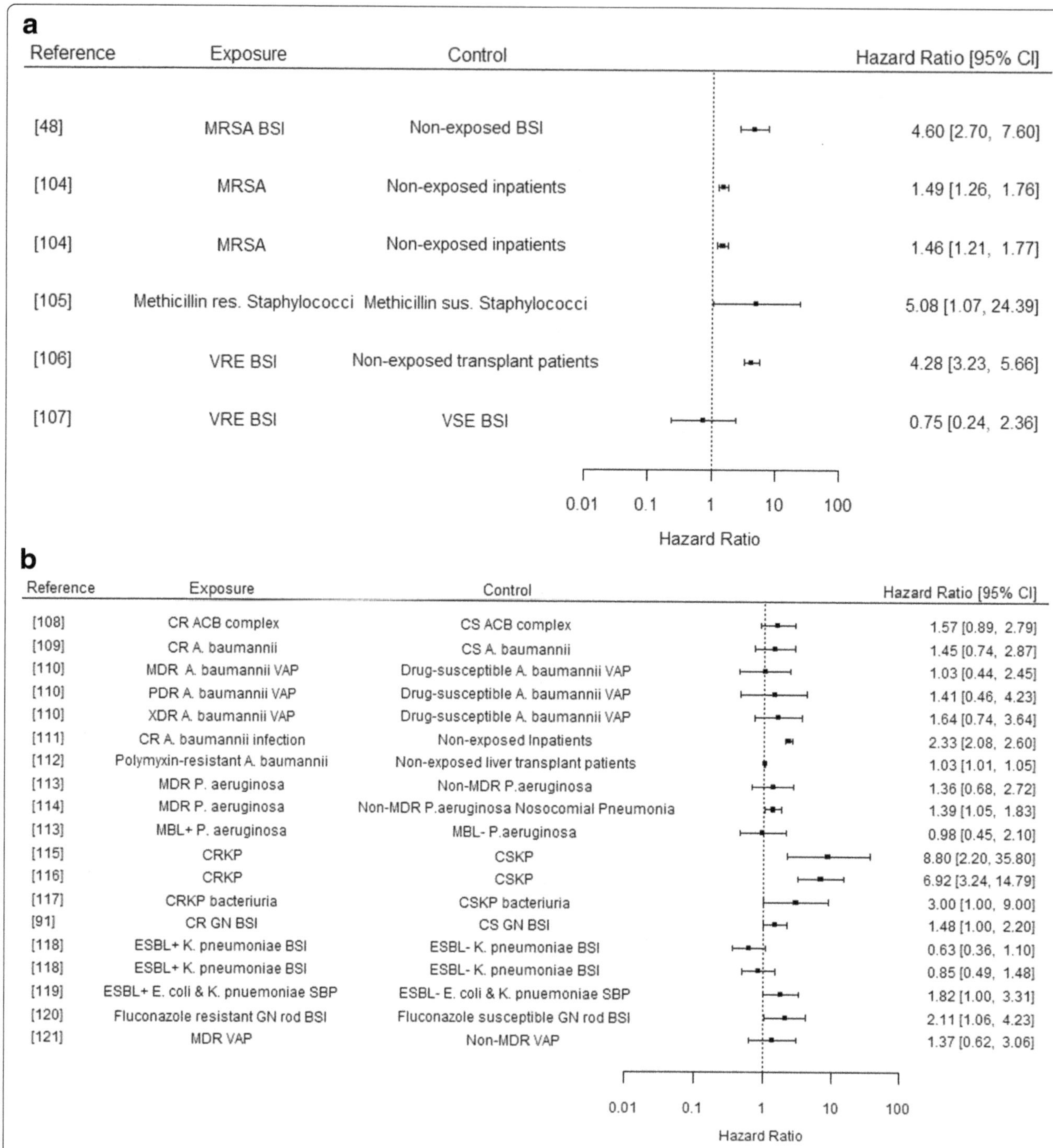

Fig. 3 Hazard Ratios of Mortality Outcomes for Resistant Infections. Results presented are from studies utilising Cox proportional hazards regression techniques, where 1.0 represents the point at which exposure and control experience the same event rate at any point in time. The box point represents the reported HR value, with horizontal lines representing the reported 95% Confidence Interval. Results have not been adjusted or adapted to represent sample size, and are presented grouped by genera. **a** Gram-positive Bacteria. **b** Gram-negative Bacteria. [48, 91, 104–121]

The only studies explicitly estimating the economic burden of AMR to include Gram-negative infections were those commissioned by 'The Review on Antimicrobial Resistance' (in which *Escherichia coli* and *Klebsiella pnuemoniae* were two out of six studied microbes) [1, 15, 55]. These modelling studies, which utilised economic modelling techniques, provided the largest estimates of cost (though of six resistant microbes), estimating over

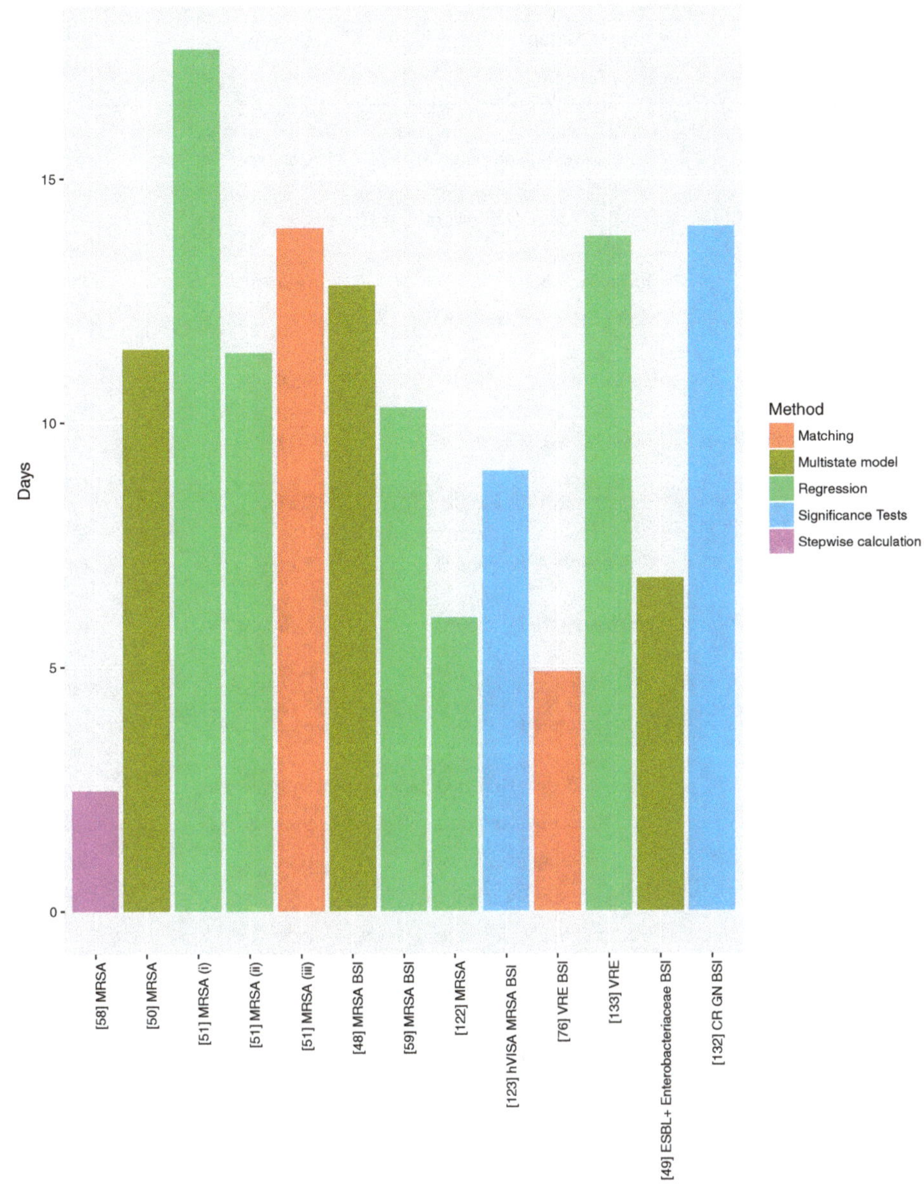

Fig. 4 Estimates of Excess Length of Stay of Hospital/ICU Stay Caused by Antimicrobial Resistance. (i) - (iii) denote different methods used in a single study [48–51, 58, 59, 76, 122, 123, 132 ,133]

$14 billion to over $3 trillion (2013 USD) in loss to global GDP by 2050 [15, 55]. Whilst the studies which utilised multistate modelling techniques (including decision tree analysis) or stepwise calculations, estimated national costs for a specific resistance type to range from over $20,000 per MRSA bloodstream infection case to over $7 billion per year attributable to community acquired MRSA in the United States (Table 4) [56, 57].

Quality of included studies

For the outcomes and exposures tested relevant to this review, 199 studies were considered cohort, 1 case-control and 13 modelling studies, whereby the stated quality checklists were then applied. One additional study was a survey-based qualitative study and was not quality assessed [54]. Median quality scores (with interquartile range (IQR)) for health, healthcare system and economic burden studies were 0.67 (0.56-0.67), 0.56 (0.46-0.67) and 0.53 (0.44-0.60) respectively. Within all perspectives, quality rarely exceeded 0.75. Notably there was a lack of economic burden studies and their median quality score was lower than that of the health and healthcare system studies (Fig. 5).

Table 3 Excess Healthcare system Cost Estimates of Antimicrobial Resistance

Study	Exposure Group	Control Group	Country	Method	Excess Cost Estimate (2013 USD)
Cost per case					
[109]	CRAB in Columbia	Carbapenem susceptible A. baumannii	Columbia	Regression	4,583[a]
[124]	ESBL+ *E. coli* & Klebsiella species UTI	ESBL- *E. coli* & Klebsiella species UTI	USA	Significance Tests	3,237[a]
[125]	ESBL+ *E.coli* BSI	ESBL- *E.coli* BSI	Germany	Matching	-2081
[49]	ESBL+ *Enterobacteriaceae* BSI	ESBL- *Enterobacteriaceae* BSI	Switzerland	Multistate model	10,154
[45]	ESBL+ UTI	ESBL- UTI	Spain	Matching & Regression	3146†
[126]	ESBL+ and/or beta-lactamases resistant UTI	Susceptible UTI	Turkey	Significance Tests	90[a]
[126]	Ciprofloxacin resistant UTI	Ciprofloxacin susceptible UTI	Turkey	Significance Tests	114[a]
[127]	MDR *A. baumannii* BSI	Susceptible *A. baumannii* BSI	Turkey	Significance Tests	15,365
[58]	MRSA	Non-exposure inpatients	Germany	Stepwise Calculations	11,878
[53]	MRSA breast abscess	MSSA breast abscess	USA	Matching	515
[128]	MRSA BSI	Non-exposure BSI	South Korea	Stepwise Calculations	5216
[129]	MRSA BSI (survivors)	Non-nosocomial-infected patients	South Korea	Matching	11,627
[129]	MRSA BSI (non-survivors)	Non-nosocomial-infected patients	South Korea	Matching	15,254
[51]	MRSA infections	Non-exposure inpatients	USA	Matching	28,553[a]
[130]	MRSA colonisation & infection	Non-exposure inpatients	USA	Matching	12,167[a]
[131]	Resistant BSI	Susceptible BSI	India	Significance Tests	912[a]
[132]	Carbapenem-resistant device associated healthcare acquired infections ICU patients	Non-"device associated healthcare acquired infections" ICU patients	Greece	Significance Tests	3,884[a]
[133]	VRE colonisation & infections	Non-exposure inpatients	Canada	Matching & Regression	18,631[a]
[76]	VRE BSI	VSE BSI	Australia	Matching & Regression	30,093[a]
[134]	VRE BSI in allo-HSCT recipients	Non-exposure in allo-HSCT recipients	USA	Significance Tests	6104
[135]	MDR TB	Non-MDR TB	Germany	Stepwise Calculations	86,321
[136]	MDR TB	Non-MDR TB	South Africa	Stepwise Calculations	6728
[137]	MDR TB	Non-MDR TB	Latvia	Regression	33291[a]
[138]	XDR and pre-XDR TB	Rifampicin-mono-resistant or MDR TB	South Africa	Stepwise Calculations	15,567
[136]	XDR TB	Non-"XDR or MDR" TB	South Africa	Stepwise Calculations	26,989
[139]	VRE BSI in leukaemia patients	Non-exposure leukaemia patients	USA	Matching	88150[a]
Per-patient per-day					
[50]	MRSA in Switzerland	Non-exposure inpatients	Switzerland	Multistate model	867
[140]	Resistant Gram-negative Bacilli infection	Susceptible Gram-negative Bacilli infection	Singapore	Matching	812

Table 3 Excess Healthcare system Cost Estimates of Antimicrobial Resistance *(Continued)*

Study	Exposure Group	Control Group	Country	Method	Excess Cost Estimate (2013 USD)
Annual cost per stated country or stated region					
[57]	MRSA	No-MRSA	USA	Multistate model	1,382,733,079
[141]	Resistant Streptococcus pneumonia	Susceptible Streptococcus pneumonia	USA	Multistate model	91,773,500
[142]	Artemisinin resistant malaria	No-"Artemisinin resistant malaria"	High endemicity region	Multistate model	32,000,000

[a]Statistically significant where *p*-value is less than 0.05

The Newcastle-Ottawa checklist criteria showed that only 54% of the total available points for adjustment/comparability of different exposure groups across all cohort studies were awarded (in all 199 studies, where two points were available per study [29]), suggesting a need for more robust analyses estimating the impact of AMR. Some of the least fulfilled quality assessment categories by studies were those that focused on representativeness of the sample utilised (18% of the appraised studies met this criteria), description/adequacy of follow-up or non-response rates (40% met this criteria) and demonstration of non-exposure before study period (8% met this criteria), across the Newcastle-Ottawa cohort quality assessment checklist (199 studies).

For the 13 studies for which the Philips checklist was utilised to assess quality, there were many indicators for which scores were generally low, including those related to descriptions of the choice of model structure and the approach to obtaining parameter values (less than 1/3 of studies obtaining the related criteria). However, of note, none of the relevant studies met the following criteria; "Have the four principal types of uncertainty been addressed?", "If not, has the omission been justified?" and "Is there evidence that the mathematical logic of the

Table 4 Excess Economic Burden Estimates of Antimicrobial Resistance

Study	Exposure Group	Control Group	Country	Method	Excess Cost Estimate (2013 USD)
Cost per case					
[135]	MDR TB	Susceptible TB	Germany	Stepwise Calculation	110,063
[135]	XDR TB	Susceptible TB	Germany	Stepwise Calculation	145,679
[143]	MDR TB	Susceptible TB	Europe	Stepwise Calculation	62,931
[143])	XDR TB	Susceptible TB	Europe	Stepwise Calculation	215,038
[56]	MRSA BSI	Non-nosocomial-infected patients	South Korea	Matching	21,832
Annual cost per stated country or stated region					
[141]	Resistant Streptococcus pneumonia	Susceptible Streptococcus pneumonia	USA	Multistate model	236,495,000
[57]	MRSA	No MRSA	USA	Multistate model	7,848,223,600
[142]	Artemisinin resistant malaria	No resistance	High endemicity regions	Decision Tree	385,000,000
Global economic cost					
[15]	Resistance globally (doubling of current infection rates and 100% resistance)	Lower rates of resistance (a 40% resistance increase from current rates)	Global	Total Factor Productivity model	14,228,000,000 less GDP produced in 2050 compared to 2050 in a scenario with lower resistance
[55]	Resistance globally (100% resistance rate)	No resistance	Global	Computable General Equilibrium model	3,158,862,360 less GDP produced in 2050 compared to 2050 with no resistance

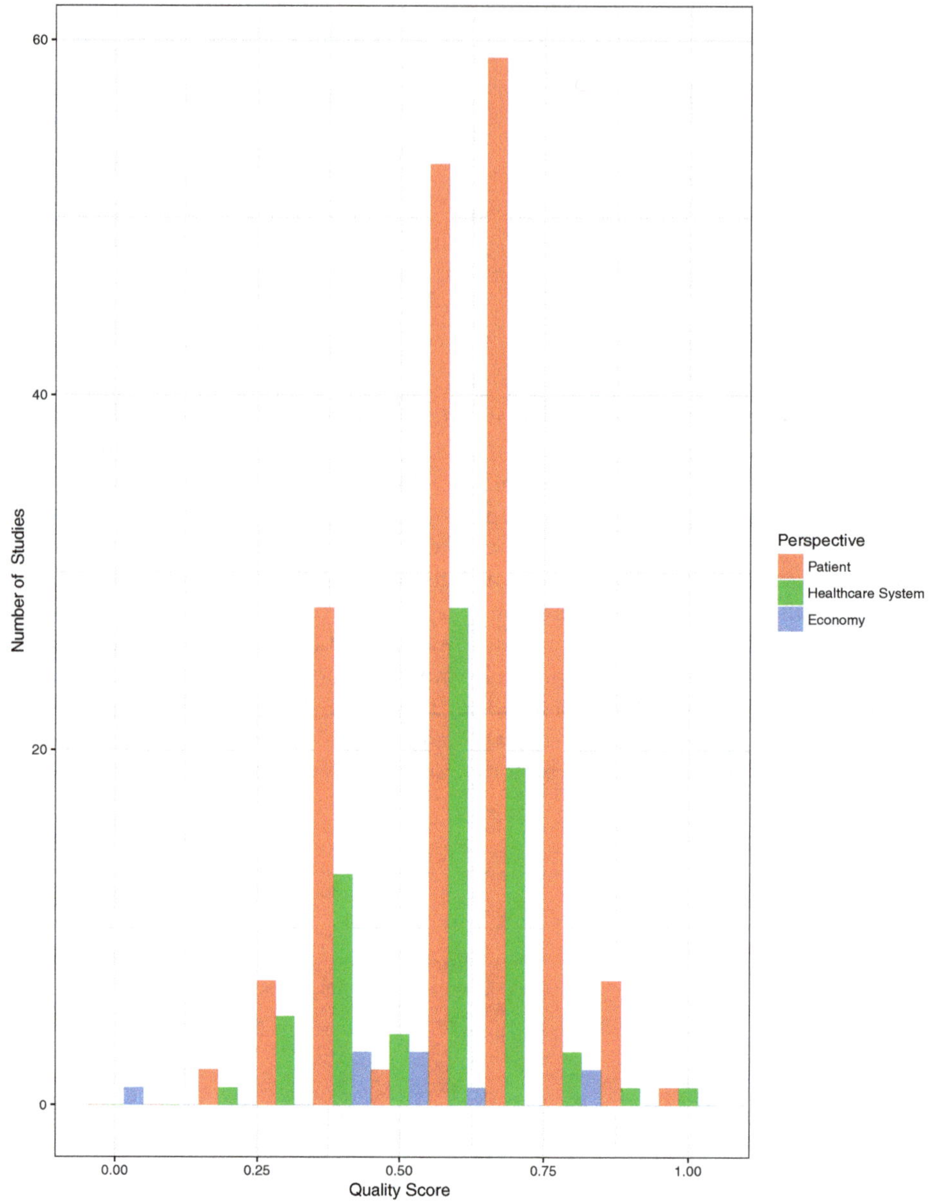

Fig. 5 Histograms of Quality Assessment Scores by Study Perspective

model has been tested thoroughly before use?" [31]. Additionally, only 23% of studies used a lifetime horizon or justified why they didn't use it and only 15% demonstrated a systematic approach to parameter selection.

Box 1: Across Perspectives: A Tuberculosis Case Study

To illustrate the importance of clarifying the perspective chosen when investigating the burden of AMR, the case of multidrug resistant (MDR-) and extensively drug resistant (XDR-) Tuberculosis (TB) will be used, as studies of this infection-type provided cost estimates (monetary costs are 2013 USD) across perspectives (for full study details refer to Additional file 1: Table S4).

Patient burden: In Peruvian adult patients, it was estimated that MDR-TB was significantly associated with mortality [HR = 7.5 (95% CI; 4.1 – 13.4)]

(Continued)

using regional network data [144]. Likewise, in American patients, using data from a national institute, XDR was found to be significantly associated with mortality [HR = 2.8 (95% CI; 1.4 – 5.4)] [145]. In South African adult patients from one hospital, both MDR and XDR were associated with increased mortality [MDR HR = 3.37, $p < 0.0001$, and XDR HR = 6.75, $p < 0.001$] [146]. All of the aforementioned studies looking into TB and mortality utilised a Cox proportional hazards approach. Another study utilised a Kaplan-Meier survival analysis methodology, and found that capromycin resistance in XDR TB was not significantly associated with mortality ($p < 0.0573$) [147]. Using Israeli patient data from a national registry, MDR was found to be significantly associated with TB-related death [OR = 2.83(95% CI; 1.70-4.72), $p < 0.001$], using a logistic regression approach [148].

Healthcare system burden: MDR-TB was estimated to cost the South African healthcare system $6728 excess per case, $33,291 total per case

(Continued)

in Latvia and $86,321 total per case in Germany using an evidence synthesis approach [135–137]. These studies included factors such as length of stay, drug costs and services consumed (varying between studies).

Economic burden: It was estimated, by evidence synthesis and stepwise calculation, that the total economic and societal burden costs per case for the original EU-15 states (i.e. healthcare system costs plus productivity loss, compared to susceptible TB) from MDR and XDR TB were $62,931 and $215,038 [143]. MDR-TB was also found to be independently associated with incurring catastrophic costs in Peruvian patients older than 15 years [OR = 1.61 (95% CI = 0.98–2.64)], whereby catastrophic costs were defined as total costs greater than or equal to 20% of household annual income. Costs included direct medical and non-medical out-of-pocket costs (such as excess transport and food) [43].

Discussion

The first aim of this review was to establish what perspectives and resulting methodologies have been used to estimate AMR burden in recent literature and to discern the impact this has on the actual estimates of burden. This review found that out of the 214 studies included, 187 studies provided an estimate of burden from the health perspective, 75 studies from the healthcare system perspective and 11 studies from the economic perspective. This review describes the large range of estimates that fall within these categories, and the methodologies used to obtain them. The most utilised methodologies were regression analysis for patient health and healthcare system burden calculations and either stepwise calculations or multistate models for economic burden estimates. An additional aim of this paper was to assess the quality of evidence for health, healthcare system and economic burden. There was a lack of economic burden studies, with the median quality score of these studies being lower than those of the health and healthcare system studies.

AMR is thought to potentially impact patient health through increasing patient mortality, though only around 50% of studies found a statistically significant impact when comparing resistant and susceptible infections. A substantial proportion of studies which used parametric regression or Cox proportional hazards techniques to estimate the impact of resistant infections in Gram-negative bacteria on mortality through OR or HR measures, had high uncertainty.

Evidence on additional length of hospital stay, a key driver of cost of infections in hospitals, was variable in terms of methodological choice and values found. A large proportion of the studies addressing length of stay in a healthcare facility did not explicitly state excess or associated length of stay, but rather estimated average length of stay for different groups and performed univariate comparisons of these averages. For those that did estimate excess length of stay, it was expected (given previous literature [28]) that multistate model length of stay estimates compared to those found using alternative methods would be more conservative. However, this review found that multistate model estimates for length of stay for MRSA infection and MRSA bloodstream infection were higher than those using stepwise analysis and regression analysis [48, 50, 58, 59]. This is likely due to the fact that the described studies were set in different countries (Australia, Germany, Switzerland and US) and were mainly single centre studies, and so less externally valid. The use of multistate modelling methods to estimate attributable health and cost burden for resistant infections has previously been recommended because standard regression techniques may overstate the attributable length of stay for hospital onset infections, thus overestimating burden of AMR [28, 60]. However, we demonstrate that very few studies took advantage of this method over the search period.

Due to the small sample of economic burden studies, no consensus on method can be stated for estimating the economic burden, though 6 out of the 11 studies did utilise evidence synthesis and stepwise approaches or multistate models. The median quality of studies quantifying the economic burden of AMR fell below those of health and healthcare system burden studies, seemingly mainly due to a lack of rigorous, transparent modelling studies which appropriately present or incorporate uncertainty.

The recent reports produced by the 'The Review on Antimicrobial Resistance' attempted to address the lack of economic burden estimates in the field of AMR [1, 15, 55]. However due to the large scope of these projects the models used provide only broad, general estimates (such as the global economic burden of AMR in general) which may be unsuitable for cost-effectiveness or resource allocation models. The review itself calls for the estimates to be developed using more data-driven approaches [1]. This type of analysis has also recently been called into question due to its lack of scientific scrutiny and transparency, questioning the methodology used [7].

Based on the results of this study, focusing on the results of the quality assessment of included studies, the following actions are recommended for future research in AMR burden;

1. Utilise data from a representative sample of the population of interest. If this is not achievable due to data limitations, create and publish a clearly defined protocol that can be utilised in other institutions. This will enable future meta-analyses to be conducted.
2. Choose an appropriate methodology that takes into account potential confounding factors (such as patient comorbidities or age) and biases (such

as time dependency bias, competing risks or non-informative censoring).
3. Describe data collection, data cleaning, follow-up, response rates and/or censoring clearly, where appropriate.
4. Estimate healthcare system and economic impact where possible.
5. If performing a mathematical or economic model, clearly describe the reasons for the chosen model structure (for example by detailing a formal health economic reasoning, including for chosen time horizon) and methods of parameterisation (with structured or systematic methods preferred). In addition, it is important to discuss how methodological, structural, heterogeneity and parameter uncertainty has been addressed (or discuss why these were not addressed).

Smith and Coast reported that estimates ranged from less than $15 to around $50,000 for additional costs per patient per episode to about $20 billion per year from the societal/economic perspective (converted to 2013 USD) [8]. This review found the healthcare system excess costs ranged from just almost non-significance to over $90 million per year, whilst economic costs ranged from just over $100,000 per case to over $3 trillion total GDP loss by 2050 (in 2013 USD). Adding to the 21 studies included in the Smith and Coast 2012 review, this review discusses the results from an additional 214 studies. This review encountered a similar result to that of Smith and Coast in terms of lack of indirect burden evidence [8]. However this review did find additional evidence on the potential secondary effects of AMR, with studies estimating the potential secondary effect of AMR on health and economic burden [1, 12].

Strengths of this review include its rigorous systematic methodology and its use of accepted quality assessment scales to present the first systematic picture of the quality of recent AMR burden estimates. This is particularly important when establishing the current evidence, as previously published review studies in this area have either been commentary pieces or have not incorporated any quality assessment across all three perspectives [8, 9, 18]. One limitation of this study is that is has a relatively short search time period. This was chosen to build upon rather than duplicate the evidence produced within a previous review, and to capture recent evidence [8]. Other limitations of the review include that the Health Related Quality of Life was not included as an outcome of interest. This was beyond the scope of this review given the very different methodologies applied in order to estimate Health Related Quality of Life burden, and that the majority of discussion of patient burden currently surrounds mortality impact.

Conclusion

This study concludes that perspective affects chosen methodology and outcome for quantifying the burden of AMR. The review finds substantially more research in patient burden and seemingly more of a consensus on the most appropriate methods to use (regression or survival techniques), in comparison to healthcare system and economic burden research. However, across patient and healthcare system burden studies, a worryingly high number of studies are utilising univariate statistical significance tests, suggesting that a high proportion of this evidence is unreliable. The review also concludes that the evidence on the economic burden of AMR is not substantial, whereby the majority of studies have not used established health economic modelling techniques or adhered well to the Philip's checklist [31]. More evidence on the secondary effect of AMR on health, healthcare system and economic burden is also needed [1, 12].

The estimates presented in this review can be used as parameter inputs in future health economics models used to inform health policy, whilst the description of previous methods used can inform future researchers' methodology choice (based on their desired perspective). The review also highlights key areas where research is needed, including multivariate, internally and externally valid health and healthcare system burden studies. This research is needed particularly for Gram-negative bacteria. Additionally, high quality economic burden and secondary burden research is needed in general. Future AMR burden research should follow the recommendations highlighted in this review, in order to increase the quality of evidence available.

Abbreviations

3GCR: Third-generation cephalosporin resistant; *A. baumannii*: *Acinetobacter baumannii*; AC: Amoxicilline-clavulanate; Allo-HSCT: Allogeneic hematopoietic stem cell transplantation; AMR: Antimicrobial Resistance; BIVR: Beta-lactam induced vancomycin resistance; BSI: Bloodstream infection; CR: Carbapenem resistant; CRAB: Carbapenem-resistant *Acinetobacter baumannii*; CRKP: Carbapenem-resistant *Klebsiella pneumoniae*; *E. coli*: *Escherichia coli*; ESBL: Extended Spectrum Beta-lactamase; EUR: Euro; GDP: Gross Domestic Product; GN: Gram-negative; HR: Hazard ratio; hVISA: Heterogeneous vancomycin-intermediate *Staphylococcus aureus*; ICU: Intensive care unit; IQR: Interquartile range; *K. pneumoniae*: *Klebsiella pneumoniae*; KPC: *Klebsiella pneumoniae* Carbapenemase; LoS: Length of stay; MBL: Metallo-beta-lactamase; MDR: Multidrug resistance; MIC: Minimum inhibitory concentration; MLSR: Macrolide-lincosamide-streptogramin resistance; MRSA: Methicillin resistant *Staphylococcus aureus*; MSSA: Methicillin susceptible *Staphylococcus aureus*; NDM-1: New Delhi Metallo-beta-lactamase-1; OR: Odds ratio; *P. aeruginosa*: *Pseudomonas aeruginosa*; PDR: Pan drug resistant; res.: Resistant; *S. aureus*: *Staphylococcus aureus*; sus.: Susceptible; TB: Tuberculosis; USD: United States Dollars; UTI: Urinary tract infection; VAP: Ventilator associated pneumonia; VRE: Vancomycin resistant *Enterococcus*; VSE: Vancomycin susceptible *Enterococcus*; XDR: Extensively drug resistant

Acknowledgements

The authors would like to acknowledge Prof Alison Holmes and Dr Ceire Costelloe for their guidance in correspondence to the nature of this review and systematic literature reviews in general.

Funding
The research was funded by the National Institute for Health Research Health Protection Research Unit (NIHR HPRU) in Healthcare Associated Infections and Antimicrobial Resistance at Imperial College London in partnership with Public Health England (PHE). The views expressed are those of the author(s) and not necessarily those of the NHS, the NIHR, the Department of Health or Public Health England. More information on HPRU and current projects can be found on http://www.imperial.ac.uk/medicine/hpru-amr.

Authors' contributions
NN, GK, JR, RA, NZ, KK and SS created the final protocol. NN performed the searches, independent reviews, data collection and data analysis. NZ, KK and SS performed the independent reviews. All authors contributed to the drafting of the final manuscript, especially in how to present the results and data interpretation. All authors read and approved the final manuscript.

Authors' information
NN is currently undertaking a PhD funded by the National Institute for Health Research Health Protection Research Unit (NIHR HPRU) in Healthcare Associated Infections and Antimicrobial Resistance.

Consent for publication
Not applicable.

Competing interests
The authors declare that they have no competing interests.

Author details
[1]National Institute for Health Research Health Protection Research Unit in Healthcare Associated Infection and Antimicrobial Resistance at Imperial College, Hammersmith Campus, London W12 0NN, UK. [2]Imperial College London, Sir Alexander Fleming Building, South Kensington Campus, London, UK. [3]Harvard University, 665 Huntington Avenue, Boston, MA 02115, USA. [4]Modelling and Economics Unit, National Infection Service, Public Health England, 61 Colindale Avenue, London NW9 5EQ, UK.

References
1. The AMR Review. Antimicrobial Resistance : Tackling a crisis for the health and wealth of nations. 2014.
2. Public Health England. English surveillance programme for antimicrobial utilisation and resistance (ESPAUR); 2014. p. 1–143.
3. Centers for Disease Control and Prevention. Antibiotic resistance threats in the United States, 2013. Current. 2013:1–114.
4. European Food Safety Authority, European Centre for Disease Prevention and Control. The European Union Summary Report on antimicrobial resistance in Antimicrobial resistance in zoonotic and indicator bacteria from humans, animals and food in the European Union in 2014. EFSA J. 2016;14:1–207.
5. Public Health England. New report shows stark effect of antibiotic resistance [Internet]. 2014. Available from: https://www.gov.uk/government/news/new-report-shows-stark-effect-of-antibiotic-resistance. [cited 15 May 2016].
6. Husereau D, Drummond M PS. Consolidated health economic evaluation reporting standards (CHEERS)—Explanation and elaboration: A report of the ISPOR health economic evaluations publication guidelines good reporting practices task force. 2013.
7. de Kraker MEA, Stewardson AJ, Harbarth S. Will 10 Million People Die a Year due to Antimicrobial Resistance by 2050? PLoS Med. 2016;13:1–6.
8. Smith R, Coast J. The economic burden of antimicrobial resistance: why it is more serious than current studies suggest. London: London School of Hygiene & Tropical Medicine; 2012.
9. De Angelis G, D'Inzeo T, Fiori B, Spanu T, Sganga G. Burden of Antibiotic Resistant Gram Negative Bacterial Infections: Evidence and Limits. J Med Microbiol Diagn. 2014;3:1–6.
10. Jacobs P, Fassbender K. The measurement of indirect costs in the health economics evaluation literature. A review. Int J Technol Assess Health Care. 1998;14:799–808.
11. Tam CC, O'Brien SJ. Economic cost of campylobacter, norovirus and rotavirus disease in the United Kingdom. PLoS One. 2016;11:1–12.
12. Teillant A, Gandra S, Barter D, Morgan DJ, Laxminarayan R. Potential burden of antibiotic resistance on surgery and cancer chemotherapy antibiotic prophylaxis in the USA: A literature review and modelling study. Lancet Infect Dis. 2015;15:1429–37.
13. Lambert ML, Suetens C, Savey A, Palomar M, Hiesmayr M, Morales I, et al. Clinical outcomes of health-care-associated infections and antimicrobial resistance in patients admitted to European intensive-care units: A cohort study. Lancet Infect Dis. 2011;11:30–8.
14. Alam MF, Cohen D, Butler C, Dunstan F, Roberts Z, Hillier S, et al. The additional costs of antibiotics and re-consultations for antibiotic-resistant Escherichia coli urinary tract infections managed in general practice. Int J Antimicrob Agents. 2009;33:255–7.
15. KPMG. The global economic impact of antimicrobial resistance. 2014.
16. Yao Z, Peng Y, Chen X, Bi J, Li Y, Ye X, et al. Healthcare associated infections of Methicillin-resistant Staphylococcus aureus: A case-control-control study. PLoS One. 2015;10:1–9.
17. Stewardson AJ, Allignol A, Beyersmann J, Graves N, Schumacher M, Meyer R, et al. The health and economic burden of bloodstream infections caused by antimicrobial-susceptible and non-susceptible Enterobacteriaceae and Staphylococcus aureus in European hospitals, 2010 and 2011: a multicentre retrospective cohort study. Eur Secur. 2016;21:1–12.
18. Gandra S, Barter DM, Laxminarayan R. Economic burden of antibiotic resistance: how much do we really know? Clin Microbiol Infect. 2014;20:973–80.
19. Cosgrove SE, Carmeli Y. The Impact of Antimicrobial Resistance on Health and Economic Outcomes. Clin Infect Dis. 2003;36:1433–7.
20. Wilton P, Smith R, Coast J, Millar M. Strategies to contain the emergence of antimicrobial resistance: a systematic review of effectiveness and cost-effectiveness. J Health Serv Res Policy. 2002;7:111–7.
21. Gallagher J. Antibiotic resistance: World on cusp of "post-antibiotic era" [Internet]. BBC. 2015. Available from: http://www.bbc.co.uk/news/health-34857015. [cited 1 Nov 2016].
22. Department of Health, Department for Environment Food and Rural Affairs. UK Five Year Antimicrobial Resistance Strategy 2013 to 2018. 2013.
23. Naylor N, Silva S, Kulasabanathan K, Atun R, Zhu N, Knight G, et al. How to estimate the burden of antimicrobial resistance: a systematic literature review [Internet]. PROSPERO. 2016. Available from: http://www.crd.york.ac.uk/PROSPERO/display_record.asp?ID=CRD42016037510. [cited 13 Jul 2016].
24. Moher D, Liberati A, Tetzlaff J, Altman DG, The PRISMA Group. Preferred Reporting Items for Systematic Reviews an Meta-Analyses: The PRISMA Statement. PLoS Med. 2009;6:1–2.
25. Naylor NR, Silva S, Kulasabanathan K, Atun R, Zhu N, Knight GM, et al. Methods for estimating the burden of antimicrobial resistance : a systematic literature review protocol. Syst Rev. 2016;5:187.
26. PubMed [Internet]. 2018. Available from: https://www.ncbi.nlm.nih.gov/pubmed/. [cited 10 Jan 2018].
27. Takizawa C, Thompson PL, Van Walsem A. Epidemiological and Economic Burden of Alzheimer ' s Disease : A Systematic Literature Review of Data across Europe and the United States of America. J Alzheimers Dis. 2015;43:1271–84.
28. Graves N, Harbarth S, Beyersmann J, Barnett A, Halton K, Cooper B. Estimating the cost of health care-associated infections: mind your p's and q's. Clin Infect Dis. 2010;50:1017–21.
29. Wells G., Shea B, O'Connell D, Peterson J, Welch V, Losos M, et al. The Newcastle-Ottawa Scale (NOS) for assessing the quality of nonrandomised studies in meta-analyses [Internet]. University of Ottawa. 2014. Available from: http://www.ohri.ca/programs/clinical_epidemiology/oxford.asp. [cited 1 Feb 2016].
30. Song J, Chung K. Observational Studies: Cohort and Case-Control Studies. Plast Reconstr Surg. 2011;126:2234–42.
31. Philips Z, Bojke L, Sculpher M, Claxton K, Golder S. Good Practice Guidelines for Decision-Analytic Modelling in Health Technology Assessment. PharmacoEconomics. 2006;24:355–71.
32. Higgins JPT, Green S. Cochrane Handbook for Systematic Reviews of Interventions Version 5.1.0 [updated March 2011]: The Cochrane Collaboration; 2011. Table 7.7.a: Formulae for combining groups
33. Rate Inflation. Historical Inflation Rates for Australia (2007 to 2017) [Internet]. 2017. Available from: http://www.rateinflation.com/inflation-rate/australia-historical-inflation-rate. [cited 10 Jan 2017].
34. Triami Media BV. Historic Inflatin - CPI inflation year pages [Internet]. inflation.eu. 2017. Available from: www.inflation.eu. [cited 12 Feb 2017].

35. UKForex. Yearly Average Rates [Internet]. 2017. Available from: www.ukforex.co.uk/forex-tools/historical-rate-tools/yearly-average-rates. [cited 12 Nov 2017].
36. Wickham H, Chang W, RStudio. ggplot2: Create Elegant Data Visualisations Using the Grammar of Graphics [Internet]. 2016. Available from: https://cran.r-project.org/package=ggplot2
37. Wickham H. The Split-Apply-Combine Strategy for Data Analysis. J Stat Softw. 2011;40:1–29.
38. Viechtbauer W. Package "metafor." 2017.
39. Bodro M, Sanclemente G, Lipperheide I, Allali M, Marco F, Bosch J, et al. Impact of antibiotic resistance on the development of recurrent and relapsing symptomatic urinary tract infection in kidney recipients. Am J Transplant. 2015;15:1021–7.
40. Qureshi ZA, Syed A, Clarke LG, Doi Y, Shields RK. Epidemiology and clinical outcomes of patients with carbapenem-resistant Klebsiella pneumoniae bacteriuria. Antimicrob Agents Chemother. 2014;58:1–18.
41. Vazirani J, Wurity S, Ali MH. Multidrug-resistant Pseudomonas aeruginosa keratitis: Risk factors, clinical characteristics, and outcomes. Ophthalmology. 2015;122:2110–4.
42. Francis JR, Blyth CC, Colby S, Fagan JM, Waring J. Multidrug-resistant tuberculosis in Western Australia, 1998–2012. Med J Aust. 2014;200:328–32.
43. Wingfield T, Boccia D, Tovar M, Gavino A, Zevallos K, Montoya R, et al. Defining Catastrophic Costs and Comparing Their Importance for Adverse Tuberculosis Outcome with Multi-Drug Resistance: A Prospective Cohort Study, Peru. PLoS Med. 2014;11:e1001675.
44. Rello J, Molano D, Villabon M, Reina R, Rita-Quispe R, Previgliano I, et al. Differences in hospital- and ventilator-associated pneumonia due to Staphylococcus aureus (methicillin-susceptible and methicillin-resistant) between Europe and Latin America: a comparison of the EUVAP and LATINVAP study cohorts. Med Intensiva. 2013;37:241–7.
45. Esteve-Palau E, Solande G, Sanchez F, Sorli L, Montero M, Guerri R, et al. Clinical and economic impact of urinary tract infections caused by ESBL-producing Escherichia coli requiring hospitalization: A matched cohort study. J Infect. 2015;71:667–74.
46. Ong SJ, Huang Y-C, Tan H-Y, Ma DHK, Lin H-C, Yeh L-K, et al. Staphylococcus aureus Keratitis: A Review of Hospital Cases. PLoS One. 2013;8:e80119.
47. Kini AR, Shetty V, Kumar AM, Shetty SM, Shetty A. Community-associated, methicillin-susceptible, and methicillin-resistant Staphylococcus aureus bone and joint infections in children. J Pediatr Orthop B. 2013;22:158–66.
48. Barnett AG, Page K, Campbell M, Martin E, Rashleigh-Rolls R, Halton K, et al. The increased risks of death and extra lengths of hospital and ICU stay from hospital-acquired bloodstream infections: a case-control study. BMJ Open. 2013;3:e003587.
49. Stewardson A, Fankhauser C, De Angelis G, Rohner P, Safran E, Schrenzel J, et al. Burden of bloodstream infection caused by extended-spectrum β-lactamase-producing enterobacteriaceae determined using multistate modeling at a Swiss University Hospital and a nationwide predictive model. Infect Control Hosp Epidemiol. 2013;34:133–43.
50. Macedo-Viñas M, De Angelis G, Rohner P, Safran E, Stewardson A, Fankhauser C, et al. Burden of meticillin-resistant Staphylococcus aureus infections at a Swiss University hospital: excess length of stay and costs. J Hosp Infect. 2013;84:132–7.
51. Nelson RE, Samore MH, Jones M, Greene T, Stevens VW, Liu CF, et al. Reducing Time-dependent Bias in Estimates of the Attributable Cost of Health Care-associated Methicillin-resistant Staphylococcus aureus Infections: A Comparison of Three Estimation Strategies. Med Care. 2015;53:827–34.
52. Leistner R, Gürntke S, Sakellariou C, Denkel LA, Bloch A, Gastmeier P, et al. Bloodstream infection due to extended-spectrum beta-lactamase (ESBL)-positive K. pneumoniae and E. coli: an analysis of the disease burden in a large cohort. Infection. 2014;42:991–7.
53. Branch-Elliman W, Lee GM, Golen TH, Gold HS, Baldini LM, Wright SB. Health and Economic Burden of Post-Partum Staphylococcus aureus Breast Abscess. PLoS One. 2013;8:1–7.
54. Morris MD, Quezada L, Bhat P, Moser K, Smith J, Perez H, et al. Social, Economic, and Psychological Impacts of MDR-TB Treatment in Tijuana, Mexico: A Patient's Perspective. Int J Tuberc Lung Dis. 2013;17:954–60.
55. Taylor J, Hafner M, Yerushalmi E, Smith R, Bellasio J, Vardavas R, et al. Estimating the economic costs of antimicrobial resistance. 2014.
56. Lee JY, Chong YP, Kim T, Hong HL, Park SJ, Lee ES, et al. Bone and joint infection as a predictor of community-acquired methicillin-resistant Staphylococcus aureus bacteraemia: A comparative cohort study. J Antimicrob Chemother. 2014;69:1966–71.
57. Lee BY, Singh A, David MZ, Bartsch SM, Slayton RB, Huang SS, et al. The economic burden of community-associated methicillin-resistant Staphylococcus aureus (CA-MRSA). Clin Microbiol Infect. 2013;19:528–36.
58. Hübner C, Hübner NO, Hopert K, Maletzki S, Flessa S. Analysis of MRSA-attributed costs of hospitalized patients in Germany. Eur J Clin Microbiol Infect Dis. 2014;33:1817–22.
59. Shorr AF, Zilberberg MD, Micek ST, Kollef MH. Outcomes associated with bacteremia in the setting of methicillin-resistant Staphylococcus aureus pneumonia: a retrospective cohort study. Crit Care. 2015;19:312.
60. Graves N, Weinhold D, Roberts JA. Correcting for bias when estimating the cost of hospital-acquired infection: an analysis of lower respiratory tract infections in non-surgical patients. Health Econ. 2005;14:755–61.
61. Rieg S, Jonas D, Kaasch AJ, Porzelius C, Peyerl-Hoffmann G, Theilacker C, et al. Microarray-Based Genotyping and Clinical Outcomes of Staphylococcus aureus Bloodstream Infection: An Exploratory Study. PLoS One. 2013;8:e71259.
62. Manandhar S, Pai G, Gidwani H, Nazim S, Buehrle D, Shutt KA, et al. Does Staphylococcus aureus Bacteriuria Predict Clinical Outcomes in Patients With Bacteremia? Analysis of 274 Patients With Staphylococcus aureus Blood Stream Infection. Infect Dis Clin Pract. 2016;24:151–4.
63. Theodorou P, Lefering R, Perbix W, Spanholtz TA, Maegele M, Spilker G, et al. Staphylococcus aureus bacteremia after thermal injury: The clinical impact of methicillin resistance. Burns. 2013;39:404–12.
64. Cobos-Carrascosa E, Soler-Palacín P, Nieves Larrosa M, Bartolomé R, Martín-Nalda A, Antoinette Frick M, et al. Staphylococcus aureus Bacteremia in Children. Pediatr Infect Dis J. 2015;34:1329–34.
65. Hernández C, Feher C, Soriano A, Marco F, Almela M, Cobos-Trigueros N, et al. Clinical characteristics and outcome of elderly patients with community-onset bacteremia. The Journal of infection. 2014;70:135–43.
66. Okada Y, Hosono M, Sasaki Y, Hirai H, Suehiro S. Preoperative increasing C-reactive protein affects the outcome for active infective endocarditis. Ann Thorac Cardiovasc Surg. 2014;20:48–54.
67. Yavuz SŞ, Şensoy A, Çeken S, Deniz D, Yekeler I. Methicillin-resistant Staphylococcus aureus infection: An independent risk factor for mortality in patients with poststernotomy mediastinitis. Med Princ Pract. 2014;23:517–23.
68. Sakoda Y, Ikegame S, Ikeda-Harada C, Takakura K, Kumazoe H, Wakamatsu K, et al. Retrospective analysis of nursing and healthcare-associated pneumonia: Analysis of adverse prognostic factors and validity of the selection criteria. Respiratory Investigation. 2014;52:114–20.
69. Takata T, Miyazaki M, Futo M, Hara S, Shiotsuka S, Kamimura H, et al. Presence of both heterogeneous vancomycin-intermediate resistance and β-lactam antibiotic-induced vancomycin resistance phenotypes is associated with the outcome in methicillin-resistant Staphylococcus aureus bloodstream infection. Scand J Infect Dis. 2013;45:203–12.
70. Hu H-C, Kao K-C, Chiu L-C, Chang C-H, Hung C-Y, Li L-F, et al. Clinical outcomes and molecular typing of heterogenous vancomycin-intermediate Staphylococcus aureus bacteremia in patients in intensive care units. BMC Infect Dis. 2015;15:444.
71. Lee H-Y, Chen C-L, Liu S-Y, Yan Y-S, Chang C-J, Chiu C-H. Impact of Molecular Epidemiology and Reduced Susceptibility to Glycopeptides and Daptomycin on Outcomes of Patients with Methicillin-Resistant Staphylococcus aureus Bacteremia. PLoS One. 2015;10:e0136171.
72. Lee JK, Lee J, Park YS, Lee CH, Yim JJ, Yoo CG, et al. Clinical manifestations of pneumonia according to the causative organism in patients in the intensive care unit. Korean J Intern Med. 2015;30:829–36.
73. Hope R, Blackburn RM, Verlander NQ, Johnson A, Kearns A, Hill R, et al. Vancomycin MIC as a predictor of outcome in MRSA bacteraemia in the UK context. J Antimicrob Chemother. 2013;68:2641–7.
74. Tadros M, Williams V, Coleman BL, McGeer AJ, Haider S, Lee C, et al. Epidemiology and Outcome of Pneumonia Caused by Methicillin-Resistant Staphylococcus aureus (MRSA) in Canadian Hospitals. PLoS One. 2013;8:4–11.
75. Castón JJ, González-Gasca F, Porras L, Illescas S, Romero MD, Gijón J. High vancomycin minimum inhibitory concentration is associated with poor outcome in patients with methicillin-susceptible Staphylococcus aureus bacteremia regardless of treatment. Scand J Infect Dis. 2014;46:783–6.
76. Cheah ALY, Spelman T, Liew D, Peel T, Howden BP, Spelman D, et al. Enterococcal bacteraemia: Factors influencing mortality, length of stay and costs of hospitalization. Clin Microbiol Infect. 2013;19:E181–9.
77. Kang C-I, Song J-H, Kim SH, Chung DR, Peck KR, Thamlikitkul V, et al.

Association of levofloxacin resistance with mortality in adult patients with invasive pneumococcal diseases: a post hoc analysis of a prospective cohort. Infection. 2013;41:151–7.
78. Fu Q, Ye H, Liu S. Risk factors for extensive drug-resistance and mortality in geriatric inpatients with bacteremia caused by Acinetobacter baumannii. Am J Infect Control. 2015;43:857–60.
79. Kitazono H, Rog D, Sa G, Nm C, Acinetobacter RGE. Acinetobacter baumannii infection in solid organ transplant recipients. Clin Transpl. 2015: 227–32.
80. Park SY, Choo JW, Kwon SH, Yu SN, Lee EJ, Kim TH, et al. Risk Factors for Mortality in Patients with Acinetobacter baumannii Bacteremia. Infect Chemother. 2013;45:325–30.
81. De Jager P, Chirwa T, Naidoo S, Perovic O, Thomas J. Nosocomial outbreak of New Delhi metallo-Beta-lactamase-1-producing Gram-negative bacteria in South Africa: A case-control study. PLoS One. 2015;10:1–12.
82. Zhang HT, Liu H. Laboratory-based evaluation of MDR strains of Pseudomonas in patients with acute burn injuries. Int J Clin Exp Med. 2015;8:16512–9.
83. Samonis G, Vardakas KZ, Kofteridis DP, Dimopoulou D, Andrianaki AM, Chatzinikolaou I, et al. Characteristics, risk factors and outcomes of adult cancer patients with extensively drug-resistant Pseudomonas aeruginosa infections. Infection. 2014;42:721–8.
84. Theodorou P, Thamm O, Perbix W, Phan V. Pseudomonas aeruginosa bacteremia after burn injury: The impact of multiple-drug resistance. J Burn Care Res. 2013;34:649–58.
85. Micek ST, Kollef MH, Torres A, Chen C, Rello J, Chastre J, et al. Pseudomonas aeruginosa Nosocomial Pneumonia: Impact of Pneumonia Classification. Infect Control Hosp Epidemiol. 2015;36:1190–7.
86. Keddy KH, Sooka A, Musekiwa A, Smith AM, Ismail H, Tau NP, et al. Clinical and microbiological features of salmonella meningitis in a South African Population, 2003-2013. Clin Infect Dis. 2015;61:S272–82.
87. Tumbarello M, Trecarichi EM, De Rosa FG, Giannella M, Giacobbe DR, Bassetti M, et al. Infections caused by KPC-producing Klebsiella pneumoniae: Differences in therapy and mortality in a multicentre study. J Antimicrob Chemother. 2014;70:2133–43.
88. Capone A, Giannella M, Fortini D, Giordano A, Meledandri M, Ballardini M, et al. High rate of colistin resistance among patients with carbapenem-resistant Klebsiella pneumoniae infection accounts for an excess of mortality. Clin Microbiol Infect. 2013;19:E23–30.
89. Hussein K, Raz-Pasteur A, Finkelstein R, Neuberger A, Shachor-Meyouhas Y, Oren I, et al. Impact of carbapenem resistance on the outcome of patients' hospital-acquired bacteraemia caused by Klebsiella pneumoniae. J Hosp Infect. 2013;83:307–13.
90. Biehle LR, Cottreau JM, Thompson DJ, Filipek RL, O'Donnell JN, Lasco TM, et al. Outcomes and risk factors for mortality among patients treated with carbapenems for klebsiella spp. bacteremia. PLoS One. 2015;10:6–13.
91. Andria N, Henig O, Kotler O, Domchenko A, Oren I, Zuckerman T, et al. Mortality burden related to infection with carbapenem-resistant Gram-negative bacteria among haematological cancer patients: A retrospective cohort study. J Antimicrob Chemother. 2015;70:3146–53.
92. Papadimitriou-Olivgeris M, Marangos M, Fligou F, Christofidou M, Sklavou C, Vamvakopoulou S, et al. KPC-producing Klebsiella pneumoniae enteric colonization acquired during intensive care unit stay: the significance of risk factors for its development and its impact on mortality. Diagn Microbiol Infect Dis. 2013;77:169–73.
93. Abernethy JK, Johnson AP, Guy R, Hinton N, Sheridan EA, Hope RJ. Thirty day all-cause mortality in patients with Escherichia coli bacteraemia in England. Clin Microbiol Infect. 2015;21:251. e1-251.e8
94. Bergin SP, Thaden JT, Ericson JE, Cross H, Messina J, Clark RH, et al. Neonatal Escherichia coli Bloodstream Infections: Clinical Outcomes and Impact of Initial Antibiotic Therapy. Pediatr Infect Dis J. 2015;34:933–6.
95. Denis B, Lafaurie M, Donay JL, Fontaine JP, Oksenhendler E, Raffoux E, et al. Prevalence, risk factors, and impact on clinical outcome of extended-spectrum beta-lactamase-producing Escherichia coli bacteraemia: A five-year study. Int J Infect Dis. 2015;39:1–6.
96. Kim S-H, Kwon J-C, Choi S-M, Lee D-G, Park SH, Choi J-H, et al. Escherichia coli and Klebsiella pneumoniae bacteremia in patients with neutropenic fever: factors associated with extended-spectrum β-lactamase production and its impact on outcome. Ann Hematol. 2013;92:533–41.
97. Rodríguez-Baño J, Mingorance J, Fernández-Romero N, Serrano L, López-Cerero L, Pascual A. Outcome of bacteraemia due to extended-spectrum β-lactamase-producing Escherichia coli: Impact of microbiological determinants. J Infect. 2013;67:27–34.
98. Ha YE, Kang C-Il, Cha MK, Park SY, Wi YM, Chung DR, et al. Epidemiology and clinical outcomes of bloodstream infections caused by extended-spectrum β-lactamase-producing Escherichia coli in patients with cancer. Int J Antimicrob Agents. 2015;42:403–9.
99. Hernandez C, Cobos-Trigueros N, Feher C, Morata L, De La Calle C, Marco F, et al. Community-onset bacteraemia of unknown origin: clinical characteristics, epidemiology and outcome. Eur J Clin Microbiol Infect Dis. 2014;33:1973–80.
100. Seboxa T, Amogne W, Abebe W, Tsegaye T, Azazh A, Hailu W, et al. High mortality from blood stream infection in Addis Ababa, Ethiopia, is due to antimicrobial resistance. PLoS One. 2015;10:1–14.
101. Chaulk J, Carbonneau M, Qamar H, Keough A, Chang HJ, Ma M, et al. Third-generation cephalosporin-resistant spontaneous bacterial peritonitis: a single-centre experience and summary of existing studies. Can J Gastroenterol Hepatol. 2014;28:83–8.
102. Huh K, Kang CI, Kim J, Cho SY, Ha YE, Joo EJ, et al. Risk factors and treatment outcomes of bloodstream infection caused by extended-spectrum cephalosporin-resistant Enterobacter species in adults with cancer. Diagn Microbiol Infect Dis. 2014;78:172–7.
103. Haeusler GM, Mechinaud F, Daley AJ, Starr M, Shann F, Connell TG, et al. Antibiotic-resistant Gram-negative Bacteremia in Pediatric Oncology Patients—Risk Factors and Outcomes. Pediatr Infect Dis J. 2013;32:723–6.
104. Nelson RE, Stevens VW, Jones M, Samore MH, Rubin MA. Health care associated methicillin-resistant Staphylococcus aureus infections increases the risk of postdischarge mortality. Am J Infect Control. 2015;43:38–43.
105. Nitta H, Beppu T, Itoyama A, Higashi T, Sakamoto K, Nakagawa S, et al. Poor outcomes after hepatectomy in patients with ascites infected by methicillin-resistant staphylococci. Journal of Hepatobiliary-Pancreatic Sciences. 2015; 22:166–76.
106. Tavadze M, Rybicki L, Mossad S, Avery R, Yurch M, Pohlman B, et al. Risk factors for vancomycin-resistant enterococcus bacteremia and its influence on survival after allogeneic hematopoietic cell transplantation. Bone Marrow Transplant. 2014;49:1310–6.
107. Cho S-Y, Lee D-G, Choi S-M, Kwon J-C, Kim S-H, Choi J-K, et al. Impact of vancomycin resistance on mortality in neutropenic patients with enterococcal bloodstream infection: a retrospective study. BMC Infect Dis. 2013;13:504.
108. Chusri S, Chongsuvivatwong V, Rivera JI, Silpapojakul K, Singkhamanan K, McNeil E, et al. Clinical Outcomes of Hospital-Acquired Infection with Acinetobacter nosocomialis and Acinetobacter pittii. Antimicrob Agents Chemother. 2014;58:4172–9.
109. Lemos EV, de la Hoz FP, Alvis N, Einarson TR, Quevedo E, Castañeda C, et al. Impact of carbapenem resistance on clinical and economic outcomes among patients with Acinetobacter baumannii infection in Colombia. Clin Microbiol Infect. 2014;20:174–80.
110. Inchai J, Pothirat C, Bumroongkit C, Limsukon A, Khositsakulchai W, Liwsrisakun C. Prognostic factors associated with mortality of drug-resistant Acinetobacter baumannii ventilator-associated pneumonia. Journal of Intensive Care. 2015;3:9.
111. Henig O, Weber G, Hoshen MB, Paul M, German L, Neuberger A, et al. Risk factors for and impact of carbapenem-resistant Acinetobacter baumannii colonization and infection: matched case-control study. Eur J Clin Microbiol. 2015;34:2063–8.
112. Freire MP, Van Der Heijden IM, do Prado GVB, Cavalcante LS, Boszczowski I, Bonazzi PR, et al. Polymyxin use as a risk factor for colonization or infection with polymyxin-resistant *Acinetobacter baumannii* after liver transplantation. Transpl Infect Dis. 2014;16:369–78.
113. Willmann M, Kuebart I, Marschal M, Schröppel K, Vogel W, Flesch I, et al. Effect of metallo-β-lactamase production and multidrug resistance on clinical outcomes in patients with Pseudomonas aeruginosa bloodstream infection: a retrospective cohort study. BMC Infect Dis. 2013;13:515.
114. Micek ST, Wunderink RG, Kollef MH, Chen C, Rello J, Chastre J, et al. An international multicenter retrospective study of Pseudomonas aeruginosa nosocomial pneumonia: Impact of multidrug resistance. Crit Care. 2015;19:219.
115. Simkins J, Muggia V, Cohen HW, Minamoto GY. Carbapenem-resistant *Klebsiella pneumoniae* infections in kidney transplant recipients: a case-control study. Transpl Infect Dis. 2014;16:775–82.
116. Pereira MR, Scully BF, Pouch SM, Uhlemann A-C, Goudie S, Emond JE, et al.

Risk factors and outcomes of carbapenem-resistant Klebsiella pneumoniae infections in liver transplant recipients. Liver Transpl. 2015;21:1511–9.

117. Pouch SM, Kubin CJ, Satlin MJ, Tsapepas DS, Lee JR, Dube G, et al. Epidemiology and outcomes of carbapenem-resistant Klebsiella pneumoniae bacteriuria in kidney transplant recipients. Transpl Infect Dis. 2015;17:800–9.
118. Gürntke S, Kohler C, Steinmetz I, Pfeifer Y, Eller C, Gastmeier P, et al. Molecular epidemiology of extended-spectrum beta-lactamase (ESBL)-positive Klebsiella pneumoniae from bloodstream infections and risk factors for mortality. J Infect Chemother. 2014;20:817–9.
119. Kim MJ, Song K-H, Kim N-H, Choe PG, Park WB, Bang JH, et al. Clinical outcomes of spontaneous bacterial peritonitis due to extended-spectrum beta-lactamase-producing Escherichia coli or Klebsiella pneumoniae: a retrospective cohort study. Hepatol Int. 2014;8:582–7.
120. Miles-Jay A, Butler-Wu S, Rowhani-Rahbar A, Pergam SA. Incidence rate of fluoroquinolone resistant gram-negative rod bacteremia among allogeneic hematopoietic cell transplant patients during an era of levofloxacin prophylaxis. Biol Blood Marrow Transplant. 2015;257:539–45.
121. Tedja R, Nowacki A, Fraser T, Fatica C, Griffiths L, Gordon S, et al. The impact of multidrug resistance on outcomes in ventilator-associated pneumonia. Am J Infect Control. 2014;42:542–5.
122. Issler-Fisher AC, McKew G, Fisher OM, Harish V, Gottlieb T, Maitz PKM. Risk factors for, and the effect of MRSA colonization on the clinical outcomes of severely burnt patients. Burns. 2015;41:1212–20.
123. Casapao AM, Leonard SN, Davis SL, Lodise TP, Patel N, Goff DA, et al. Clinical Outcomes in Patients with Heterogeneous Vancomycin-Intermediate Staphylococcus aureus Bloodstream Infection. Antimicrob Agents Chemother. 2013;57:4252–9.
124. MacVane SH, Tuttle LO, Nicolau DP. Impact of extended-spectrum β-lactamase-producing organisms on clinical and economic outcomes in patients with urinary tract infection. J Hosp Med. 2014;9:232–8.
125. Leistner R, Bloch A, Sakellariou C, Gastmeier P, Schwab F. Costs and length of stay associated with extended-spectrum β-lactamase production in cases of Escherichia coli bloodstream infection. J Glob Antimicrob Resist. 2014;2:107–9.
126. Sozen H, Caylak S, Cetinkaya M, Citil BE, Sahins C, Deliktas H, et al. Clinical and Economic Outcomes Associated with Urinary Tract Infections Caused by Extended Spectrum Beta-lactamase Producing Bacteria in a Tertiary Care Hospital. Stud Ethnomed. 2015;9:173–9.
127. Gulen TA, Guner R, Celikbilek N, Keske S, Tasyaran M. Clinical importance and cost of bacteremia caused by nosocomial multi drug resistant acinetobacter baumannii. Int J Infect Dis. 2015;38:32–5.
128. Joo E-JJ, Peck KRR, Ha YEE, Kim Y-SS, Song Y-GG, Lee S-SS, et al. Impact of acute kidney injury on mortality and medical costs in patients with meticillin-resistant Staphylococcus aureus bacteraemia: a retrospective, multicentre observational study. J Hosp Infect. 2013;83:300–6.
129. Kim C-J, Kim H-B, Oh M, Kim YYK, Kim A, Oh S-H, et al. The burden of nosocomial staphylococcus aureus bloodstream infection in South Korea: a prospective hospital-based nationwide study. BMC Infect Dis. 2014;14:590.
130. Nelson RE, Jones M, Liu C-F, Samore MH, Evans ME, Graves N, et al. The Impact of Healthcare-Associated Methicillin-Resistant Staphylococcus Aureus Infections on Post-Discharge Healthcare Costs and Utilization. Infect Control Hosp Epidemiol. 2015;36:534–42. 9p
131. Chandy SJ, Naik GS, Balaji V, Jeyaseelan V, Thomas K, Lundborg CS. High cost burden and health consequences of antibiotic resistance: The price to pay. J Infect Dev Ctries. 2014;8:1096–102.
132. Apostolopoulou E, Zikos D, Tselebis A, Drosatou X, Steganidis E, Xristodoulou A, et al. Clinical outcomes and economic variables in critically ill patients with bloodstream infections. Health Sci J. 2014;8
133. Lloyd-Smith P, Younger J, Lloyd-Smith E, Green H, Leung V, Romney MG. Economic analysis of vancomycin-resistant enterococci at a Canadian hospital: assessing attributable cost and length of stay. J Hosp Infect. 2013; 85:54–9.
134. Ford CD, Lopansri BK. Gazdik M a, Snow GL, Webb BJ, Konopa KL, et al. The clinical impact of vancomycin-resistant Enterococcus colonization and bloodstream infection in patients undergoing autologous transplantation. Transpl Infect Dis. 2015;17:688–94.
135. Diel R, Nienhaus A, Lampenius N, Rüsch-Gerdes S, Richter E. Cost of multi drug resistance tuberculosis in Germany. Respir Med. 2014;108:1677–87.
136. Pooran A, Pieterson E, Davids M, Theron G, Dheda K. What is the Cost of Diagnosis and Management of Drug Resistant Tuberculosis in South Africa? PLoS One. 2013;8:e54587.
137. Miller TTL, Cirule A, Wilson FA, Holtz TH, Riekstina V, Cain KP, et al. The value of effective public tuberculosis treatment: an analysis of opportunity costs associated with multidrug resistant tuberculosis in Latvia. Cost Eff Resour Alloc. 2013;11:9.
138. Cox H, Ramma L, Wilkinson L, Azevedo V, Sinanovic E. Cost per patient of treatment for rifampicin-resistant tuberculosis in a community-based programme in Khayelitsha, South Africa. Trop Med Int Health. 2015;20:1337–45.
139. Ford CD, Lopansri BK, Haydoura S, Snow G, Dascomb KK, Asch J, et al. Frequency, risk factors, and outcomes of vancomycin-resistant Enterococcus colonization and infection in patients with newly diagnosed acute leukemia: different patterns in patients with acute myelogenous and acute lymphoblastic leukemia. Infect Control Hosp Epidemiol. 2015;36:47–53.
140. Vasudevan A, Memon B, Mukhopadhyay A, Li J, Tambyah P. The costs of nosocomial resistant gram negative intensive care unit infections among patients with the systemic inflammatory response syndrome- a propensity matched case control study. Antimicrob Resist Infect Control. 2015;4:3.
141. Reynolds C, Finkelstein J, Ray G, Moore M, Huang S. Attributable healthcare utilization and cost of pneumoniae due to drug-resistant Streptococcus pneumoniae: a cost analysis. Antimicrob Resist Infect Control. 2014;3:16.
142. Lubell Y, Dondorp A, Guérin PJ, Drake T, Meek S, Ashley E, et al. Artemisinin resistance – modelling the potential human and economic costs. Malar J. 2014;13:452.
143. Diel R, Vandeputte J, De Vries G, Stillo J, Wanlin M, Nienhaus A. Costs of tuberculosis disease in the European Union: A systematic analysis and cost calculation. Eur Respir J. 2014;43:554–65.
144. Chung-Delgado K, Guillen-Bravo S, Revilla-Montag A, Bernabe-Ortiz A. Mortality among MDR-TB cases: Comparison with drug-susceptible tuberculosis and associated factors. PLoS One. 2015;10:1–10.
145. Ershova JV, Kurbatova EV, Moonan PK, Cegielski JP. Mortality Among Tuberculosis Patients With Acquired Resistance to Second-line Antituberculosis Drugs–United States, 1993-2008. Clin Infect Dis. 2014;59: 465–72.
146. Gandhi NR, Brust JCM, Moodley P, Weissman D, Heo M, Ning Y, et al. Minimal diversity of drug-resistant Mycobacterium tuberculosis strains, South Africa. Emerg Infect Dis. 2014;20:426–33.
147. O'Donnell MR, Pillay M, Pillay M, Werner L, Master I, Wolf A, et al. Primary capreomycin resistance is common and associated with early mortality in patients with extensively drug-resistant tuberculosis in KwaZulu-Natal, South Africa. J Acquir Immune Defic Syndr. 2015;69:536–43.
148. Shuldiner J, Leventhal A, Chemtob D, Mor Z. Mortality of tuberculosis patients during treatment in israel, 2000-2010. Int J Tuberc Lung Dis. 2014; 18:818–23.

17

Extended spectrum beta-lactamase mediated resistance in carriage and clinical gram-negative ESKAPE bacteria: a comparative study between a district and tertiary hospital in South Africa

Raspail Carrel Founou[1,2*], Luria Leslie Founou[1,3] and Sabiha Yusuf Essack[1]

Abstract

Background: Gram-negative ESKAPE bacteria are increasingly implicated in several difficult-to-treat infections in developed and developing countries. They are listed by the World Health Organization as resistant bacteria of critical priority in research.

Objectives: To determine the risk factors, prevalence, phenotypic profiles, genetic diversity and clonal relatedness of extended-spectrum β-lactamase (ESBL)-producing multi-drug resistant (MDR) Gram-negative ESKAPE bacteria in the faecal carriage and clinical samples from patients in an urban, tertiary and a rural, district hospital in uMgungundlovu District, KwaZulu-Natal, South Africa.

Methods: This study took place in a district and tertiary hospital during a two-months period from May to June 2017 in uMgungundlovu district, South Africa. Rectal swabs collected from hospitalized patients, at admission, after 48 h and at discharge (whenever possible) formed the carriage sample while clinical isolates routinely processed in the microbiological laboratory during the sampling period were also collected and formed the clinical sample. Gram-negative ESKAPE bacteria were screened for ESBL production on selective MacConkey agar and confirmed using ROSCO kits. Minimum inhibitory concentrations were determined, and real-time and multiplex polymerase chain reaction were used to ascertain the presence of bla_{CTX-M} group-1-2-9, bla_{CTX-M} group 8/25, bla_{SHV}, bla_{TEM}, $bla_{OXA-1-like}$, bla_{KPC}, bla_{VIM}, bla_{IMP}, bla_{GES} and AmpC genes. Genomic fingerprinting was also performed using ERIC-PCR. Risk factors for ESBL-mediating MDR Gram-negative ESKAPE colonization were ascertained by univariate and multivariate logistic regression analyses.

(Continued on next page)

* Correspondence: czangue@yahoo.fr
[1]Antimicrobial Research Unit, School of Health Sciences, College of Health Sciences, University of KwaZulu-Natal, Durban 4000, South Africa
[2]Department of Clinical Microbiology, Centre of Expertise and Biological Diagnostic of Cameroon, (CEDBCAM), Yaoundé, Cameroon
Full list of author information is available at the end of the article

(Continued from previous page)

Results: Overall prevalence of carriage of ESBL-mediating MDR Gram-negative ESKAPE was 37.21% (16/43), 42.31% (11/26) and 57.14% (4/7) at admission, after 48 h and at discharge respectively. The prevalence of ESBL-mediating MDR Gram-negative ESKAPE bacteria in faecal carriage (46%) was higher than clinical samples (28%). Colonization was mainly associated with the referral from district to tertiary hospital with high statistical significance (OR: 14.40, 95% CI 0.98–210.84). $bla_{\text{CTX-M-group-9}}$, $bla_{\text{CTX-M-group-1}}$ and bla_{SHV} were the main resistance genes identified. Several patients carried more than two different isolates. A *Klebsiella pneumoniae* (K1) clone was circulating within wards and between hospitals.

Conclusion: The study highlights the high prevalence of ESBL-mediating MDR Gram-negative ESKAPE bacteria in carriage and clinical samples among hospitalized patients in uMgungundlovu, South Africa. The wide dissemination of these resistant ESKAPE bacteria in hospitals necessitates improvements in routine screening and reinforcement of infection, prevention and control measures.

Keywords: Antibiotic resistance, ESKAPE bacteria, ESBLs, Carriage, Clonality, Hospitalized patients

Introduction

The selective pressure exerted using antibiotics and aggravated by the dearth of new active substances in the current therapeutic pipeline has led to a considerable increase in antibiotic resistance (ABR) worldwide [1, 2]. A small group of bacteria, i.e., *Enterococcus spp., Staphylococcus aureus, Klebsiella pneumoniae, Acinetobacter baumannii, Pseudomonas aeruginosa* and *Enterobacter spp.*, termed "ESKAPE" due to their ability to escape the activity of and develop high levels of resistance to multiple antibiotics, have recently gained global attention [3–5]. Of the six infamous ESKAPE pathogens, the four Gram-negative bacteria, i.e., *K. pneumoniae, A. baumannii, P. aeruginosa*, and *Enterobacter spp.*, have been associated with four major types of multi-drug resistance (MDR), namely extended-spectrum β-lactamase (ESBL)-producing *K. pneumoniae* and *Enterobacter spp.*, carbapenemase-producing *A. baumannii* and metallo-β-lactamase producing *P. aeruginosa* (MBL-PA) which limit therapeutic options and negatively affect clinical outcomes [3–6]. Several resistance genes have been associated with the emergence of ESBL-mediating MDR Gram-negative ESKAPE bacteria globally. The bacterial production of enzyme hydrolysing antibiotics, particularly β-lactam antibiotics, is the most common mechanism of resistance in Gram-negative ESKAPE. Beta-lactamase enzymes have emerged following chromosomal mutation and acquisition of resistance genes carried on diverse mobile genetic elements (MGEs) such as plasmids, integrons, insertion sequences, transposons, genomic islands and bacteriophages [7]. The common transferability of resistance amongst bacteria will likely be associated with increasing rates of MDR infections and carriage, although some gaps remain as to the dissemination of multi-drug resistant bacteria in the community and among hospitalized patients.

MDR is increasingly being detected in numerous Gram-negative bacteria because of the extensive antibiotic use in communities and hospitals. Despite considerable efforts for their containment, ESBL-mediating multi-drug resistant Gram-negative ESKAPE bacteria are increasingly implicated in several difficult-to-treat infections in both developed and developing countries [5, 6, 8, 9] and were recently listed by the World Health Organization (WHO) as resistant bacteria of critical priority in research [3, 7, 8, 10]. Hospitals remain the main reservoir while immune-compromised patients such as those suffering from diabetes, chronic lung, kidney and cardiovascular diseases and cancers are the most affected. Whilst a better understanding on the impact of faecal carriage of ESBL-mediated resistance to Gram-negative ESKAPE bacteria is required, carriage is recognized as a potential risk for transmission and on subsequent development of infections especially in healthcare settings in developing countries due to inadequate infection, prevention and control measures.

In the African continent, antimicrobial resistance issue in general and MDR particularly, has not been adequately illustrated yet due limited financial resources. Knowledge of the burden of multidrug-resistant bacteria in South Africa could thus be valuable both to raise awareness on the necessity to prevent the spread of resistant infections in communities and hospitals, and to ameliorate empirical antibiotic therapy and clinical practice. This study seeks to compare the prevalence of faecal carriage of ESBL-mediated MDR Gram-negative ESKAPE bacteria among patients hospitalized in an urban, tertiary and a rural, district hospital in uMgungundlovu District, South Africa. In addition, the study is an attempt to provide insight into the risk factors associated with this carriage. Finally, the study assesses the phenotypic and genotypic characteristics and clonal relatedness of carriage and clinical ESBL-mediated MDR Gram-negative ESKAPE bacteria.

Materials and methods

Study population and settings

This study was conducted in a rural, district and urban, tertiary hospital, encoded for ethical reasons as H1 and

H2, respectively, during 2 months from May 2017 to June 2017 in uMgungundlovu district, South Africa. The district hospital (H1) represents the smallest level of hospital and provides four services including obstetrics and gynaecology, paediatrics and child health, general surgery and general medicine with 141 beds. In contrast, the tertiary hospital (H2) offers several specialties, receives referral patients according to a nationally agreed referral plan and has approximately 505 beds.

Patient enrolment and questionnaire survey

Total sampling was performed for the recruitment of participants i.e. all patients older than 18 years old, hospitalized in medical or surgical ward of the hospitals H1 and H2, and willing to participate were included in the study. Oral and written informed consent was obtained from all study participants after explanation of the procedure and purpose of the study. Patient information was gleaned from questionnaires completed by patients and data from patient records. Information was codified prior to analysis to maintain confidentiality.

Sample collection

Sample collection took place in both surgical and general medical wards during a two-month period, 1 month at each of the hospitals. Rectal swabs that were collected aseptically with Amies swabs from symptomatic in-patients, at three-time points, at admission, after 48 h and at discharge (whenever possible) formed the carriage sample. Isolates from symptomatic patients originating from tissue, blood, urine, intravenous catheters, and sputum routinely processed in the microbiological laboratory during the sampling period formed the clinical sample.

Definitions of terms

The specimen (blood, urine, sputum, tissue, intravenous catheter tips, fluid/aspirate and superficial swab) collected for diagnostic purpose from a symptomatic hospitalized patient was considered clinical sample. The clinical isolates were recovered from clinical samples obtained from patients hospitalized in various units of the selected hospitals. In contrast, carriage sample was the rectal swab collected from hospitalized patients at different time-points (admission, after 48 h and at discharge) out of diagnostic tests performed at hospitals.

Laboratory analysis

Identification of gram-negative ESKAPE bacteria

During the sample collection, all rectal swabs were cultured onto MacConkey agar with and without cefotaxime (2 mg/L). After incubation for 18-24 h at 37 °C, each morphotype growing on MacConkey with cefotaxime (MCA + CTX) was subjected to Gram staining, catalase and oxidase tests, followed by biochemical identification with API 20E (bioMérieux, Marcy l'Etoile, France) and Vitek® 2 System (bioMérieux, Marcy l'Etoile, France) using the GN card according to the manufacturer's instructions. Pure colonies were stored into Tryptone Soya Broth supplemented with 30% glycerol at – 20 °C for future use.

Phenotypic screening

All growing colonies were phenotypically screened for ESBL, AmpC, KPC, MBL, and OXA-48 production using ROSCO DIAGNOSTICA (Taastrup, Denmark) using 0.5 McFarland on Mueller-Hinton agar according to the manufacturer's instructions.

Antimicrobial susceptibility testing

Minimum inhibitory concentrations (MICs) were determined via broth microdilution for all presumptive ESBLs and/or AmpCs, and/or MBL producers. Ampicillin, cefoxitin, cefuroxime, cefotaxime, ceftazidime, meropenem, imipenem, ertapenem, amikacin, gentamicin, ciprofloxacin, tigecycline, tetracycline, doxycycline, nitrofurantoin, and colistin constituted the antibiotic panel for carriage isolates. The Vitek® 2 System and Vitek® 2 Gram-negative Susceptibility card (AST-N255) were used to determining the MICs of clinical isolates. The results of MIC tests were interpreted according to the European Committee on Antimicrobial Susceptibility Testing (EUCAST) breakpoints [11] and the MDR which is the resistance to three or more classes of antibiotics was also assessed. *Escherichia coli* ATCC 25922, *K. pneumoniae* ATCC 700603 and *K. pneumoniae* ATCC 51503 were used as controls.

Genomic characterization

Genomic extraction

Genomic DNA of selected strains were extracted using GenElute Bacterial Genomic DNA Kit (Sigma-Aldrich, St. Louis, MO, USA) according to the manufacturer's instructions. Genomic DNA was stored at – 20 °C for future use.

Multiplex polymerase chain reaction (M-PCR)

The isolates were subjected to molecular testing using conventional and M-PCR assays to identify $bla_{\text{CTX-M}}$ group 8/25 ($bla_{\text{CTX-M-gp8/25}}$), bla_{SHV}, bla_{TEM}, $bla_{\text{OXA-1-like}}$, $bla_{\text{OXA-48}}$, bla_{KPC}, bla_{VIM}, bla_{IMP} and bla_{GES} genes as previously described [12] (Additional file 1: Table S1).

Real-time polymerase chain reaction (RT-PCR)

RT-PCR was performed to ascertain bla_{AmpC}, $bla_{\text{CTX-M-group-1}}$ ($bla_{\text{CTX-M-gp1}}$), $bla_{\text{CTX-M-group-2}}$ ($bla_{\text{CTX-M-gp2}}$) and $bla_{\text{CTX-M-group-9}}$ ($bla_{\text{CTX-M-gp9}}$) resistance genes. Results were analysed on a programmable automate QuantStudio5™ (Applied Biosystems, CA, USA) using the Taqman Universal Master Mix 2× (Applied Biosystems, CA, USA) and ready-made assays (Thermo Scientific, CA, USA). Thermal temperature running conditions were as follows: UNG activation at 50 °C for 2 min, initial denaturation at 95 °C for 10 min, 30 cycles of denaturation at 95 °C for 10 s, annealing/extension at 60 °C for 1 min and a final extension at 60 °C for 30 s. The results were interpreted with QuantStudio™ design and analysis software version 1.4 (Applied Biosystems, CA, USA).

Genomic fingerprinting

Enterobacterial Repetitive Intergenic Consensus-Polymerase Chain Reaction (ERIC-PCR) was used to establish the link of different strains within and between hospitals, wards, carriage and clinical samples as well as across sampling points. The primers ERIC1 5'ATGTAAGCTC CTGGGGATTCAC3' and ERIC2 5'AAGTAAGTGAC TGGGGTGAGCG3' [13] were used and PCR reactions were carried out in a 10 µl volume containing 5 µl of Dream*Taq* Green Polymerase Master Mix 2X (Thermo Fisher Scientific, Johannesburg, South Africa), 2.8 µl of nuclease free water, 0.1 µl of each primer (100 µM), and 2 µl of DNA template. The reactions were carried out with the following cycling conditions: initial denaturation at 94 °C for 3 min, 30 cycles consisting of a denaturation step at 94 °C for 30 s, annealing at 50 °C for 1 min, extension at 65 °C for 8 min, a final extension step at 65 °C for 16 min and final storage at 4 °C. The generated amplicons were resolved by horizontal electrophoresis on 1.5% (wt/vol) Tris-Borate-EDTA (Merck, Germany) agarose gels together with the Quick-load®1-kb (Biolabs, New England) and run in an electric field of 110 V for 2 h 30 min. Electrophoresis gels were visualized by a UV light trans-illuminator, images were captured using a Gel Doc™ XR+ system (BioRad Laboratories, CA, Foster City, USA) and analysed by Image Lab™ Software (version 4.0, BioRad Laboratories, CA, Foster City, USA).

ERIC-PCR profiles were normalized using the Quick-load®1-kb (Biolabs, New England) DNA molecular weight marker as the external standard. For cluster analysis, data were exported to Bionumerics software (version 7.6, Applied Maths, TX, USA). Strains were allocated to different clusters by calculating the similarity coefficient from the homology matrix using the Jaccard method. Dendrograms were constructed based on the average linkages of the matrix and using the Unweighted Pair-Group Method (UPGMA). Optimization and band tolerance were set at 1% (version 7.6, Applied Maths, TX, USA) and 80% similarity cut-off was used to define clusters.

Data analysis

Data was coded and entered on an Excel spreadsheet (Microsoft Office 2016) and analysed using STATA (version 14.0, STATA Corporation, TX, USA). Risk factors for ESBL-mediating MDR Gram-negative ESKAPE colonization were ascertained by univariate and multivariate logistic regression analyses. Prevalence of MDR carriage was compared between categories (viz. hospital, ward and time-point) using the chi-square and Fisher's exact test as appropriate. A p-value < 0.05 was regarded as statistically significant.

Results

Population characteristics

A total of 75 hospitalized patients were contacted, amongst whom, 45 (60%) agreed to participate, answered the questionnaire and provided samples. Out of the 45 patients enrolled, faecal carriage was collected from 21 female and 24 were males, and the district hospital ($n = 27$) accounted more participant than the tertiary hospital ($n = 18$). The main reasons of hospitalization were cancer, cellulitis, hypoglycaemia, renal failure, diabetes, breath disorder, surgery and wound, in both hospitals. The patient's follow-up rate was 96%, 58% and 16% of rectal swabs collected at admission, after 48 h and at discharge, respectively.

The overall prevalence of carriage was 37.21% (16/43), 42.31% (11/26) and 57.14% (4/7) at admission, after 48 h and at discharge, respectively, with males being more colonized than females as were patients referred from another hospital (Table 1). Patients in the tertiary hospital were more likely to be colonized by MDR ESKAPE bacteria at admission (50%) and discharge (66.66%) than those of the district hospital (Table 1). Furthermore, patients admitted to the general medical ward were more colonized in the district hospital at all time-points whereas, in the tertiary hospital, the prevalence in the surgical ward was higher at admission and discharge. In parallel, the prevalence of MDR ESKAPE bacteria in faecal carriage (46%) was higher than clinical samples (28%).

Risk factors for MDR gram-negative ESKAPE bacteria carriage

Patients referred from the district to the tertiary hospital had an increased the risk of being colonized by resistant bacteria at admission (OR = 9, 95% CI 4.68–17.30) and after 48 h (OR = 4; 95% CI 1.50–10.66, Table 2). Similarly, the gender (male) increases the odds of being colonized at admission and after 48 h in district hospital (Table 2).

The multivariate analysis further confirmed that referral from district to tertiary hospital was significantly associated with MDR Gram-negative ESKAPE bacteria at admission (OR = 14.40, 95% CI 1. 0.98–210.84) and after 48 h (OR = 5.72, 95% CI 0.17–189.00) as was the gender for these two time-points in the district hospital (Table 3).

Table 1 Fecal carriage of resistant Gram-negative ESKAPE bacteria isolated from hospitalized patients in a rural district and a tertiary urban hospital

Variables	District Rural Hospital $n = 27$						Tertiary Urban Hospital $n = 18$					
	Admission, (%)	*p*	After 48 h, (%)	*p*	At discharge, (%)	P	Admission, (%)	*p*	After 48 h, (%)	*p*	At discharge, (%)	*P*
Overall	29.63	....	47.05	.....	50	....	50	...	33.33	...	66.66	...
Socio-demographic factors												
Gender												
Female	21.4	0.333	33	0.229	50	....	40	0.590	50	0.571	50	0.386
Male	38.4		63		0		55		29		100	
Clinical history												
Previous hospitalization (within one year)												
Yes	13	0.206	0	0.012	0	0.248	20	0.106	25	0.635	100	0.386
No	37		67		66.67		64		40		50	
Antibiotic use (during hospital stay)												
Yes	27.78	0.766	33.33	0.402	50	1.000	33	0.522	33	1.000	100	0.386
No	33.33		54.55		50		54		33		50	
Transferred from another hospital												
Yes	100	0.116	0	...	0	....	75	0.046	50	0.343	100	0.386
No	27		47		50		25		20		50	
Hospital ward												
Medicine	40	0.187	56	0.457	50	1.000	40	0.590	40	0.635	50	0.386
Surgery	17		38		50		55		25		100	

Out of the 45 patients enrolled, some refused rectal sampling, some were discharged or transferred after 48 h, while other could not be sampled due to their condition, leading to variability in number

Prevalence of MDR gram-negative ESKAPE bacteria

Out of 159 non-duplicates resistant Gram-negative bacteria isolated, 31 (19.50%) were MDR Gram-negative ESKAPE bacteria of which 21 (67.74%) were clinical isolates (11 tissue, 2 bloods, 3 urines, 3 intravenous catheters, 2 sputum) obtained after 48 h from hospitalized patients (15 males and 6 females) with symptomatic infections in different departments (medicine, surgery, intensive care units). Ten (32.26%) MDR Gram-negative ESKAPE bacteria were isolated from the rectal swab of in-patients (6 females, 4 males). In the district hospital, seven isolates were identified, five (71.43%) in carriage and two (28.57%) in clinical samples. *K. pneumoniae* ($n = 2$) and *E. aerogenes* ($n = 2$) were the main bacterial species isolated in carriage samples while *E. cloacae* ($n = 2$) was the sole clinical isolates. In contrast, in the tertiary hospital, five (20.83%) isolates were identified in carriage and 19 (79.16%) in clinical samples. The main pathogen identified in carriage was *E. aerogenes* ($n = 2$) while *P. aeruginosa* ($n = 7$) and *A. baumannii* ($n = 7$) were the main clinical isolates.

Table 2 Risk factors associated with faecal carriage of ESBL-producing Gram-negative ESKAPE bacteria (Univariate Logistic regression)

Variables	District hospital		Tertiary hospital	
	Admission	After 48 h	Admission	After 48 h
	OR (95% CI)	OR (95% CI)	OR (95% CI)	OR (95% CI)
Gender (F or M)	2.29 (0.42–12.50)	3.33 (0.45–24.44)	1.8 (0.21–15.40)	0.4 (0.16–10.02)
Antibiotic use (Yes or No)	1.3 (0.23–7.32)	0.42 (0.05–3.31)	0.43 (0.03–5.98)	1
Co-morbidity	1.05 (0.61–1.83)	1.03 (0.48–2.24)	1.05 (0.61–1.83)	1.03 (0.48–2.24)
Previous hospitalization	0.24 (0.02–2.40)	1	0.14 (0.01–1.76)	0.5 (0.03–8.95)
Transferred from another hospital	1	1	9 (0.93–86.52)	4 (0.21–75.67)
Ward (Medicine or Surgery)	0.3 (0.05–1.88)	0.48 (0.07–3.35)	1.8 (0.21–15.40)	0.5 (0.03–8.95)

Table 3 Predictive risk factors associated with fecal carriage of MDR Gram-negative ESKAPE bacteria in a district and tertiary hospital (Multivariate Logistic regression)

Variables	District Hospital		Tertiary Hospital	
	Admission; OR (95% CI)	After 48 h; OR (95% CI)	Admission; OR (95% CI)	After 48 h; OR (95% CI)
Gender (F or M)	7.12 (0.54–93.75)	3.61 (0.34–37.83)	1.21 (0.09–15.61)	0.29 (0.005–16.27)
Antibiotic use (Yes or No)	4.73 (0.28–80.57)	0.93 (0.08–11.40)	0.26 (0.007–9.01)	0.41 (0.009–17.46)
Transferred from another hospital	1	1	14.40 (0.98–210.84)	5.72 (0.17–189.00)
Hospital Ward (Medicine or Surgery)	0.08 (0.004–1.39)	0.42 (0.05–3.81)	2.09 (0.10–42.29)	1.14 (0.03–49.14)

Antimicrobial resistance profiles

In the tertiary hospital, especially in the medical ward, isolates expressed high resistance to ampicillin (100%), cefuroxime (100%) and cefotaxime (100%) in both carriage and clinical samples (Table 4). Similarly, in the surgical ward of the same hospital, clinical samples showed high resistance to ampicillin (100%), cefuroxime (100%), cefotaxime (88%), cefoxitin (88%), and nitrofurantoin (55%) while the unique carriage isolate was resistant to all the panel of antibiotics tested.

In the district hospital, the isolate identified in carriage samples in the surgical ward displayed maximum resistance (100%) to all antibiotics except colistin while those detected in medical ward exhibited high level of resistance to ampicillin (100%), cefuroxime (100%), cefotaxime (100%), ceftazidime (100%), cefoxitin (100%), amikacin (100%), gentamicin (100%), nitrofurantoin (100%) and tigecycline (100%) (Table 4).

Genetic diversity of isolated MDR strains

Overall, the predominant ESBL genes were $bla_{CTX\text{-}M\text{-}gp9}$ (90%, 28/31), $bla_{CTX\text{-}M\text{-}gp1}$ (71%, 22/31), bla_{SHV} (42%, 13/31), $bla_{CTX\text{-}M\text{-}gp8/25}$ (36%, 11/31), $bla_{OXA\text{-}1\text{-}Like}$ (29%, 9/31) and bla_{TEM} (23%, 7/31) for both carriage and clinical samples. In the tertiary hospital, $bla_{CTX\text{-}M\text{-}gp9}$ (100%), $bla_{CTX\text{-}M\text{-}gp1}$ (87.5%), bla_{KPC} (75%) and bla_{VIM} (50%) were the main resistance genes detected in *A. baumannii* while *K. pneumoniae* strains harboured mainly $bla_{CTX\text{-}M\text{-}gp8/25}$ (66.6%), bla_{TEM} (66.6%), bla_{SHV} (66.6%), $bla_{CTX\text{-}M\text{-}gp9}$ (50%) and $bla_{CTX\text{-}M\text{-}gp1}$ (50%) (Table 5). It is noteworthy to mention that all isolates harboured at least two resistance genes and a maximum of seven genes were detected in one *E. aerogenes* (G702R2B5) isolate (Fig. 1b). In the district hospital, $bla_{CTX\text{-}M\text{-}gp9}$ (100%), bla_{SHV} (100%), and bla_{TEM} (100%) were the predominant genes in *K. pneumoniae* whereas $bla_{CTX\text{-}M\text{-}gp9}$ (100%), $bla_{OXA\text{-}1\text{-}Like}$ (50%), $bla_{CTX\text{-}M\text{-}gp1}$ (50%) and $bla_{CTX\text{-}M\text{-}gp8/25}$ (50%) were the main genes identified in *E. cloacae* (Table 5).

Genomic fingerprint

ERIC-profiles revealed some associations within species and suggest a likely transmission of resistant ESKAPE bacteria across patients, wards and hospitals (Additional file 2: Table S2). For *K. pneumoniae*, one main cluster showing high genetic similarities was observed (Fig. 1a). *K. pneumoniae* strains A111R1B2 and A105R2B2 detected among two patients at admission for the former and after 48 h for the latter, in the medical ward of the district hospital showed 100% of similarity and shared common ancestors with one carriage and three clinical strains isolated in the tertiary hospital (Fig. 1a and Additional file 2: Table S2). Similarly, one pair of *E. aerogenes*, A105R1B5 and G702R1B5 isolated from two patients in the medical ward of the district and tertiary hospital, both at admission, also exhibited 100% of similarity and shared a common ancestor with another strain G702R2B5 collected after 48 h (Fig. 1b). Although, *A. baumannii* (Fig. 1c) and *P. aeruginosa* (Fig. 1d) were more genetically diverse, some isolates shared a common ancestor within and between the carriage and clinical samples.

Discussion

The overall prevalence of carriage at admission was 37.21% (16/43) and we found that 42.31% (11/26) and 57.14% (4/7) were still MDR ESKAPE carriers after 48 h and at discharge. Notwithstanding the small sample size, our results showed that the carriage of MDR Gram-negative ESKPAPE bacteria increased with the hospital length of stay. Our results are consistent with a Norwegian prospective cohort study carried out from 2009 to 2011 investigating the risk factors for and duration of prolonged faecal carriage of ESBL-producing *K. pneumoniae* amongst patients with community acquired urinary tract infections which revealed high prevalence of ESBL faecal carriage (ranging from 15 to 61%) at six different time points [14].

At hospital level, the rate of carriage at admission in the district hospital (30%) compared with the tertiary hospital (50%) suggests that patients admitted to the tertiary hospital are likely to be more colonized by MDR Gram-negative ESKAPE bacteria than those of the district healthcare facility (Table 1). Our findings could be explained by the fact that all patients admitted to this level of the hospital are generally transferred from lower level healthcare facilities of the South African health system. This is further confirmed by the increased odds of being colonized in the univariate and multivariate analysis.

Table 4 Resistance to selected antibiotics in ESBL-producing Gram-negative ESKAPE bacteria isolated from carriage and clinical samples in a district and tertiary hospital

Antibiotics	Tertiary hospital								District hospital					
	Medical ward				Surgical ward				Medical ward				Surgical ward	
	Carriage		Clinical		Carriage		Clinical		Carriage		Clinical		Carriage	
	MIC (μg/ml) range	No. resistant isolates (%)	MIC (μg/ml) range	No. resistant isolates (%)	MIC (μg/ml) range	No. resistant isolates (%)	MIC (μg/ml) range	No. resistant isolates (%)	MIC (μg/ml) range	No. resistant isolates (%)	MIC (μg/ml) range	No. resistant isolates (%)	MIC (μg/ml) range	No. resistant isolates (%)
Ampicillin	≥512	4 (100)	≥32	11 (100)	≥512	1 (100)	16–32	8 (100)	≥512	4 (100)	16- ≥ 32	2 (100)	≥512	1 (100)
Cefoxitin	8–512	3 (75)	4	7 (64)	16	1 (100)	8- ≥ 64	7 (88)	128 ≥ 512	4 (100)	≥64	2 (100)	≥512	1 (100)
Cefuroxime	≥512	4 (100)	≥64	11 (100)	128	1 (100)	8–64	8 (100)	256 ≥ 512	4 (100)	16- ≥ 64	2 (100)	≥512	1 (100)
Cefotaxime	≥512	4 (100)	≥64	11 (100)	128	1 (100)	1- ≥ 64	7 (88)	32- ≥ 512	4 (100)	< 1–32	2 (100)	≥512	1 (100)
Ceftazidime	512	4 (100)	≥64	8 (73)	256	1 (100)	1- ≥ 64	4 (50)	32- ≥ 512	4 (100)	≤1–16	2 (100)	≥512	1 (100)
Meropenem	0.5–2	2(50)	0.25	3 (27)	2	1 (100)	0.25 ≥ 16	4 (50)	0.25–16	2 (50)	0.25	0 (0)	16	1 (100)
Imipenem	4–8	4 (100)	0.25	3 (27)	16	1 (100)	0.5- ≥ 16	3 (37.3)	2–32	2 (50)	0.25–1	0 (0)	64	1 (100)
Ertapenem	1–2	4 (100)	0.5	0 (0)	16	1 (100)	≤0.5	0 (0)	0.25–8	3 (75)	0.5	0 (0)	64	1 (100)
Amikacin	8–128	4 (100)	8	2 (18)	64	1 (100)	2- ≥ 64	4 (50)	8–128	2 (100)	2	0 (0)	≥512	1 (100)
Gentamicin	128	4 (100)	≥16	8 (73)	8	1 (100)	1- ≥ 16	4 (50)	4–16	4 (100)	1	0 (0)	≥512	1 (100)
Ciprofloxacin	64–512	4 (100)	≥4	6 (55)	32	1 (100)	0.25- ≥ 4	5 (45)	0.5–64	3 (75)	≤0.25	0 (0)	32	1 (100)
Tigecycline	16–64	4 (100)	1	4 (36)	16	1 (100)	0.5- ≥ 8	3 (37.3)	2–64	4 (100)	1	0 (0)	8	1 (100)
Nitrofurantoin	≥512	4 (100)	128	9 (82)	≥512	1 (100)	≥512	6 (55)	≥512	4 (100)	16- ≥ 512	0 (0)	≥512	1 (100)
Colistin	8–512	4 (100)	0.5	0 (0)	8	1 (100)	≤0.5	0(0)	0(0)	0(0)	≤0.5	0 (0)	≤0.5	0

Table 5 Resistance genes in ESBL-producing Gram-negative ESKAPE bacteria

Bacteria	No. of strains, *n* = 31 (%)	Resistance genes, *n* (%)									
		AmpC	TEM	SHV	CTX-M group-1	CTX-M group-9	CTX-M Group 8/25	IMP	VIM	KPC	OXA-1-like
Tertiary hospital (*n* = 24)											
K. pneumoniae	6 (25)	2 (33.3)	4 (66.6)	4 (66.6)	3 (50)	3 (50)	4 (66.6)	1 (16.6)	1 (16.6)	1 (16.6)	2 (33.33)
A. baumannii	8 (33.3)	3 (37.5)	/	3 (37.5)	7 (87.5)	8 (100)	/	/	4 (50)	6 (75)	2 (25)
P. aeruginosa	7 (29.5)	1 (14.28)	/	/	7 (100)	7 (100)	/	/	/	/	/
E. aerogenes	2 (8.33)	2 (100)	/	2 (100)	/	2 (100)	2 (100)	/	/	/	2 (100)
E. cloacae	1 (4.16)	/	/	/	1 (100)	1 (100)	1 (100)	1 (100)	/	1 (100)	/
District hospital (n = 7)											
K. pneumoniae	2 (28.57)	/	2 (100)	2 (100)	1 (50)	2 (100)	1 (50)	/	/	/	2 (33.33)
P. aeruginosa	1 (14.28)	/	/	/	1 (100)	1 (100)	/	/	/	/	/
E. aerogenes	2 (28.57)	1 (50)	1 (50)	1 (50)	1 (50)	2 (100)	2 (100)	/	/	/	/
E. cloacae	2 (28.57)	1 (50)	/	1 (50)	1 (50)	2 (100)	1 (50)	/	/	/	1 (50)

Similarly, at discharge, patients of the tertiary hospital (67%) were more colonized than those of the district hospital (50%). This could be explained by the complexity of cases associated with invasive medical procedures and greater antibiotic use in the tertiary hospital. However, after 48 h, the prevalence of carriage was higher in patients in the district hospital (47%) compared with the tertiary hospital (33%) intimating. This contrast could point out sub-optimal infection prevention and control measures in this level of healthcare setting. Besides, tertiary hospital with its more complicated cases and subsequent higher antibiotic use would have likely created greater selection pressure for resistance, but an anomalously greater resistance was observed in carriage samples in the district hospital. The small sample numbers preclude nonetheless definitive conclusions about carriage rates and resistance patterns.

The prevalence of MDR Gram-negative ESKAPE bacteria in faecal carriage (46%) was higher than that of clinical samples (28%) during the study period. Faecal carriage of resistant bacteria has been demonstrated to precede infections and consequently, such high prevalence of asymptomatic faecal carriage is of critical significance. Our results concur with a study from France where the prevalence of MDR Gram-negative bacilli isolated from stool samples was higher than that of clinical samples during a non-outbreak situation in a French Hospital [15]. They are however higher than a report from Mahomed and Coovadia (2014) which demonstrated 4.7% of faecal carriage of ESBL producing *Enterobacteriaceae* amongst children from the community in KwaZulu-Natal, South Africa [16]. Our findings may be an underestimation because of different diagnostic, stewardship practices, preference for empirical treatment and budget constraints such that not every infection generates a microbiological sample.

During the two-months period, 21 clinically relevant MDR Gram-negative ESKAPE bacteria out of 74 isolates were identified in both hospitals. Moreover, the prevalence of MDR *A. baumannii* and *P. aeruginosa* were 41.61% (10 out of 21 MDR Gram-negative ESKAPE bacteria) and 33.33% (7 out of 21 MDR Gram-negative ESKAPE bacteria) in clinical samples, respectively. The isolation of three *A. baumannii* strains, cluster A1, from tissue of three different patients (ED01498924, ED01498793, ED01498924) in surgery, consolidate the likely dissemination of this cluster within this ward in the tertiary hospital (Additional file 2: Table S2 and Fig. 1c).

In carriage samples, MDR *K. pneumoniae* and *Enterobacter spp.* were the predominant bacteria in both hospitals. This is consistent with a South African study where *K. pneumoniae* was the main pathogen identified in stool samples of children from the community of KwaZulu-Natal, South Africa [16]. Similarly, a 68% prevalence of ESBL-producing *Enterobacteriaceae* faecal carriage was shown amongst Egyptian patients with community-acquired gastrointestinal complaints [17].

An interesting finding was the inter-hospital and inter-patient spread of *K. pneumoniae* (cluster K1) in carriage, which were isolated from two patients (A105R2B2 and A111R1B2) hospitalized in general medicine in district hospital, sharing common ancestor with a patient (G702R3B2) from tertiary hospital (Additional file 2: Table S2). Interestingly, the isolated strains were identified in the medical ward and at different time-points, confirming the dissemination of this cluster across hospitals. In addition, *K. pneumoniae* strains from the same cluster (K1) were detected in urine (ED01500733) and sputum (ED01502268) of clinically ill patients hospitalized in intensive care unit (ICU) and medical ward in the tertiary hospital, respectively. This suggests that

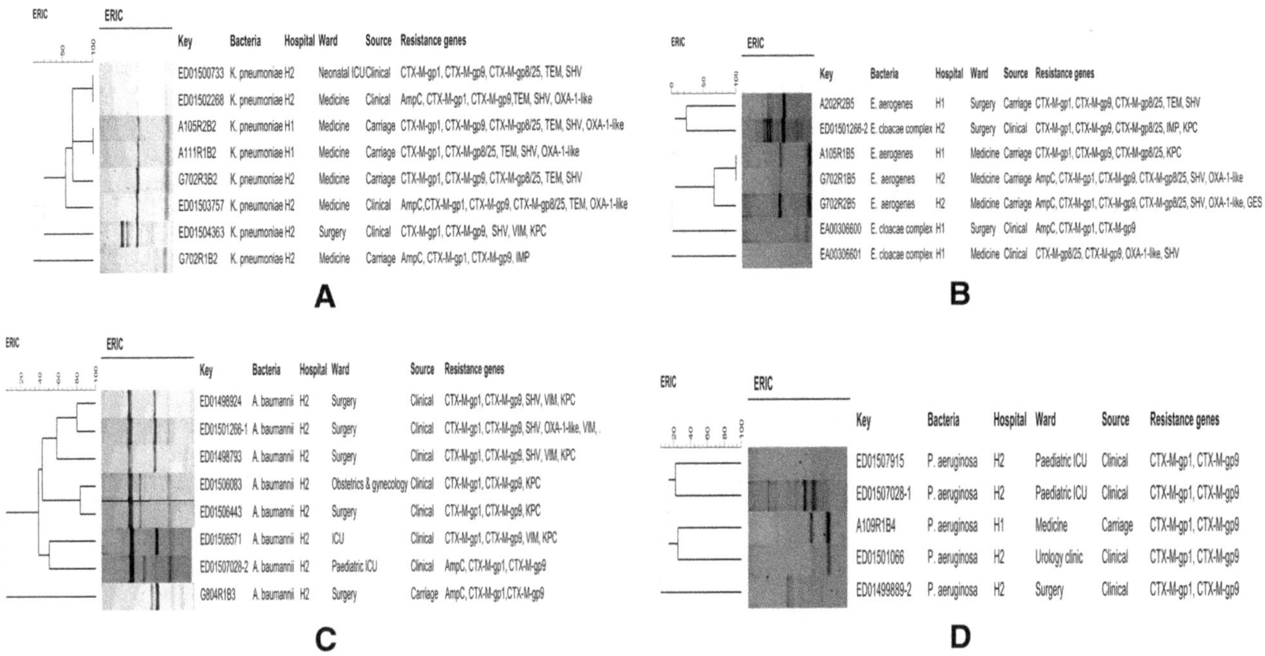

Fig. 1 Dendrograms of ESBL-producing of Gram-negative ESKAPE bacteria isolated from carriage and clinical samples from hospitalized patients. **a** *K. pneumoniae*, (**b**) *E. aerogenes* and *cloacae*, (**c**) *A. baumannii*, (**d**) *P. aeruginosa*

the *K. pneumoniae* K1 strains is circulating within wards and hospitals, and consequently could probably be source of nosocomial infections in hospitals.

Two patients, A105R1B5 and G702R1B5 also carried *Enterobacter spp.* (cluster E2) at admission in both district and tertiary hospitals, specifically in the medical wards (Additional file 2: Table S2) intimating the emergence of these strains in the community with subsequent entry into the district hospital, as the first level of care, and followed by spread to the tertiary hospital through referral. This result is consistent with our analyses which demonstrated that in the district hospital, the main risk factors were antibiotic use and gender while the referral and hospital ward were the principal risk factors at tertiary level (Tables 2 and 3).

Overall, the predominant ESBLs detected in carriage were $bla_{CTX\text{-}M\text{-}gp9}$ (90%), bla_{SHV} (60%), $bla_{CTX\text{-}M\text{-}gp1}$(50%), bla_{TEM} (40%) and $bla_{OXA\text{-}1\text{-}like}$ (40%). CTX-M is predominantly reported in community-acquired infections which would be more prevalent in the district hospital as the first level of care. These results are consistent with global reports. For instance, $bla_{CTX\text{-}M\text{-}group}$ were recently observed in adults in a community in Netherlands and ambulatory patients in Egypt with both gastrointestinal complaints [17, 18]. Similarly, studies from Guinee-Bissau, Niger, Gabon and Tanzania, reported high prevalence of ESBL faecal carriage with $bla_{CTX\text{-}M}$, bla_{TEM} and bla_{SHV} being the main genes identified [19–21]. The prevalence of AmpC was also higher in carriage (40%) compared to clinical samples (23.80%). Finally, carbapenemases were identified in clinical samples for in these hospitals, specifically, KPC and VIM in clinical *A. baumannii* isolates as well as IMP in a carriage *K. pneumoniae* isolate. An *E. aerogenes* isolate further showed bla_{GES} along with $bla_{CTX\text{-}M\text{-}gp1}$, $bla_{CTX\text{-}M\text{-}gp9}$, $bla_{CTX\text{-}M\text{-}gp8/25}$, bla_{SHV} and $bla_{OXA\text{-}1\text{-}like}$ in a carriage sample. The faecal carriage of MDR Gram-negative ESKAPE bacteria appears to be a source of cross-transmission between patients. The substantial genetic similarity within and between carriage and clinical isolates as well as wards and hospital settings reveal their potential implications in future outbreak situations that may occur either in hospitals or in communities. Efforts should thus be made amongst communities and asymptomatic patients for better containment of antibiotic resistance dissemination.

Gender, antibiotic use, type of healthcare settings and referral from another hospital were the main risk factors identified. These results suggest that routine screening for MDR Gram-negative ESKAPE bacteria at admission should be implemented, and infection, prevention and control measures reinforced to prevent potential outbreaks by these resistant pathogens [22].

Conclusion

This study highlights the high prevalence of ESBL-mediating MDR Gram-negative ESKAPE bacteria in carriage and clinical samples among hospitalized patients in uMgungundlovu. It is imperative to implement regular screening and surveillance of MDR Gram-negative ESKAPE bacteria in communities and hospitals, to monitor epidemiological changes, ascertain socio-economic impact and inform antibiotic treatment. These screening and surveillance measures coupled with strict infection prevention and control programmes and antimicrobial stewardship programmes (ASP) are essential to address antibiotic resistance in these settings.

Acknowledgments
The authors would like to express their profound gratitude to Professor Mlisana Koleka, Dr. Sumayya Haffejee and Mrs. Nadira Moodley of the National Health Laboratory of South Africa for their collaboration and for providing us with clinical strains. The Infection, Prevention and Control officers, Mrs. Thandi Masango, Mrs. Jennifer Grace Green and Mrs. Zelda Reddy, are also gratefully acknowledged for their considerable assistance during the sample collection in both hospitals.

Funding
This work was supported by the Antimicrobial Research Unit (ARU) and a scholarship awarded to R.C. Founou and L.L. Founou by the College of Health Sciences (CHS) of the University of KwaZulu-Natal. The National Research Foundation funded this study through the NRF Incentive Funding for Rated Researchers (Grant No. 85595), the NRF Competitive Grant for Rated Researchers (Grant no.: 106063) and the DST/NRF South African Research Chair in Antibiotic Resistance and One Health (Grant No. 98342) awarded to SY Essack. Any opinions, findings and conclusions, or recommendations expressed in this study are those of the authors, and therefore do not represent the official position of the funders. The funders had no role in the study design, data collection and analysis, preparation of the manuscript nor decision to publish.

Authors' contributions
RF co-conceptualized the study, undertook sample collection, laboratory and statistical analyses, prepared tables and figures, interpreted results and drafted the manuscript. LF undertook sample collection and laboratory analyses and vetted the results. SE co-conceptualized the study, undertook vetting of the results and critically reviewed the manuscript. All authors read and approved the manuscript.

Consent for publication
Not applicable.

Competing interests
Professor Essack is a member of the Global Respiratory Infection Partnership sponsored by an unrestricted educational grant from Reckitt and Benckiser. All other authors declare that there is no competing financial interest.

Author details
[1]Antimicrobial Research Unit, School of Health Sciences, College of Health Sciences, University of KwaZulu-Natal, Durban 4000, South Africa. [2]Department of Clinical Microbiology, Centre of Expertise and Biological Diagnostic of Cameroon, (CEDBCAM), Yaoundé, Cameroon. [3]Department of Food Safety and Environmental Microbiology, Centre of Expertise and Biological Diagnostic of Cameroon, (CEDBCAM), Yaoundé, Cameroon.

References
1. O'Neill J. Tackling drug-resistant infections globally: final report and recommendations. Rev Antimicrob Resist. 2016.
2. World Health Organization. Antimicrobial resistance global report on surveillance. Geneva: World Health Organization; 2014.
3. Rice LB. Federal funding for the study of antimicrobial resistance in nosocomial pathogens: no eskape. J Infect Dis. 2008;197(8):1079–81.
4. Almasaudi SB. *Acinetobacter spp.* as nosocomial pathogens: epidemiology and resistance features. Saudi J Biol Sci. 2016; In Press. doi: https://doi.org/10.1016/j.sjbs.2016.02.009.
5. Pedleton JN, Gorman SP, Gilmore BF. Clinical relevance of the ESKAPE pathogens. Expert Rev Anti-Infect Ther. 2013;11(3):297–308.
6. Lim C, Takahashi E, Hongsuwan M, Wuthiekanun V, Thamlikitkul V, Hinjoy S, Day NP, Peacock SJ, Limmathurotsakul D. Epidemiology and burden of multidrug-resistant bacterial infection in a developing country. elife. 2016;5. https://doi.org/10.7554/eLife.18082.
7. Dantas G, Sommer MOA. How to fight Back against antibiotic resistance. Am Sci. 2014;102:42–51.
8. Slavcovici A, Maier C. Antimicrobial resistance of ESKAPE-pathogens in culture-positive pneumonia. FARMACIA. 2015;63(2):201–5.
9. Founou RC, Founou LL, Essack SY. Clinical and economic impact of antibiotic resistance in developing countries: a systematic review and meta-analysis. PLoS One. 2017;12(12):e0189621.
10. World Health Organization. Global priority list of antibiotic-resistance Bacteria to guide research, discovery, and development of new antibiotics. Geneva: World Health Organization; 2017.
11. EUCAST. Breakpoint tables for interpretation of MICs and zone diameters. 2017. Available from http://www.eucast.org/clinical_breakpoints/.
12. Dallenne C, Costa AD, Decre D, Favier C, Arlet G. Development of a set of multiplex PCR assays for the detection of genes encoding important b-lactamases in Enterobacteriaceae. J Antimicrob Chemother. 2010;65(3):490–5. https://doi.org/10.1093/jac/dkp498.
13. Versalovic J, Koeuth T. Distribution of repetitive DNA sequences in eubacteria and application to fingerprinting of bacterial genomes. Nucleic Acids Res. 1991;19(24):6823–31.
14. Jorgensen SB, Soraas A, Sundsfjord A, Liestøl K, Leegaard TM, Jenum PA. Faecal carriage of extended spectrum beta-lactamase producing *Escherichia coli* and *Klebsiella pneumoniae* after urinary tract infection - a three-year prospective cohort study. PLoS One. 2017;12(3):e0173510.
15. Vidal-Navarro L, Pfeiffer C, Bouziges N, Sotto A, Lavigne JP. Faecal carriage of multidrug-resistant gram-negative bacilli during a non-outbreak situation in a French university hospital. J Antimicrob Chemother. 2010;65(11):2455–8. https://doi.org/10.1093/jac/dkq333.
16. Mahomed S, Coovadia MY. Faecal carriage of extended Spectrum Beta-lactamase producing *Escherichia coli* and *Klebsiella pneumoniae* in children from the community of Kwadedangendlale, KwaZulu-Natal, South Africa. Int J Infect Control. 2014;11(3):1–8. https://doi.org/10.3396/ijic.v11i3.14391.
17. Abdallah HM, Alnaiemi N, Reuland EA, Wintermans BB, Koek A, Abdelwahab AM, Samy A, Abdelsalam KW, Vandenbroucke-Grauls CMJE. Faecal carriage of extended-spectrum β-lactamase- and carbapenemase-producing *Enterobacteriaceae* in Egyptian patients with community-onset gastrointestinal complaints: a hospital -based cross-sectional study. Antimicrob Resist Infect Control. 2017;6(1):62. https://doi.org/10.1186/s13756-017-0219-7.
18. Reuland EA, Naiemi N, Kaiser AM, Heck M, Kluytmans JA, Savelkoul PH, Elders PJ, Vandenbroucke-Grauls CM. Prevalence and risk factors for carriage of ESBL-producing *Enterobacteriaceae* in Amsterdam. J Antimicrob Chemother. 2016;71(4):1076–82. https://doi.org/10.1093/jac/dkv441.
19. Isendahl J, Turlej-Rogacka A, Manjuba C, Rodrigues A, Giske CG, Nauclér P. Fecal carriage of ESBL-producing *E. coli* and *K. pneumoniae* in children in Guinea-Bissau: a hospital-based cross-sectional study. PLoS One. 2012;7:e51981.
20. Woerther PL, Angebault C, Jacquier H, Hugede HC, Janssens AC, Sayadi S, El Mniai A, Armand-Lefèvre L, Ruppé E, Barbier F, Raskine L, Page AL, Rekeneire DN, Andremont A. Massive increase, spread, and exchange of extended spectrum beta-lactamase-encoding genes among intestinal *Enterobacteriaceae* in hospitalized children with severe acute malnutrition in Niger. Clin Infect Dis. 2011;53(7):677–85. https://doi.org/10.1093/cid/cir522.
21. Schaumburg F, Alabi A, Kokou C, Grobusch MP, Köck R, Kaba H, Becker K, Adegnika AA, Kremsner PG, Peters G, Mellmann A. High burden of extended-spectrum beta-lactamase-producing *Enterobacteriaceae* in Gabon. J Antimicrob Chemother. 2013;68(9):2140–3. https://doi.org/10.1093/jac/dkt164.

18

Continuous increase of vancomycin resistance in enterococci causing nosocomial infections in Germany

Cornelius Remschmidt[1,2*], Christin Schröder[1,2], Michael Behnke[1,2], Petra Gastmeier[1,2], Christine Geffers[1,2] and Tobias Siegfried Kramer[1,2]

Abstract

Background: Enterococci are frequent pathogens causing nosocomial infections in Germany. Infections due to strains with vancomycin resistance are high when compared with other European states. Therefore, the study aimed to describe the recent progression of nosocomial infections due to vancomycin-resistant enterococci (VRE) in Germany.

Methods: We analyzed data from two components of the German national nosocomial infection surveillance system for the period 2007–2016. For primary bloodstream infections (BSIs) and urinary tract infections (UTIs) we used data from intensive care units and for surgical site infections (SSIs) data from surgical departments. In a sensitivity analysis, we considered only data from participants that participated continuously from 2007 to 2016 ("core group"). We calculated proportions of VRE among all nosocomial enterococcal infections with 95% confidence intervals (95% CIs) and trends over time. A multivariable logistic regression was used to compare occurrence of VRE proportions among German federal states.

Results: Enterococcal infections from 857 ICUs and 1119 surgical departments were analyzed. On ICUs, the proportion of vancomycin resistance in enterococci causing nosocomial infections significantly increased for BSIs from 5.9 to 16.7% and for UTIs from 2.9 to 9.9%; for surgical site infections, the proportion of VRE increased from 0.9 to 5.2% ($P < 0.001$ for all). In the core group, the increase of VRE was more pronounced in ICUs (BSIs: 5.5 to 21.6%; UTIs: 2 to 11.2%) but was not seen in surgical departments (SSIs: 1.5 to 2.8%). Compared with the most populous German federal state North Rhine Westphalia, enterococcal infections in Hesse (Odds Ratio (OR) 2.3, 95% CI 1.7–3.1), Saxony (OR 2.5, 95% CI 1.8–3.5) and Thuringia (OR 1.9, 95% CI 1.4–2.6) were more likely to be caused by vancomycin-resistant strains.

Conclusion: In Germany, the proportion of VRE in nosocomial infection due to enterococci is still increasing. It remains unclear, why a large variation in the proportion of VRE exists between German federal states.

Keywords: Vancomycin-resistant enterococci, Multiresistant, Surveillance, Epidemiology

* Correspondence: cornelius.remschmidt@charite.de
[1]Institute of Hygiene and Environmental Medicine, Charité – University Medicine Berlin, Hindenburgdamm 27, 12203 Berlin, Germany
[2]German National Reference Centre for Surveillance of Nosocomial Infections (NRZ), Hindenburgdamm 27, 12203 Berlin, Germany

Background

Vancomycin-resistant enterococci (VRE) have emerged as important multiresistant pathogens causing nosocomial infections [1, 2]. Infections with VRE are associated with increased length of stay and excess in-hospital mortality and therefore pose a rising public health threat [3]. In 2017, the World Health Organization identified VRE as one of the most important resistant bacteria in their "Global Priority list of antibiotic-resistant bacteria list" [4].

According to the 2016 surveillance report of the European Antimicrobial Resistance Network (EARS-Net), a significant increasing trend for VRE between 2013 and 2016 was not identified among invasive isolates for the EU/EEA population-weighted mean percentage [5]; however, in seven out of 30 participating countries a significant increase of VRE was observed. Ireland (VRE rate of 44.1%), Greece (27.9%), Slovakia (26.4%), Poland (25.2%) and Hungary (22.5%) showed the highest resistance rates in the EARS-Net 2016 report, if only countries with more than 100 reported isolates were considered. In Germany, the proportion of VRE among invasive *Enterococcus (E.) faecium* isolates was 12.1% and comparable with the EU/EEA mean.

Previously, we observed a dramatic increase of the proportion of VRE among blood-stream infections and surgical site infections between 2007 and 2012 [6]. Therefore, the objective of this study was to investigate the recent development of different nosocomial infections caused by VRE in Germany by using data from the large German national nosocomial infection surveillance system.

Methods

We analyzed data that were recorded into two surveillance components of the German national nosocomial infection surveillance system (Krankenhaus-Infektions-Surveillance-System, KISS) between 2007 and 2016. Detailed information on KISS and its above-mentioned components have been described elsewhere [7]. Briefly, data on nosocomial primary blood stream-infections (BSI) and nosocomial urinary tract-infections (UTIs) on intensive care units (ICUs) were recorded in the ICU component of KISS (ICU-KISS). Data on nosocomial surgical site infections (SSIs) on surgical departments were recorded in OP-KISS. Infections were documented according to definitions by the CDC [8]. In KISS, enterococcal infections are not documented on a species level. Therefore, the term VRE is defined as all infections due to enterococci resistant against vancomycin regardless of the underlying mechanism or species.

Ethics and data protection

We analyzed aggregated and anonymous data that are collected by the participating hospitals in accordance with the German "Protection against Infection Act" §23. Therefore, ethical approval by an institutional board was not necessary.

Statistical analysis

We pooled data recorded in ICU-KISS and OP-KISS and analyzed the proportion of VRE for each type of infection (BSI, UTI, SSI) by dividing the number of enterococcal infections resistant against vancomycin by the number of all enterococcal infections multiplied by 100. 95% confidence intervals (CIs) were calculated. Data were univariate tested for a yearly linear trend by using Cochrane-Armitage-test [6].

A multivariable logistic regression was used to compare VRE proportions among German federal states. In addition to the risk factor federal state, the following potential confounders were considered: year of the surgical procedure, gender and age group for the patient (0–50, 51–65, 66–70 and 71–120 years), type of hospital (university hospital, other hospital), season, type of ICU or type of surgical department, and hospital size (400 beds and ≥ 400 beds). Stepwise forward-backward selection was used to derive the final logistic regression model. Parameters were entered into the model at a significance level of $P \leq 0.05$ and were removed at $P > 0.05$. Odds Ratios (OR) with 95% CIs were calculated.

Since not all hospitals reported data for the entire study period, we conducted a sensitivity analysis in which only hospitals were included that had reported data continuously from 2007 to 2016 for at least 6 month per year ("core group"). *P*-values less than 0.05 were considered statistically significant.

All analyses were performed with R 3.4.3 [R Core Team (2013); R Foundation for statistical computing, Vienna, Austria] and SAS 9.4 (SAS Institute Inc., Cary, NC, USA).

Results

Between 2007 and 2016 a total of 1121 ICUs and 1412 surgical departments from all German federal states reported data on nosocomial infections to ICU-KISS and OP-KISS, respectively (Table 1). Of those, 12,659 infections were due to enterococcus species. Overall, the proportion of VRE increased from 1.4% in 2007/2008 to 10% in 2015/2016 (Fig. 1). In BSI, the proportion of VRE increased from 5.9 to 16.7% ($P < 0.001$). Among UTIs and SSIs, the proportion of VRE increased from 2.9 to 9.9% ($P < 0.001$) and from 0.9 to 5% ($P < 0.001$), respectively (Table 2).

According to our sensitivity analysis, 218 ICUs and 174 surgical wards reported data continuously on an annual basis (core group). Overall, the core group showed a comparable increase regarding the proportion of VRE from 4 to 10%; however, the increase in the core group

Table 1 ICUs and surgical departments providing VRE infection data for 2007–16 per year from the German national nosocomial infection surveillance system (KISS)

Year/number (*n*)	2007/08	2009/10	2011/12	2013/14	2015/16	Total[a]
Number (*n*) of ICUs	465	533	645	764	857	1121
Number (*n*) of surgical departments	432	558	681	919	1119	1412
Nosocomial enterococcal infections						
Total number (*N*) of nosocomial enterococcal infections	2047	2559	2253	2639	3161	12,659
Number of VRE infections, *n* (% (n/N))	79 (3.9)	106 (4.1)	143 (6.4)	187 (7.1)	318 (10.1)	833 (6.6)
Total number (*N*) of enterococcal infections on ICUs	1520	1927	1574	1700	1929	8650
Number of VRE infections on ICUs, *n* (% (n/N))	74 (4.9)	90 (4.7)	119 (7.6)	158 (9.3)	229 (11.9)	670 (7.8)
Total number (*N*) of nosocomial enterococcal infections in surgical wards	527	637	679	939	1232	4009
Number of nosocomial VRE infections in surgical wards, *n* (% (n/N))	5 (1.0)	16 (2.5)	24 (3.5)	30 (3.2)	57 (4.6)	132 (3.3)

ICU intensive care unit, *VRE* vancomycin-resistant enterococci; [a] Total number of ICUs/surgical departments that reported data for at least 6 month in any year

was more pronounced in BSIs and UTIs whereas the proportion of VRE among SSI showed only a small increase (Fig. 2). VRE proportions increased significantly in primary BSI from 5.5 to 21.6% ($P < 0.001$) and in UTI from 2 to 11.2% ($P = 0.001$).

Regarding differences in the proportion of VRE among German federal states, we found that proportion of VRE infections were > 10% in the 6 federal states of Berlin, Hesse, Saarland, Saxony-Anhalt, Saxony and Thuringia, all of which are in the center of Germany (Fig. 3). Compared with the most populous federal state North Rhine Westphalia, enterococcal infections in Hesse (OR 2.3, 95% CI 1.7–3.1), Saxony (OR 2.5, 95% CI 1.8–3.5) and Thuringia (OR 1.9, 95% CI 1.4–2.6) were more likely to be caused by VRE. Additionally, the final multivariable logistic regression indicated that type of hospital (university hospital vs. non-university hospital: OR 2.1, 95% CI 1.7–2.5), type of ICU (internal medicine ICU vs. non-internal medicine ICU: OR: 1.8 (95% CI 1.5–2.2) and calendar year (OR 1.1, 95% CI 1.1–1.2) statistically significant increased the chance for VRE.

Discussion

Our analysis of the German national nosocomial infection surveillance system revealed a continuous increase of VRE proportions in nosocomial infections caused by enterococci in Germany between 2007 and 2016. This development has become even more apparent since our last report [6].

The results on VRE are concordant with other reports from Germany. Behnke et al. showed in two consecutive national point prevalence studies that vancomycin resistance in *E. faecium* causing nosocomial infections increased from 10.2% in 2011 to 23.1% in 2016 [9, 10]. Another study which analyzed data on antibiotic consumption and antimicrobial resistance in German ICUs

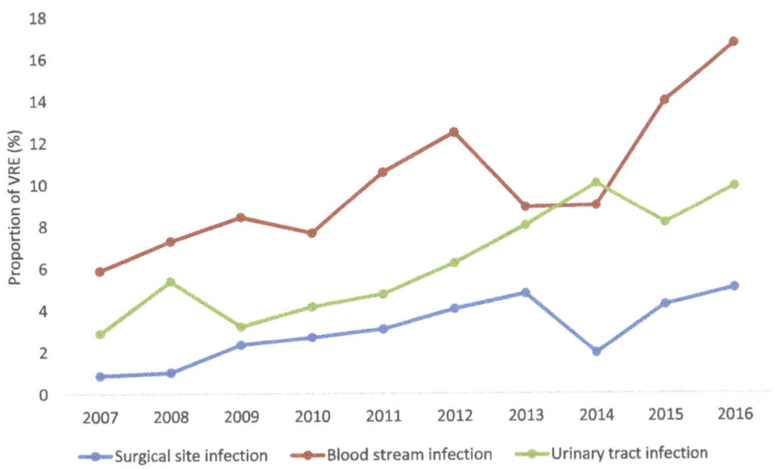

Fig. 1 Time trend for percentage of vancomycin-resistant entercoccal (VRE) infections according to the German national nosocomial infection surveillance system (KISS), by infection site

Table 2 Data on nosocomial infections due to Enterococci for 2007–16 per year from the German national nosocomial infection surveillance system (KISS), by infection site

Year	Surgical site infections			Bloodstream infections			Urinary tract infections		
	Enterococci (*n*)	VRE (*n*)	Proportion in % (95% CI)	Enterococci (*n*)	VRE (*n*)	Proportion in % (95% CI)	Enterococci (*n*)	VRE (*n*)	Proportion in % (95% CI)
2007	231	2	0.87 (0.15, 2.83)	170	10	5.88 (3.03, 10.23)	450	13	2.89 (1.62, 4.78)
2008	296	3	1.01 (0.26, 2.73)	206	15	7.28 (4.29, 11.47)	540	29	5.37 (3.69, 7.52)
2009	301	7	2.33 (1.02, 4.55)	273	23	8.42 (5.55, 12.18)	591	19	3.21 (2.00, 4.88
2010	336	9	2.68 (1.31, 4.86)	261	20	7.66 (4.88, 11.38)	627	26	4.15 (2.78, 5.93)
2011	357	11	3.08 (1.63, 5.29)	303	32	10.56 (7.46, 14.41)	379	18	4.75 (2.93, 7.26)
2012	322	13	4.04 (2.26, 6.63)	265	33	12.45 (8.88, 16.85)	434	27	6.22 (4.22, 8.80)
2013	420	20	4.76 (3.02, 7.13)	338	30	8.88 (6.18, 12.27)	462	37	8.01 (5.79, 10.76)
2014	519	10	1.93 (0.98, 3.41)	335	30	8.96 (6.24, 12.38)	439	44	10.02 (7.47, 13.10)
2015	615	26	4.23 (2.84, 6.05)	409	57	13.94 (10.83, 17.55)	504	41	8.13 (5.98, 10.77)
2016	617	31	5.02 (3.50, 6.97)	437	73	16.70 (12.39, 18.90)	496	49	9.88 (7.48, 12.75)

VRE vancomycin-resistant enterococci

found a continuous increase in resistance against vancomycin in *E. faecium* between 2001 and 2016 [11]. Finally, comparable results were found in the national antimicrobial resistance surveillance project [12], where detection of *E. faecium* derived from blood-cultures has increased by up to 50% in recent years and proportion of isolates resistant against vancomycin increased to 11.9% [13].

Interestingly, the recent report by the EARS-net described a high but stable situation regarding the proportion of VRE among *E. faecium* isolates of 12.1% in Germany, which is comparable with the European population weighted mean of 11.8% for 2016 [5]. These differences might be caused by the following reasons. (i) In EARS-Net, a static representative sample of hospitals from defined regions deliver rates of BSI from all wards based on laboratory results whereas in KISS a continuously growing sample of hospitals and individual wards report different types of infections (UTIs, SSIs and BSIs). However, even when considering only ICUs that continuously reported data on BSI we observed a continuous increase of VRE. (ii) As compared to EARS-net, we considered not only BSI but also surgical site infections and urinary tract infections. However, when only BSI were analysed in our study, the increase in the last 3 years has been particularly pronounced and differences to EARS-Net data remain unclear. (iii) Antimicrobial susceptibility testing (AST) in many microbiological laboratories Germany was performed according to Clinical & Laboratory Standards Institute (CLSI) while EARS-net uses EUCAST-standards only [14]. This potentially could influence vancomycin resistance rates especially in low and medium-level resistance due to differing recommended AST methods and clinical breakpoints [15].

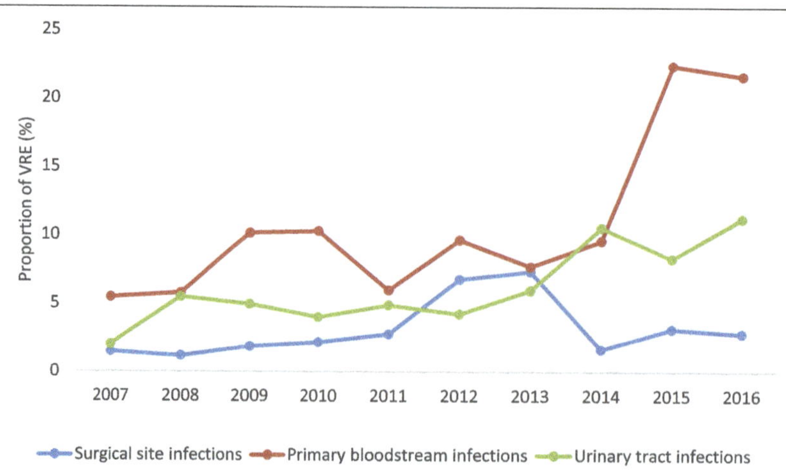

Fig. 2 Time trend for percentage of vancomycin-resistant enterococcal (VRE) infections according to the German national nosocomial infection surveillance system (KISS), by infection site. Data from wards that participated continuously from 2007 to 2016 ("core group")

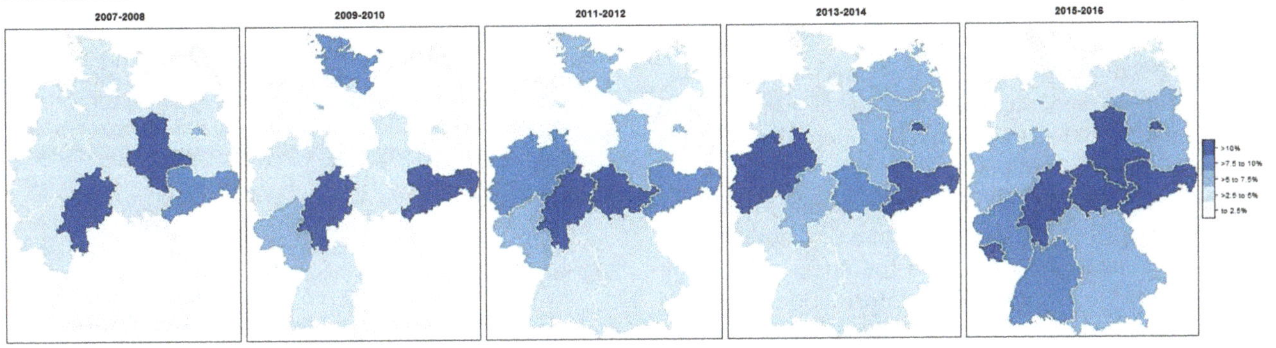

Fig. 3 Distribution of the proportion of vancomycin-resistant entercoccal (VRE) infections among German federal states according to data from the German national nosocomial infection surveillance system (KISS) 2007–2016

Risk factors that have been described for VRE colonization or infections are long periods of hospitalization, hemodialysis, immunosuppression as well as close proximity to patients infected or colonized with VRE [16]. The fact that enterococci are able to survive on environmental surfaces for long periods of time [16, 17] highlights the importance of adherence to hand hygiene practice to prevent transmission. But despite improved adherence to hand-hygiene and successful reduction of nosocomial infections in Germany [18, 19], VRE continues to gain importance when compared to other multidrug resistant gram-positive organisms [11].

Increased antibiotic consumption has been advocated as another important risk factor that influence spread of VRE [16, 20, 21]. Many reports have established an indirect or direct link between appearance of VRE and the consumption of certain antimicrobial groups but the connection probably is more complex [21]. Exposure to substances with a broad gram-negative and anerobic microbiological spectrum, but no coverage against *E. faecium* are believed to facilitate the colonization of the GI-tract with VRE [22]. Particularly carbapenems [20], 3rd generation cephalosporins [23] but also penicillin's with beta-lactamase inhibitors such as piperacillin/tazobactam [24] are likely to trigger this process. In Germany, cephalosporins are now the most commonly prescribed in German primary care [25] and might have triggered VRE-selection in the outpatient setting already. This would highlight the need of antibiotic stewardship not only in the inpatient but also in the outpatient setting [26, 27]. Interestingly, a recent meta-analysis has not found a direct influence of measures within in-hospital antimicrobial stewardship and the occurrence of VRE; however, the number of included studies was limited [28].

Although differences of VRE are obviously among European countries [5], only few studies have assessed regional differences of VRE within the same country. In a Canadian study, in which the molecular epidemiology of VRE from invasive samples from the National Nosocomial Infection Surveillance Program (CNISP) was analyzed found an increase of VRE in western and central Canada [29]. The authors assumed that the clonal spread of certain sequence types might have been in part responsible for these findings, although a reliable explanation was not possible. Kullar et al. evaluated regional variations on VRE across blood, urine and wound sources in United States Hospitals 2015 and found significant differences among US states [30]. A potential explanation for these results was not discussed.

The reasons for the regional differences in our study are also unclear and possible reasons for higher VRE rates in the center of Germany are difficult to explain and are likely to be multifactorial [6]. One possible explanation might be regional variations in antibiotic usage in the ambulatory and/or the inpatient setting; for example, a large population-based study found among German federal states differences in outpatient antibiotic prescription rates [25] of fluoroquinolones and cephalosporines, substances that might influence VRE selection process [1, 16, 22]. Other reasons for the regional differences that have been discussed are differences in the proportion of VRE in the environment (e.g. higher proportion of VRE in farm animals) or the spread of new or clonal VRE strain in certain areas [6]. However, Willems et al. found genetic differences in hospital-acquired VRE isolates and community-acquired or animal isolates which makes an association between the environment and increased VRE rates in German ICUs unlikely [31].

Some limitations have to be acknowledged: (i) Since fulfillment of case criteria depends on diagnostic sampling and documentation there is a risk for underdetection of cases. However, using proportions of VRE for all nosocomial infections caused by enterococci might have reduce confounding effects for changes in the bacteriological diagnostic over time, since only pathogen-derived infections were included. (ii) We did not record below a genus level of enterococci; therefore, we were unable to rule out an increase of Enterococcus spp. with intrinsic glycopeptide resistance. However, this is less likely since national and international sources have reported an increase vancomycin-resistant *E. faecium*, while infections due to vancomycin-resistant *E. faecalis* and Enterococcus spp. with intrinsic glycopeptid resistance e.g. *E. gallinarum* remain rare [2, 32]. (iii) Since we used surveillance definitions to determine infections, in some cases of UTIs the identified VRE might have been a contamination rather than the infection-causing pathogen. (iv) Finally, we had no information regarding strain characteristics, therefore local or regional outbreaks cannot be excluded.

Conclusion

To proportion of vancomycin-resistant enterococcal infections has emerged as a relevant threat for patients and the healthcare system in Germany. Particularly the increasing rate of VRE in blood stream infections pose a serious threat for patients. Although specific recommendations and efforts regarding prevention of nosocomial infections, transmission of VRE and improvement in antimicrobial prescription are in place in Germany, the proportion of VRE continues to increase. To this end, implementation of effective strategies are necessary in order to reduce the spread of VRE.

Abbreviations

95% CI: 95% confidence interval; BSI: Blood stream infection; ICU: Intensive care unit; OR: Odds ratio; SSI: Surgical site infection; UTI: Urinary tract infection;; VRE: Vancomycin-resistant enterococcus

Authors' contributions

CR, PG, CG and TSK were responsible for the study design. PG supervised the study. MB and CS were responsible for data collection and data cleaning. CS conducted the statistical analysis. All authors interpreted the data, gave important intellectual content and revised the manuscript critically. All authors read and approved the final manuscript.

Competing interests

The authors declare that they have no competing interests.

References

1. O'Driscoll T, Crank CW. Vancomycin-resistant enterococcal infections: epidemiology, clinical manifestations, and optimal management. Infect Drug Resist. 2015;8:217–30.
2. Werner G, Coque TM, Hammerum AM, Hope R, Hryniewicz W, Johnson A, Klare I, Kristinsson KG, Leclercq R, Lester CH, et al. Emergence and spread of vancomycin resistance among enterococci in Europe. Euro Surveill. 2008;13(47). https://www.eurosurveillance.org/content/10.2807/ese.13.47.19046-en.
3. Chiang HY, Perencevich EN, Nair R, Nelson RE, Samore M, Khader K, Chorazy ML, Herwaldt LA, Blevins A, Ward MA, et al. Incidence and outcomes associated with infections caused by vancomycin-resistant enterococci in the United States: systematic literature review and meta-analysis. Infect Control Hosp Epidemiol. 2017;38(2):203–15.
4. World Health Organization (WHO): Global priority list of antibiotic-resistant bacteria to guide research, discovery, and development of new antibiotics. Available at http://www.who.int/medicines/publications/WHO-PPL-Short_Summary_25Feb-ET_NM_WHO.pdf?ua=1. Accessed 03 Mar 2017. 2017.
5. European Centre for Disease Prevention and Control: Antimicrobial resistance surveillance in Europe 2016. Annual report of the European antimicrobial resistance surveillance network (EARS-net). Stockholm: ECDC. 2018.
6. Gastmeier P, Schroder C, Behnke M, Meyer E, Geffers C. Dramatic increase in vancomycin-resistant enterococci in Germany. J Antimicrob Chemother. 2014;69(6):1660–4.
7. Gastmeier P, Sohr D, Schwab F, Behnke M, Zuschneid I, Brandt C, Dettenkofer M, Chaberny IF, Ruden H, Geffers C. Ten years of KISS: the most important requirements for success. J Hosp Infect. 2008;70(Suppl 1):11–6.
8. Horan TC, Andrus M, Dudeck MA. CDC/NHSN surveillance definition of health care-associated infection and criteria for specific types of infections in the acute care setting. Am J Infect Control. 2008;36(5):309–32.
9. Nationales Referenzzentrum für nosokomiale Infektionen: Deutsche nationale Punkt-Prävalenzerhebung zu nosokomialen Infektionen und Antibiotika-Anwendung 2016; Abschlussbericht. Access at http://www.nrz-hygiene.de/fileadmin/nrz/download/pps2016/PPS_2016_Abschlussbericht_20.07.2017.pdf. Last Accessed 20 Mar 2018. 2016.
10. Behnke M, Aghdassi SJ, Hansen S, Diaz LAP, Gastmeier P, Piening B. The prevalence of nosocomial infection and antibiotic use in German hospitals. Dtsch Arztebl Int. 2017;114(50):851–7.
11. Remschmidt C, Schneider S, Meyer E, Schroeren-Boersch B, Gastmeier P, Schwab F. Surveillance of antibiotic use and resistance in intensive care units (SARI). Dtsch Arztebl Int. 2017;114(50):858–65.
12. Noll I, Schweickert B, Abu Sin M, Feig M, Claus H, Eckmanns T. Antimicrobial resistance in Germany. Four years of antimicrobial resistance surveillance (ARS). Bundesgesundheitsblatt Gesundheitsforschung Gesundheitsschutz. 2012;55(11–12):1370–6.
13. Klare IBJ, Koppe U, Abu Sin M, Eckmanns T, Werner G. Eigenschaften, Häufigkeit und Verbreitung von Vancomycin-resistenten Enterokokken (VRE) in Deutschland – Update 2015/2016. Epid Bull. 2017;46:519–27. https://doi.org/10.17886/EpiBull-2017-063. 2017
14. European Society of Clinical Microbiology and Infectious Diseases: The European Committee on Antimicrobial Susceptibility Testing - EUCAST. Available at http://www.eucast.org/. Last Access 20 Mar 2018. 2017.
15. Hegstad K, Giske CG, Haldorsen B, Matuschek E, Schonning K, Leegaard TM, Kahlmeter G, Sundsfjord A, Nordic ASTVREDSG. Performance of the EUCAST disk diffusion method, the CLSI agar screen method, and the Vitek 2 automated antimicrobial susceptibility testing system for detection of clinical isolates of enterococci with low- and medium-level VanB-type vancomycin resistance: a multicenter study. J Clin Microbiol. 2014;52(5):1582–9.
16. Arias CA, Murray BE. The rise of the enterococcus: beyond vancomycin resistance. Nat Rev Microbiol. 2012;10(4):266–78.
17. McDermott H, Skally M, O'Rourke J, Humphreys H, Fitzgerald-Hughes D. Vancomycin-resistant enterococci (VRE) in the intensive care unit in a nonoutbreak setting: identification of potential reservoirs and epidemiological associations between patient and environmental VRE. Infect Control Hosp Epidemiol. 2018;39(1):40–5.
18. Wetzker W, Walter J, Bunte-Schonberger K, Schwab F, Behnke M, Gastmeier P, Reichardt C. Hand rub consumption has almost doubled in 132 German hospitals over 9 years. Infect Control Hosp Epidemiol. 2017;38(7):870–2.
19. Gastmeier P, Geffers C, Herrmann M, Lemmen S, Salzberger B, Seifert H, Kern W, Fatkenheuer G. Nosocomial infections and infections with multidrug-resistant pathogens - frequency and mortality. Dtsch Med Wochenschr. 2016;141(6):421–6.
20. Remschmidt C, Behnke M, Kola A, Pena Diaz LA, Rohde AM, Gastmeier P, Schwab F. The effect of antibiotic use on prevalence of nosocomial vancomycin-resistant enterococci- an ecologic study. Antimicrob Resist Infect Control. 2017;6:95.
21. Harbarth S, Cosgrove S, Carmeli Y. Effects of antibiotics on nosocomial epidemiology of vancomycin-resistant enterococci. Antimicrob Agents Chemother. 2002;46(6):1619–28.
22. Donskey CJ, Chowdhry TK, Hecker MT, Hoyen CK, Hanrahan JA, Hujer AM, Hutton-Thomas RA, Whalen CC, Bonomo RA, Rice LB. Effect of antibiotic therapy on the density of vancomycin-resistant enterococci in the stool of colonized patients. N Engl J Med. 2000;343(26):1925–32.
23. Fridkin SK, Edwards JR, Courval JM, Hill H, Tenover FC, Lawton R, Gaynes RP, McGowan JE Jr, Intensive Care Antimicrobial Resistance Epidemiology P, the National Nosocomial Infections Surveillance System H. The effect of

vancomycin and third-generation cephalosporins on prevalence of vancomycin-resistant enterococci in 126 U.S. adult intensive care units. Ann Intern Med. 2001;135(3):175–83.

24. Stiefel U, Pultz NJ, Donskey CJ. Effect of carbapenem administration on establishment of intestinal colonization by vancomycin-resistant enterococci and Klebsiella pneumoniae in mice. Antimicrob Agents Chemother. 2007; 51(1):372–5.
25. Batzing-Feigenbaum J, Schulz M, Schulz M, Hering R, Kern WV. Outpatient Antibiotic Prescription. Dtsch Arztebl Int. 2016;113(26):454–9.
26. Dyar OJ, Beovic B, Vlahovic-Palcevski V, Verheij T, Pulcini C, on behalf of E. How can we improve antibiotic prescribing in primary care? Expert Rev Anti-Infect Ther. 2016;14(4):403–13.
27. McNulty C, Hawking M, Lecky D, Jones L, Owens R, Charlett A, Butler C, Moore P, Francis N. Effects of primary care antimicrobial stewardship outreach on antibiotic use by general practice staff: pragmatic randomized controlled trial of the TARGET antibiotics workshop. J Antimicrob Chemother. 2018;73(5):1423–32.
28. Baur D, Gladstone BP, Burkert F, Carrara E, Foschi F, Dobele S, Tacconelli E. Effect of antibiotic stewardship on the incidence of infection and colonisation with antibiotic-resistant bacteria and Clostridium difficile infection: a systematic review and meta-analysis. Lancet Infect Dis. 2017; 17(9):990–1001.
29. McCracken M, Wong A, Mitchell R, Gravel D, Conly J, Embil J, Johnston L, Matlow A, Ormiston D, Simor AE, et al. Molecular epidemiology of vancomycin-resistant enterococcal bacteraemia: results from the Canadian nosocomial infection surveillance program, 1999-2009. J Antimicrob Chemother. 2013;68(7):1505–9.
30. Kullar RM, S.; Tabak, YP.; Deryke CA.; Johannes RS.; Sarpong EM.; Gupta V.;: Regional and Source Variations in Vancomycin-Resistant Enterococci Rates in United States Hospitals 2015. Open Forum Infectious Diseases, 3, Issue suppl_1, 2016, 307. 2016.
31. Willems RJ, Top J, van Schaik W, Leavis H, Bonten M, Siren J, Hanage WP, Corander J. Restricted gene flow among hospital subpopulations of enterococcus faecium. MBio. 2012;3(4):e00151–12.
32. Klare I, Witte W, Wendt C, Werner G. Vancomycin-resistant enterococci (VRE). Recent results and trends in development of antibiotic resistance. Bundesgesundheitsblatt Gesundheitsforschung Gesundheitsschutz. 2012; 55(11–12):1387–400.

Carbapenem non-susceptibility of *Klebsiella pneumoniae* isolates in hospitals from 2011 to 2016, data from the German Antimicrobial Resistance Surveillance (ARS)

Uwe Koppe[1*], Anja von Laer[3], Lars E. Kroll[2], Ines Noll[1], Marcel Feig[1], Marc Schneider[1], Hermann Claus[1], Tim Eckmanns[1] and Muna Abu Sin[1]

Abstract

Background: Carbapenem resistance in *Klebsiella pneumoniae* is of significant public health concern and recently spread across several countries. We investigated the extent of carbapenem non-susceptibility in *K. pneumoniae* isolates in Germany.

Methods: We analysed 2011–2016 data from the German Antimicrobial Resistance Surveillance (ARS) System, which contains routine data of antimicrobial susceptibility testing from voluntarily participating German laboratories. *Klebsiella pneumoniae* isolates tested resistant or intermediate against an antibiotic were classified as non-susceptible.

Results: We included 154,734 isolates from 655 hospitals in the analysis. Carbapenem non-susceptibility in *K. pneumoniae* isolates was low in Germany 0.63% (95% CI 0.51–0.76%). However, in continuously participating hospitals the number of *K. pneumoniae* isolates almost doubled and we found evidence for a slowly increasing trend for non-susceptibility (OR = 1.20 per year, 95% CI 1.09–1.33, $p < 0.001$). Carbapenem non-susceptibility was highest among isolates from patients aged 20–39 in men but not in women. Moreover, carbapenem non-susceptibility was more frequently reported for isolates from tertiary care, specialist care, and prevention and rehabilitation care hospitals as well as from intensive care units. Co-resistance of carbapenem non-susceptible isolates against antibiotics such as tigecycline, gentamicin, and co-trimoxazole was common. Co-resistance against colistin was 13.3% (95% CI 9.8–17.9%) in carbapenem non-susceptible isolates.

Conclusion: Carbapenem non-susceptibility in *K. pneumoniae* isolates in Germany is still low. However, it is slowly increasing and in the light of the strong increase of *K. pneumoniae* isolates over the last year this poses a significant challenge to public health. Continued surveillance to closely monitor trends as well as infection control and antibiotic stewardship activities are necessary to preserve treatment options.

Keywords: *Klebsiella pneumoniae*, Carbapenem, Surveillance, Antimicrobial, Resistance

* Correspondence: koppeu@rki.de
[1]Department of Infectious Disease Epidemiology, Robert Koch Institute, Seestr. 10, 13353 Berlin, Germany
Full list of author information is available at the end of the article

Background

Klebsiella (K.) pneumoniae is a gram negative pathogen in the family of *Enterobacteriaceae*. It is able to acquire a wide array of antimicrobial resistance (AMR) genes and can cause severe healthcare- associated infections [1, 2]. Infections with carbapenem non-susceptible *K. pneumoniae* are associated with higher mortality and the World Health Organization classified carbapenem-resistant *K. pneumoniae* as a critical priority pathogen for research and development [3, 4]. Carbapenem resistance has been emerging world-wide over the last years with local differences in frequency and mechanisms of resistance [1]. The prevalence of carbapenem non-susceptible *K. pneumoniae* strongly increased in countries of Southern Europe such as Greece and Italy [5]. Germany has experienced local outbreaks of carbapenem-resistant *K. pneumoniae* and other resistant *Enterobacteriaceae* [6, 7]. The German National Reference Centre for multidrug-resistant gram-negative bacteria analyses carbapenem non-susceptible *K. pneumoniae* strains that are submitted for further analysis and confirmation. In a recent analysis, carbapenemases could be identified in 50,9% of carbapenem-resistant *K. pneumoniae* isolates with OXA-48 being the most prevalent [8]. In a recent study in a German academic tertiary care centre, OXA-48 was detected in 19 of 28 carbapenem-resistant *K. pneumoniae* isolates [9].

A pivotal element in the prevention and control of carbapenem-resistant *K. pneumoniae* is the regular and ongoing surveillance of colonizations and infections in order to inform infection control measures in hospitals [10].

The Antimicrobial Resistance Surveillance (ARS) is the national surveillance system for AMR in Germany [11]. Since 2008, microbiological laboratories across Germany voluntarily participate and submit data from routine antimicrobial susceptibility testing to ARS. AMR data for selected pathogens are accessible on the ARS website (https://ars.rki.de). In addition, the surveillance system contributes data to the European Antimicrobial Resistance Surveillance Network (EARS-Net) and to the Global Antimicrobial Resistance Surveillance System (GLASS) at the World Health Organization [5].

In 2016, a national statutory surveillance system for carbapenem non-susceptibility was implemented in Germany. However, information on changes in carbapenem resistance over the recent years is scarce. The objective of our study was to analyse trends and risk-factors for carbapenem non-susceptibility of *K. pneumoniae* isolates in Germany as well as co-resistance of carbapenem non-susceptible isolates to other commonly used antibiotics.

Methods

Study design and data source

We undertook an observational cross-sectional study to analyse carbapenem non-susceptibility of *K. pneumoniae* isolates in hospitals in Germany.

Data on antimicrobial susceptibility testing are obtained from ARS. Participating laboratories share their data on routine antimicrobial susceptibility testing (AST) of microbiological samples from hospitals and medical practices [11]. Participation is voluntary for the laboratories and can change over time. The sample of hospitals and medical practices providing data to ARS is organised by laboratory clusters. The geographical distribution of the hospitals contributing data to the study is shown in Additional file 1: Appendix S2. The identity of the hospitals and medical practices is kept confidential. Data on patients is anonymised.

The laboratories identify bacteria from specimens sent in from hospitals or medical practices and determine the zone diameters or minimum inhibitory concentrations (MIC) of routinely used antibiotics (e.g. with microdilution, gradient or disk diffusion). Based on international guidelines (e.g. by the European Committee on Antimicrobial Susceptibility Testing (EUCAST)), the zone diameter or MIC are used for the interpretative results "susceptible" (S), "intermediate" (I), or "resistant" (R) against the tested antibiotic.

All participating laboratories are accredited to perform pathogen identification and antimicrobial susceptibility testing. Data are checked for plausibility during the data transmission process and are validated by the laboratories annually for completeness and consistency.

Outcomes and covariates

The main outcome of the study is the proportion of carbapenem non-susceptible *K. pneumoniae* isolates in relation to all *K. pneumoniae* isolates tested for carbapenem resistance. An isolate is considered non-susceptible against an antibiotic if the susceptibility test results are interpreted as "resistant" (R) or "intermediate" (I). Age was converted into a categorical variable for the analysis (< 1, 1–19, 20–39, 40–49, 50–59, 60–69, 70–79, and 80+ years). The specimen types were grouped as follows: swabs (swabs from eye, nose, throat, ear, tongue, and urogenital sites as well as intraoperative swabs and other/unspecified swabs), blood (blood cultures), puncture (tissue biopsy, cerebrospinal fluid, and aspirate from pleural cavity, abscess, ascites, or joint puncture, other punctures), urine (urine samples), wound (swabs from wounds and abscesses), respiratory (bronchial lavage, bronchial secretions, sputum, tracheal secretion, other respiratory samples), other (dialysate, ejaculate, catheters, other). To analyse for seasonality, a categorical variable was created according to the month in which the isolate was obtained: January – March, April – June, July – September, October – December. The geographic regions were grouped as follows: Northwest (Bremen, Hamburg, Lower Saxony, Schleswig-Holstein), West (North Rhine-Westphalia), Southwest (Baden-Wuerttemberg,

Hesse, Rhineland-Palatinate, Saarland), Southeast (Bavaria, Saxony, Thuringia), and Northeast (Berlin, Brandenburg, Mecklenburg-West Pomerania, Saxony-Anhalt). Several variables on the county level of the hospital were also included in the analysis: counties were divided into "rural" or "city" based on a list from the Federal Agency for Cartography and Geodesy [12, 13]. Moreover, the social deprivation index per county was derived from the German Index of Socioeconomic Deprivation (GISD) [14, 15]. The GISD uses nine indicators from publicly available administrative datasets. It is based on factor analysis for indexing and weighting of the indicators to the three latent dimensions education, occupation and income. For the analysis, a categorical variable was created dividing the counties by social deprivation index into quintiles with 1 indicating the lowest deprivation and 5 the highest. In addition, the density of hospital beds per 10.000 inhabitants was also included on a county level. For the analysis a categorical variable was created dividing the counties by hospital bed densities into quartiles.

Analysed risk factors include age and sex of the patient, hospital care level (Secondary Care, Tertiary Care, Specialist Care, Prevention and Rehabilitation Care, other), type of care (intensive, normal hospital ward, other), clinical speciality (surgery and related, internal medicine, other), specimen type, region, county type (rural, city), social deprivation index of the county where the hospital is located, hospital beds per 10.000 inhabitants in the county where the hospital is located as well as year and quarter when the isolate was obtained.

In- and exclusion criteria of *K. pneumoniae* isolates

In the analysis, we focused on materials that are most likely derived from clinical samples, so isolates labelled as screening samples, anal swabs, and stool samples were excluded. We excluded isolates without susceptibility testing. In order to avoid bias from repeated testing, we only included the first isolate per patient per quarter in the analysis irrespective of the specimen type. If several isolates from one patient were tested on the same day we selected the most relevant isolate for the analysis according to this priority: isolate tested non-susceptible against at least one carbapenem > isolate tested against at least one carbapenem > isolate not tested against at least one carbapenem.

Statistical analysis

The distribution of baseline characteristics of the *K. pneumoniae* isolates was analysed using percentages and 95% confidence intervals (95% CI) for categorical variables accounting for clustering on the hospital level. Continuous variables were analysed as means with standard deviations if normally distributed and as median with interquartile ranges if non-normally distributed.

Carbapenem non-susceptibility was defined as the proportion of non-susceptible isolates in relation to all tested isolates in the analysis and expressed in percentage and 95% confidence intervals accounting for clustering on the hospital level. An isolate was considered non-susceptible to at least one carbapenem if it was tested as intermediate or resistant against meropenem, imipenem, or ertapenem.

Risk factors for carbapenem non-susceptibility were analysed using univariable and multivariable multilevel (hierarchical) mixed-effects logistic regression models with random intercepts, accounting for clustering on the county and hospital level. Mixed models allow calculating intraclass correlation coefficients for the random intercepts, to quantify variance on different levels [16]. *P*-values were calculated using Wald tests. For the multivariable model, year, quarter, age and sex of patient, hospital care level, type of care, clinical speciality, specimen type, region, county type, county deprivation index, and hospital beds per 10,000 inhabitants were included. Isolates with missing data in any of these variables were not included in the uni- and multivariable regression models (full case analysis).

For the analysis of carbapenem non-susceptibility over time, a univariable multilevel (hierarchical) mixed-effects logistic regression model was calculated with year as a continuous variable. Only isolates from hospitals that continuously contributed data from 2011 to 2016 were included in the analysis. The *p*-value was derived from a Wald test.

Sensitivity analyses

Not all isolates have been tested for resistance against all three carbapenems (meropenem, imipenem, and ertapenem) and we conducted a sensitivity analysis restricted to isolates that were tested against all three carbapenems.

Differences in EUCAST and CLSI breakpoints might lead to different interpretations of carbapenem non-susceptibility. Consequently, in some cases an isolate might have been categorized as "sensitive" according to one standard and as "intermediate" (i.e. non-susceptible) according to the other standard. Since the use of standards changes over time, this could have affected our results over time. To address this issue, we performed sensitivity analyses for changes in carbapenem non-susceptibility over time: 1) restricted to isolates evaluated according to EUCAST since this is the most commonly used standard in our surveillance data; 2) excluding isolates categorized as "intermediate" to one or more carbapenems and not "resistant" to any carbapenem because for some isolates the classification as "sensitive" or "intermediate" might depend on the standard used.

Resistance against some antibiotics is not routinely tested (e.g. colistin), but only when resistance against other antibiotics is found. Since this can introduce bias into the analysis, we conducted a sensitivity analysis for these antibiotics by restricting the analysis to isolates from laboratories that routinely test ≥90% of all isolates against the respective antibiotic.

Results

Of the 394,637 *K. pneumoniae* isolates in the database we excluded screening isolates, isolates without antimicrobial testing, repeated isolates of the same patient within one quarter, and isolates from outpatients. We included 154,734 isolates between 2011 and 2016 from 655 hospitals in the analysis (Fig. 1).

The median period of data availability per hospital was 2.0 years (IQR: 1.7–4.0 years). Out of all hospitals, 96 had continuous participation in our surveillance system between 2011 and 2016 (45,995 isolates). Hospitals contributing data to the analysis were distributed across Germany with clusters in Schleswig-Holstein, North Rhine-Westphalia, and Baden-Wuerttemberg (Additional file 1: Appendix S2). Over time more hospitals contributed data and the number of isolates strongly increased (Additional file 1: Appendix S3). Interestingly, the number of isolates from continuously participating hospitals almost doubled. Most participating hospitals and included isolates were from the western region in Germany. Further information on the distribution of isolates across subgroups can be found in Additional file 1: Appendices S3 and S4.

Antimicrobial susceptibility testing results were interpreted according to guidelines from the EUCAST for most isolates (76.2%). Other interpretation guidelines used were from the Clinical & Laboratory Standards Institute (CLSI, 15.4%), the German Institute for Standardization (DIN, 7.2%), or no information on interpretation guidelines was given (1.1%). Interpretation of the results according to EUCAST guidelines strongly increased over time (Additional file 1: Appendix S5).

Out of the 154,734 *K. pneumoniae* isolates, 99.9% were tested against at least one carbapenem (Table 1).

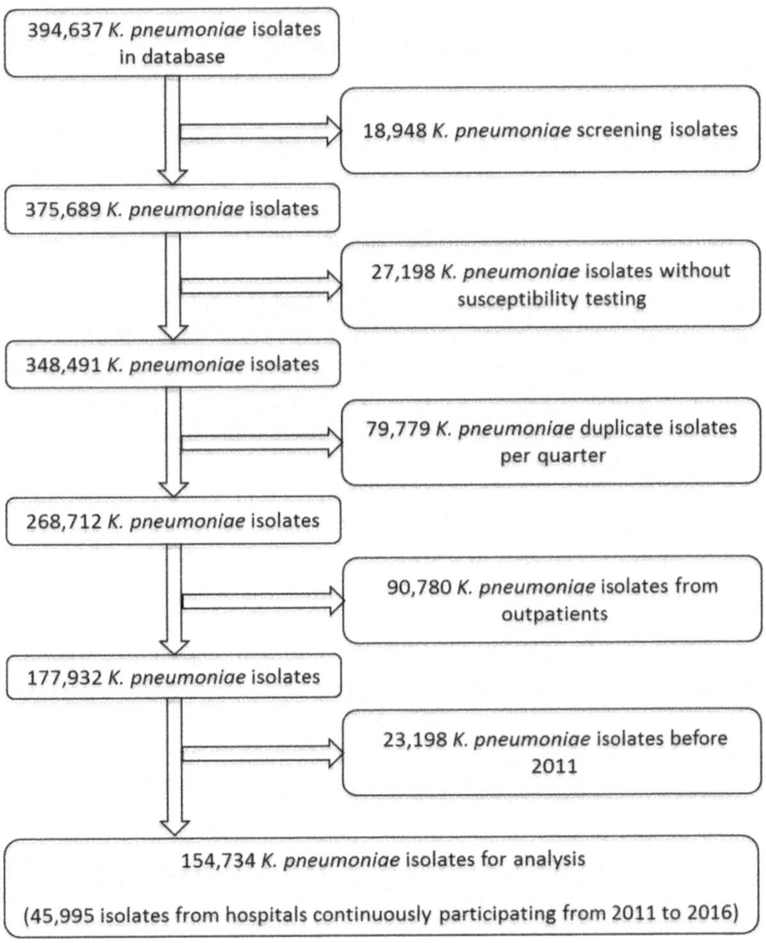

Fig. 1 Selection of *K. pneumoniae* isolates from ARS database for the analysis, 2011–2016

Table 1 Carbapenem non-susceptibility of *K. pneumoniae* isolates in Germany 2011–2016 (n = 154,734)

Tested carbapenem	Number of isolates tested (% of all isolates)	Isolates tested "susceptible" (% with 95% CI)[a]	Isolates tested "intermediate" (% with 95% CI)[a]	Isolates tested "resistant" (% with 95% CI)[a]	Isolates tested "non-susceptible" (% with 95% CI)[a]
Meropenem	150,746 (97.4%)	99.58% (99.49, 99.65%)	0.09% (0.07, 0.12%)	0.33% (0.27, 0.40%)	0.42% (0.35, 0.51%)
Imipenem	150,114 (97.0%)	99.62% (99.54, 99.69%)	0.11% (0.09, 0.14%)	0.27% (0.22, 0.34%)	0.38% (0.31, 0.46%)
Ertapenem	56,560 (36.6%)	98.95% (98.68, 99.16%)	0.11% (0.08, 0.16%)	0.94% (0.74, 1.2%)	1.05% (0.84, 1.32%)
At least one carbapenem[b]	154,524 (99.9%)	99.37% (99.24, 99.49%)	0.11% (0.08, 0.13%)	0.52% (0.42, 0.64%)	0.63% (0.51, 0.76%)

[a] 95% CI calculated accounting for clustering on hospital level
[b]Meropenem, imipenem or ertapenem

The proportion of isolates non-susceptible against at least one carbapenem was 0.63% (95% CI 0.51–0.76%). In detail, 0.11% (95% CI 0.08–0.13%) of the isolates were tested intermediate against at least one carbapenem and 0.52% (95% CI 0.42–0.64%) were tested resistant. Almost all isolates were tested against meropenem and imipenem, whereas susceptibility against ertapenem was tested in only about a third of the isolates. The proportion of non-susceptible isolates was higher for ertapenem than meropenem or imipenem. A sensitivity analysis restricted to isolates tested against all three carbapenems yielded comparable results (Additional file 1: Appendix S6).

Isolates found non-susceptible to meropenem or imipenem were often non-susceptible against the two other carbapenems as well (Table 2).

Interestingly, only about half of the isolates tested non-susceptible against ertapenem were also found to be non-susceptible against meropenem or imipenem. A sensitivity analysis restricted to isolates that had been tested against all three carbapenems yielded similar results (Additional file 1: Appendix S7). In addition, we found that out of the 501 isolates tested non-susceptible against both imipenem and meropenem, 139 (27.7%) were tested as intermediate against one or both of these substances.

Non-susceptibility of isolates against at least one carbapenem increased from 0.35% in 2011 to 0.78% in 2016 (Table 3).

Since the number of the participating hospitals changes over time, we restricted the analysis to 96 hospitals that continuously contributed data to the analyses between 2011 and 2016. In these hospitals carbapenem non-susceptibility appears to be stable until 2013 and then increased over the following years. We found evidence for an increasing trend of carbapenem non-susceptibility in the continuously participating hospitals (OR = 1.20 per year, 95% CI 1.09–1.33, $p < 0.001$). The sensitivity analyses 1) restricted to isolates evaluated according to EUCAST and 2) excluding isolates labelled as "intermediate" to one or more carbapenems and not "resistant" to any carbapenem yielded similar results (Additional file 1: Appendix S8).

In uni- and multivariable analyses for risk factors associated with carbapenem non-susceptibility, we could observe that isolates collected from men were more likely to be non-susceptible against at least one carbapenem than isolates from women (Table 4 and Additional file 1: Appendix S9).

Isolates from tertiary care, specialist care, and prevention and rehabilitation care hospitals were more likely to be non-susceptible against at least one carbapenem (Table 4). In addition, isolates from patients in intensive care units were also associated with a greater risk of carbapenem non-susceptibility. Compared to isolates from urine cultures, isolates from swabs, wounds, and other materials also were more likely to be non-susceptible. We found some evidence that isolates from the region "West" had the highest risk of non-susceptibility against at least one carbapenem in multivariable analyses. We found no association of quarter, clinical speciality, county type, social deprivation index, and hospital beds per 10,000 inhabitants with the outcome.

Table 2 Cross-resistance of *K. pneumoniae* isolates non-susceptible against one carbapenem to other tested carbapenems

	Additional non-susceptibility (R + I) against		
Non-susceptibility (R + I) against	Meropenem	Imipenem	Ertapenem
Meropenem (n = 634)	–	501/619 (80.9%)	299/314 (95.2%)
Imipenem (n = 569)	501/562 (89.1%)	–	252/272 (92.6%)
Ertapenem (n = 596)	252/591 (42.6%)	299/590 (50.7%)	–

R resistant, *I* intermediate

Table 3 Non-susceptibility of *K. pneumoniae* isolates against at least one carbapenem

		Percentage non-susceptible (R + I) against at least one carbapenem[a] (95%CI)[b]	
Year	Number of hospitals	All hospitals	Continuously participating hospitals ($n = 96$)
2011	180	0.35% (0.18%; 0.69%)	0.30% (0.17%; 0.51%)
2012	306	0.46% (0.31%; 0.68%)	0.27% (0.17%; 0.41%)
2013	363	0.49% (0.36%; 0.67%)	0.28% (0.18%; 0.45%)
2014	266	0.74% (0.53%; 1.04%)	0.78% (0.46%; 1.33%)
2015	372	0.66% (0.54%; 0.80%)	0.56% (0.35%; 0.89%)
2016	418	0.78% (0.58%; 1.06%)	0.53% (0.35%; 0.81%)

R resistant, *I* intermediate, *CI* confidence interval
[a]Meropenem, imipenem or ertapenem
[b]95% CI calculated accounting for clustering on hospital level

In the multivariable hierarchical logistical regression model accounting for clustering between counties and hospitals, the intraclass cluster coefficient for the variance of carbapenem non-susceptibility between counties was 5.9% and between hospitals 11.8%. Overall, 17.8% of the variance observed was attributable to clustering by county and hospital.

When analysed according to age groups, isolates derived from patients 20–39 years had the highest proportion of non-susceptible isolates (1.17, 95%CI 0.79–1.71%) (Additional file 1: Appendix S9). A stratification of carbapenem non-susceptibility across age groups according to sex showed that the increase in non-susceptibility in the younger age groups affected only isolates from men whereas isolates from women had a decreased chance for carbapenem non-susceptibility in both uni- and multivariable analyses (p for interaction < 0.001) (Fig. 2, Additional file 1: Appendix S10). Moreover, this pattern remained unchanged in analyses excluding isolates from gynaecology / obstetric wards or excluding isolates from urine samples (Additional file 1: Appendix S10).

For the 966 isolates non-susceptible to at least one carbapenem, we investigated co-resistance to other antibiotics (Table 5).

Non-susceptibility against penicillin/beta-lactamase inhibitor combinations, 3rd generation cephalosporins, fluoroquinolones, and nitrofurantoin was high. For tigecycline, fosfomycin, gentamicin, and co-trimoxazole non-susceptibility was found in about half of the isolates. Non-susceptibility was lowest for colistin / polymyxins with 13.3% (95% CI 9.8–17.9%). To investigate selective testing, we restricted the analyses to isolates from laboratories that tested at least 90% of their isolates against the respective antibiotic. The proportion of non-susceptible isolates remained similar to the overall analysis. Out of the 966 isolates non-susceptible to at least one carbapenem, 143 were tested against all antibiotics listed in Table 5 (14.8%). Two of those isolates were tested non-susceptible against all the above mentioned antibiotics, indicating pan-resistant *K. pneumoniae* isolates. In addition, we found 119 isolates that were potentially pan-resistant, i.e. they were tested non-susceptible to the above mentioned antibiotics where investigated, but susceptibility testing results were not available for all these antibiotics.

Discussion

In this study using routinely collected data on antimicrobial susceptibility testing we found that carbapenem non-susceptibility in *K. pneumoniae* isolates was 0.63% (95% CI 0.51–0.76%) and slowly increasing (OR = 1.20 per year, 95% CI 1.09–1.33, $p < 0.001$). Carbapenem non-susceptibility increased across younger age groups in isolates from men but not from women. Co-resistance against antibiotics of last resort for the treatment of patients with multi-drug resistant bacterial infections was common.

Carbapenem resistance has increased strongly over the last years in some regions, e.g. the United States, China, and southern European countries [5, 17, 18]. In contrast, the proportion of carbapenem non-susceptible isolates in Germany is still low and only slowly increasing. However, we found that the absolute numbers of *K. pneumoniae* isolates from continuously participating hospitals almost doubled from 2011 to 2016, which indicates a growing public health burden concerning *K. pneumoniae* in general and carbapenem non-susceptible *K. pneumoniae* in particular.

The absolute number of *K. pneumoniae* isolates was highest in the older age groups, which is in accordance with the literature [19, 20]. However, upon stratification by age and sex, it is striking that the proportion of carbapenem non-susceptibility is highest in isolates from younger male patients (ages 20–39) and lowest in female patients of the same age groups. Since we do not have further patient-based information available, we can only speculate on the reasons. This effect might be related to differences in patient-based risk factors between men and women at this age. Since we analysed only isolates from hospitals, it is possible that many women in this age group might enter the hospital for child birth while they have a good health status and few risk factors for

Table 4 Analysis of risk factors associated with carbapenem non-susceptibility of *K. pneumoniae* isolates

	Univariable analysis of risk factors associated with carbapenem non-susceptibility		Multivariable analysis of risk factors associated with carbapenem non-susceptibility	
	OR (95% CI)[a]	*p*-value[b]	OR (95% CI)[c]	*p*-value[b]
Year				
2011	1	–	1	–
2012	1.00 (0.64, 1.57)	0.994	0.99 (0.63, 1.56)	0.964
2013	1.29 (0.84, 1.99)	0.239	1.30 (0.85, 2.01)	0.229
2014	1.78 (1.16, 2.75)	0.009	1.84 (1.19, 2.84)	0.006
2015	1.87 (1.23, 2.86)	0.004	1.99 (1.29, 3.05)	0.002
2016	2.00 (1.32, 3.05)	0.001	2.10 (1.38, 3.22)	0.001
Quarter				
Jan - Mar	1	–	1	–
Apr - Jun	1.14 (0.93, 1.40)	0.217	1.13 (0.92, 1.39)	0.248
Jul - Sept	1.07 (0.87, 1.31)	0.515	1.06 (0.87, 1.30)	0.553
Oct - Dec	1.05 (0.86, 1.30)	0.618	1.07 (0.87, 1.31)	0.542
Age (years)				
< 1	0.49 (0.21, 1.11)	0.089	0.26 (0.11, 0.61)	0.002
1–19	2.28 (1.45, 3.58)	< 0.001	1.67 (1.06, 2.66)	0.029
20–39	2.87 (2.17, 3.79)	< 0.001	2.38 (1.78, 3.18)	< 0.001
40–49	1.88 (1.33, 2.64)	< 0.001	1.49 (1.05, 2.10)	0.025
50–59	2.10 (1.63, 2.70)	< 0.001	1.62 (1.26, 2.10)	< 0.001
60–69	1.73 (1.37, 2.18)	< 0.001	1.35 (1.06, 1.71)	0.013
70–79	1.57 (1.28, 1.94)	< 0.001	1.33 (1.08, 1.65)	0.007
80+	1	–	1	–
Sex				
Male	1.81 (1.57, 2.10)	< 0.001	1.57 (1.35, 1.83)	< 0.001
Female	1	–	1	–
Hospital Care Level				
Secondary Care	1	–	1	–
Tertiary Care	3.52 (2.02, 6.11)	< 0.001	2.68 (1.55, 4.66)	< 0.001
Specialist Care	2.16 (1.39, 3.37)	0.001	2.44 (1.57, 3.78)	< 0.001
Prevention and Rehabilitation Care	1.92 (0.93, 3.98)	0.078	2.22 (1.09, 4.52)	0.028
Other	0.91 (0.26, 3.21)	0.886	1.03 (0.29, 3.61)	0.966
Type of care				
Intensive care unit	2.58 (2.20, 3.03)	< 0.001	2.37 (1.98, 2.84)	< 0.001
Normal hospital ward	1	–	1	–
Other	1.96 (1.26, 3.06)	0.003	1.69 (1.08, 2.64)	0.022
Clinical specialty				
Surgery and related	1.50 (1.24, 1.82)	< 0.001	1.15 (0.94, 1.40)	0.176
Internal medicine	1	–	1	–
Other	1.50 (1.26, 1.78)	< 0.001	0.98 (0.81, 1.18)	0.821
Sample type				
Swabs	2.35 (1.94, 2.85)	< 0.001	1.87 (1.53, 2.29)	< 0.001
Blood culture	1.45 (1.01, 2.06)	0.043	1.08 (0.76, 1.56)	0.661
Puncture	1.46 (0.90, 2.37)	0.126	1.08 (0.66, 1.76)	0.769

Table 4 Analysis of risk factors associated with carbapenem non-susceptibility of *K. pneumoniae* isolates *(Continued)*

	Univariable analysis of risk factors associated with carbapenem non-susceptibility		Multivariable analysis of risk factors associated with carbapenem non-susceptibility	
	OR (95% CI)[a]	*p*-value[b]	OR (95% CI)[c]	*p*-value[b]
Urine	1	–	1	–
Wound	1.90 (1.49, 2.41)	< 0.001	1.45 (1.13, 1.87)	0.003
Respiratory	2.07 (1.69, 2.53)	< 0.001	1.21 (0.97, 1.51)	0.093
Other	3.01 (1.98, 4.58)	< 0.001	2.11 (1.37, 3.23)	< 0.001
Region				
Northwest	1	–	1	–
West	1.70 (0.93, 3.14)	0.087	1.73 (0.98, 3.06)	0.057
Southwest	1.03 (0.55, 1.93)	0.922	1.01 (0.55, 1.84)	0.983
Southeast	1.10 (0.55, 2.20)	0.783	0.89 (0.46, 1.71)	0.721
Northeast	1.57 (0.74, 3.33)	0.241	1.43 (0.69, 2.98)	0.336
County Type				
Rural	1	–	1	–
City	1.34 (0.93, 1.92)	0.119	1.17 (0.74, 1.84)	0.508
Counties by Social Deprivation Index				
1 (lowest deprivation)	1	–	1	–
2	1.29 (0.68, 2.44)	0.444	1.29 (0.70, 2.36)	0.412
3	0.96 (0.51, 1.82)	0.897	0.88 (0.47, 1.64)	0.687
4	0.84 (0.44, 1.61)	0.609	0.79 (0.42, 1.47)	0.452
5 (highest deprivation)	0.99 (0.53, 1.84)	0.971	0.91 (0.49, 1.69)	0.758
Hospital Beds per 10.000 inhabitants				
8.2–57.2	1	–	1	–
57.3–71.5	0.96 (0.59, 1.56)	0.870	0.87 (0.53, 1.42)	0.577
71.6–90.9	0.82 (0.51, 1.33)	0.431	0.62 (0.36, 1.08)	0.093
91.0–219.0	1.49 (0.94, 2.36)	0.087	1.01 (0.58, 1.77)	0.969

Isolates from patients with missing values on the variables were not included in the analysis
CI confidence interval, *OR* odds ratio
[a]Hierarchical Logistic Regression model accounting for clustering within counties and hospitals
[b]Wald test
[c]Hierarchical Logistic Regression model accounting for clustering within counties and hospitals adjusting for year, quarter age, sex, hospital care level, type of care, clinical specialty, sample type, region, county type, social deprivation index, and hospital beds per 10,000 inhabitants

carbapenem non-susceptibility. Men of the same age group, however, might potentially have more severe reasons for being in the hospital and thus potentially exhibit more risk factors to acquire carbapenem non-susceptible strains. However, sensitivity analyses excluding isolates from potentially healthier patients (from gynaecology / obstetric wards or from urine samples) still showed the same pattern of non-susceptibility and could not explain the observed disparity. Further studies with clinical information are needed to investigate this issue.

Other identified risk factors associated with carbapenem non-susceptibility include isolates from tertiary care, specialist care, and prevention and rehabilitation care hospitals as well as from ICU wards. These findings are in accordance with the literature [20–25] and can be attributed to patients with severe co-morbidities and risk factors for acquiring resistant bacteria. We did not find an association with social deprivation status of the county where the hospital is located and carbapenem non-susceptibility even though social deprivation is associated with poorer health outcomes. It would be interesting to investigate the impact of social deprivation on the patients' level, which is, however, not available in our surveillance data.

The findings of our study yield valuable information for infection control practices. While measures according to international guidelines including hand hygiene, contact precautions, patient isolation and environmental cleaning are recommended for all health institutions dealing with carbapenem-resistant strains [10], our results highlight that carbapenem non-susceptible isolates

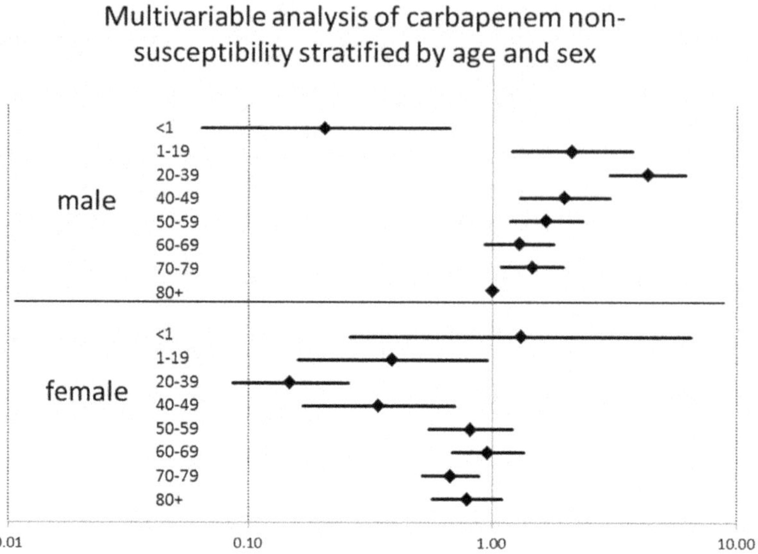

Fig. 2 Multivariable analysis for carbapenem non-susceptibility of *K. pneumoniae* isolates stratified by age and sex, Germany 2011–2016. Hierarchical logistic regression accounting for county and hospital, Outcome: carbapenem non-susceptibility stratified by age and sex, adjusted for year, quarter, hospital care level, type of care, clinical speciality, specimen type, region, county type, social deprivation index, and hospital beds per 10,000 inhabitants

were more common in Germany in highly specialized hospitals and intensive care units. Thus, these types of hospitals and hospital units should be especially vigilant and need to implement effective surveillance and infection control measures.

Treatment options for infections with carbapenem non-susceptible *K. pneumoniae* are very limited. While isolates non-susceptible to imipenem or meropenem were mostly non-susceptible to the other two carbapenems as well, in contrast only about half of the isolates non-susceptible to ertapenem showed non-susceptibility to the other two carbapenems. Ertapenem being the more sensitive parameter for carbapenemase producing isolates has been described in the literature [26, 27]. This underlines that Ertapenem non-susceptible isolates should be tested for carbapenemases even when they are still susceptible to meropenem and imipenem. Moreover, in about one third of the isolates tested non-susceptible against imipenem or meropenem we found intermediate susceptibility against one or both substances, which would make them eligible

Table 5 Co-resistance of carbapenem non-susceptible *K. pneumoniae* isolates ($n = 966$) against other antibiotics

	Isolates from all laboratories		Isolates from laboratories that routinely test against the specified antibiotic[a]	
Tested against	Included isolates	Non-susceptible isolates, % (95%CI)[b]	Included isolates	Non-susceptible isolates, % (95%CI)[b]
Ampicillin/ Sulbactam	871	93.0% (90.3, 95.0%)	c	c
Piperacillin/ Tazobactam	950	90.7% (87.4, 93.2%)	c	c
Ceftazidime	954	88.7% (85.8, 91.0%)	c	c
Cefotaxime	908	88.3% (85.0, 91.0%)	c	c
Polymyxin/ Colistin	435	13.3% (9.8, 17.9%)	214	14.0% (8.8, 21.7%)
Tigecycline	865	56.6% (51.0, 62.1%)	709	55.6% (49.1, 61.8%)
Fosfomycin	632	47.0% (40.6, 53.5%)	319	46.7% (36.2, 57.5%)
Gentamicin	960	57.8% (53.0, 62.4%)	c	c
Co-Trimoxazole	961	62.7% (57.6, 67.6%)	c	c
Ciprofloxacin	959	82.0% (78.4, 85.0%)	c	c
Nitrofurantoin	313	82.7% (76.3, 87.7%)	99	72.7% (60.0, 82.6%)

R resistant, *I* intermediate, *CI* confidence interval
[a]Analysis restricted to laboratories that test > 90% of isolates against the specified antibiotic
[b]95% CI calculated accounting for clustering by hospital
[c]Antibiotic is routinely tested in all laboratories (> 90% of all isolates tested)

for use in combination therapy. Penicillin/beta-lactamase inhibitor combinations, 3rd generation cephalosporins, fluoroquinolones and nitrofurantoin were not suitable treatment options for most isolates owing to high proportions of non-susceptibility. Less than half of the carbapenem non-susceptible isolates were still susceptible to tigecycline or gentamicin. This is lower than in previous studies and highlights the clinical challenges of infections with carbapenem-resistant *K. pneumoniae* [19, 20, 22, 28]. Non-susceptibility against colistin was observed in 13.3% of the isolates, which is comparable to other studies. However, recent publications question the reliability of routine testing methods for colistin so that the observed result should be interpreted with caution and validated in the future [29, 30]. This is especially important since treatment of carbapenem-resistant *K. pneumoniae* can require combinations of two or three antibiotics often including colistin [28, 31–33]. In this study, we found only two isolates that were non-susceptible to all the antibiotics analysed so that limited treatment options remain for most isolates in this study. However, effective antibiotic stewardship measures should be implemented to keep carbapenem-resistance low and to preserve treatment options [34].

This study uses routine data from accredited laboratories and can base its estimates on isolates from 655 hospitals across the country. This is the first time a study of this size has been conducted in Germany and we are able to investigate even low proportions of carbapenem non-susceptibility in *K. pneumoniae* with satisfactory statistical precision. We included routine data from about one third of all hospitals in Germany [35]. The sample of hospitals is reasonably large and the estimates between a) descriptive analysis and b) regression analysis adjusting for clustering by region and hospital are comparable. Thus, we are confident that our analysis yields valid results and do not expect a major influence of selection bias.

We excluded screening isolates since these have a different probability of showing resistance than clinical isolates. However, since we do not have any clinical patient information, it is possible that some isolates, e.g. from swabs or the respiratory tract, were also derived from screening samples. Due to the study design it was not possible to account for this.

Moreover, laboratories used different guidelines to interpret their AST results (EUCAST, CLSI or DIN), which could lead to differences in qualitative interpretation of the results. Owing to those discrepancies, a small proportion of isolates with values close to the breakpoints might have been classified as "sensitive" according to one standard and "intermediate" (i.e. non-susceptible) according to the other. Since the use of EUCAST increased over time, this could have artificially influenced the trend analyses over time. However, since the sensitivity analyses restricted to EUCAST isolates or excluding isolates evaluated as "intermediate" yielded similar results as the main analysis, we do not expect this effect to have a substantial impact on our study.

Conclusions

Carbapenem non-susceptibility in *K. pneumoniae* isolates in Germany is still low but slowly increasing. Since the overall number of tested *K. pneumoniae* isolates appears to increase as well, this highlights the growing public health burden of carbapenem resistance in Germany. Continued surveillance, implementation of effective infection prevention and control measures, and sustained antibiotic stewardship efforts are necessary to address these problems.

Additional file

Additional file 1: Appendix S1. List of laboratories that participate in ARS and contributed data to this analysis. **Appendix S2.** Geographical distribution of hospitals contributing data to the analysis. **Appendix S3.** *Klebsiella pneumoniae* isolates by year and location of hospital in Germany, 2011–2016. **Appendix S4.** *Klebsiella pneumoniae* isolates by patient and hospital characteristics in Germany 2011–2016. **Appendix S5.** Numbers of *K. pneumoniae* isolates in Germany 2011–2016 included in the analysis stratified by standards used for interpretation of antimicrobial susceptibility testing. **Appendix S6.** Carbapenem non-susceptibility of *K. pneumoniae* isolates in Germany 2011–2016 that were tested against all three carbapenems. **Appendix S7.** Cross-resistance of *K. pneumoniae* isolates non-susceptible to one carbapenem to other carbapenems restricted to isolates tested against all three carbapenems, Germany 2011–2016. **Appendix S8.** Sensitivity analyses to investigate the trend of carbapenem non-susceptibility over time. **Appendix S9.** Proportions of carbapenem non-susceptibility in *K. pneumoniae* isolates across substrata, Germany 2011–2016. **Appendix S10.** Uni- and multivariable analyses for carbapenem non-susceptibility of *K. pneumoniae* isolates stratified by age and sex, Germany 2011–2016.

Abbreviations

AMR: Antimicrobial Resistance; ARS: Antimicrobial Resistance Surveillance; CI: Confidence Intervals; CLSI: Clinical & Laboratory Standards Institute; DIN: Deutsches Institut für Normung (German Institute for Standardization); EARS-Net: European Antimicrobial Resistance Surveillance Network; EUCAST: European Committee on Antimicrobial Susceptibility Testing; I: Clinically Intermediate; ICU: Intensive Care Unit; IQR: Interquartile Range; *K. pneumoniae*: *Klebsiella pneumoniae*; MIC: Minimum Inhibitory Concentration; OXA-48: Oxacillinase 48; R: Clinically Resistant; S: Clinically Susceptible

Acknowledgements

We thank all the laboratories for contributing data to this analysis. A list of all participating laboratories is provided in the Additional file 1: Appendix S1. We thank our colleagues at the Robert Koch Institute for their input during this study and our colleague Doreen Richter for her documentary support.

Funding

The analysis was conducted by internal funds of the Robert Koch Institute as a Federal Institute within the portfolio of the Ministry of Health.

Authors' contributions

UK, AVL, IN, MAS, and TE were responsible for conceptualisation of the study and formulate the research goals and aims. UK, AVL, LEK, IN, MF, MAS, and TE developed the methodology and models. UK, IN, MF, HC, and MS worked on the data curation. UK performed the statistical analysis and wrote the original draft. UK, AVL, LEK, IN, MF, MS, HC, MAS, and TE reviewed and commented the draft and gave input on editing. All authors read and approved the final manuscript.

Competing interests

The authors declare that they have no competing interests.

Author details

[1]Department of Infectious Disease Epidemiology, Robert Koch Institute, Seestr. 10, 13353 Berlin, Germany. [2]Department of Epidemiology and Health Monitoring, Robert Koch Institute, General-Pape-Strasse 62-66, 12101 Berlin, Germany. [3]Postgraduate Training for Applied Epidemiology, Department of Infectious Disease Epidemiology, Robert Koch Institute, Seestr. 10, 13353 Berlin, Germany.

References

1. Lee CR, Lee JH, Park KS, Kim YB, Jeong BC, Lee SH. Global dissemination of Carbapenemase-producing Klebsiella pneumoniae: epidemiology, genetic context, treatment options, and detection methods. Front Microbiol. 2016;7: 895.
2. Gomez-Simmonds A, Uhlemann AC. Clinical implications of genomic adaptation and evolution of Carbapenem-resistant Klebsiella pneumoniae. J Infect Dis. 2017;215:S18–27.
3. World Health Organization: WHO publishes list of bacteria for which new antibiotics are urgently needed. http://www.who.int/mediacentre/news/releases/2017/bacteria-antibiotics-needed/en/, accessed on 25.09.2017. 2017.
4. Correa L, Martino MD, Siqueira I, Pasternak J, Gales AC, Silva CV, Camargo TZ, Scherer PF, Marra AR. A hospital-based matched case-control study to identify clinical outcome and risk factors associated with carbapenem-resistant Klebsiella pneumoniae infection. BMC Infect Dis. 2013;13:80.
5. European Centre for Disease Prevention and Control. Surveillance of antimicrobial resistance in Europe 2016. Annual report of the European antimicrobial resistance surveillance network (EARS-net). In: Stockholm: ECDC; 2017.
6. Ducomble T, Faucheux S, Helbig U, Kaisers UX, Konig B, Knaust A, Lubbert C, Moller I, Rodloff AC, Schweickert B, Eckmanns T. Large hospital outbreak of KPC-2-producing Klebsiella pneumoniae: investigating mortality and the impact of screening for KPC-2 with polymerase chain reaction. J Hosp Infect. 2015;89:179–85.
7. Steinmann J, Kaase M, Gatermann S, Popp W, Steinmann E, Damman M, Paul A, Saner F, Buer J, Rath P. Outbreak due to a Klebsiella pneumoniae strain harbouring KPC-2 and VIM-1 in a German university hospital, July 2010 to January 2011. Euro Surveill. 2011;16(33).
8. Pfennigwerth N. Bericht des NRZ für gramnegative Krankenhauserreger. Epid Bull. 2017;25:229-33.
9. Katchanov J, Asar L, Klupp EM, Both A, Rothe C, Konig C, Rohde H, Kluge S, Maurer FP. Carbapenem-resistant gram-negative pathogens in a German university medical center: prevalence, clinical implications and the role of novel beta-lactam/beta-lactamase inhibitor combinations. PLoS One. 2018; 13(4):e0195757.
10. World Health Organization. Guidelines for the prevention and control of carbapenem-resistant Enterobacteriaceae, Acinetobacter baumanii and Pseudomonas aeruginosa in health care facilities. In: Geneva; 2017.
11. Noll I, Schweickert B, Abu Sin M, Feig M, Claus H, Eckmanns T. Antimicrobial resistance in Germany. Four years of antimicrobial resistance surveillance (ARS). Bundesgesundheitsblatt Gesundheitsforschung Gesundheitsschutz. 2012;55:1370–6.
12. INKAR Online - Indikatoren, Karten und Graphiken zur Raum- und Stadtentwicklung in Deutschland und in Europa [www.inkar.de]. Accessed 28 May 2018.
13. Bundesamt für Kartographie und Geodäsie: Verwaltungskarte Deutschland (Länder, Regierungsbezirke, Kreise) VG250. http://http://www.geodatenzentrum.de/auftrag1/archiv/vektor/vg250_ebenen/2016/. Accessed 28 May 2018.
14. Kroll LE, Schumann M, Hoebel J, Lampert T: Regional health differences – developing a socioeconomic deprivation index for Germany. Epidemiologie und Gesundheitsberichterstattung; 2017.
15. Kroll LS. M; Hoebel, J; Lampert, T: **Regionale Unterschiede in der Gesundheit - Entwicklung eines sozioökonomischen Deprivationsindex für Deutschland.** Journal of Health Monitoring. 2017;2:103–20.
16. Wong GY, Mason WM. The hierarchical logistic regression model for multilevel analysis. J Am Stat Assoc. 1985;80:513–24.
17. Gupta N, Limbago BM, Patel JB, Kallen AJ. Carbapenem-resistant Enterobacteriaceae: epidemiology and prevention. Clin Infect Dis. 2011;53:60–7.
18. Hu FP, Guo Y, Zhu DM, Wang F, Jiang XF, Xu YC, Zhang XJ, Zhang CX, Ji P, Xie Y, et al. Resistance trends among clinical isolates in China reported from CHINET surveillance of bacterial resistance, 2005-2014. Clin Microbiol Infect. 2016;22(Suppl 1):S9–14.
19. Guh AY, Bulens SN, Mu Y, Jacob JT, Reno J, Scott J, Wilson LE, Vaeth E, Lynfield R, Shaw KM, et al. Epidemiology of Carbapenem-resistant Enterobacteriaceae in 7 US communities, 2012-2013. Jama. 2015;314: 1479–87.
20. van Duin D, Perez F, Rudin SD, Cober E, Hanrahan J, Ziegler J, Webber R, Fox J, Mason P, Richter SS, et al. Surveillance of carbapenem-resistant Klebsiella pneumoniae: tracking molecular epidemiology and outcomes through a regional network. Antimicrob Agents Chemother. 2014;58: 4035–41.
21. Giannella M, Trecarichi EM, De Rosa FG, Del Bono V, Bassetti M, Lewis RE, Losito AR, Corcione S, Saffioti C, Bartoletti M, et al. Risk factors for carbapenem-resistant Klebsiella pneumoniae bloodstream infection among rectal carriers: a prospective observational multicentre study. Clin Microbiol Infect. 2014;20:1357–62.
22. Lin MY, Lyles-Banks RD, Lolans K, Hines DW, Spear JB, Petrak R, Trick WE, Weinstein RA, Hayden MK. The importance of long-term acute care hospitals in the regional epidemiology of Klebsiella pneumoniae carbapenemase-producing Enterobacteriaceae. Clin Infect Dis. 2013;57: 1246–52.
23. Ny P, Nieberg P, Wong-Beringer A. Impact of carbapenem resistance on epidemiology and outcomes of nonbacteremic Klebsiella pneumoniae infections. Am J Infect Control. 2015;43:1076–80.
24. Schwaber MJ, Klarfeld-Lidji S, Navon-Venezia S, Schwartz D, Leavitt A, Carmeli Y. Predictors of carbapenem-resistant Klebsiella pneumoniae acquisition among hospitalized adults and effect of acquisition on mortality. Antimicrob Agents Chemother. 2008;52:1028–33.
25. Xu A, Zheng B, Xu YC, Huang ZG, Zhong NS, Zhuo C. National epidemiology of carbapenem-resistant and extensively drug-resistant gram-negative bacteria isolated from blood samples in China in 2013. Clin Microbiol Infect. 2016;22(Suppl 1):S1–8.
26. McGettigan SE, Andreacchio K, Edelstein PH. Specificity of ertapenem susceptibility screening for detection of Klebsiella pneumoniae carbapenemases. J Clin Microbiol. 2009;47:785–6.
27. CLSI: **Performance Standards for Antimicrobial Susceptibility Testing.** 27th ed. CLSI supplement M100. Wayne, PA: Clinical and Laboratory Standards Institute; 2017 2017.
28. Tumbarello M, Trecarichi EM, De Rosa FG, Giannella M, Giacobbe DR, Bassetti M, Losito AR, Bartoletti M, Del Bono V, Corcione S, et al. Infections caused by KPC-producing Klebsiella pneumoniae: differences in therapy and mortality in a multicentre study. J Antimicrob Chemother. 2015;70:2133–43.
29. Dafopoulou K, Zarkotou O, Dimitroulia E, Hadjichristodoulou C, Gennimata V, Pournaras S, Tsakris A. Comparative evaluation of Colistin susceptibility testing methods among Carbapenem-nonsusceptible Klebsiella pneumoniae and Acinetobacter baumannii clinical isolates. Antimicrob Agents Chemother. 2015;59:4625–30.
30. Matuschek E, Åhman J, Webster C, Kahlmeter G. Evaluation of five commercial MIC methods for colistin antimicrobial susceptibility testing for gram-negative bacteria. ECCMID conference, Vienna 2017. Poster. 2017:P161. https://www.escmid.org/escmid_publications/escmid_elibrary/material/?mid=41167. Accessed 28 May 2018.
31. Capone A, Giannella M, Fortini D, Giordano A, Meledandri M, Ballardini M, Venditti M, Bordi E, Capozzi D, Balice MP, et al. High rate of colistin resistance among patients with carbapenem-resistant Klebsiella pneumoniae infection accounts for an excess of mortality. Clin Microbiol Infect. 2013;19:E23–30.
32. Gonzalez-Padilla M, Torre-Cisneros J, Rivera-Espinar F, Pontes-Moreno A, Lopez-Cerero L, Pascual A, Natera C, Rodriguez M, Salcedo I, Rodriguez-

Lopez F, et al. Gentamicin therapy for sepsis due to carbapenem-resistant and colistin-resistant Klebsiella pneumoniae. J Antimicrob Chemother. 2015; 70:905–13.
33. Stein C, Makarewicz O, Bohnert JA, Pfeifer Y, Kesselmeier M, Hagel S, Pletz MW. Three dimensional checkerboard synergy analysis of Colistin, Meropenem, Tigecycline against multidrug-resistant clinical Klebsiella pneumonia isolates. PLoS One. 2015;10:e0126479.
34. de With K, Allerberger F, Amann S, Apfalter P, Brodt HR, Eckmanns T, Fellhauer M, Geiss HK, Janata O, Krause R, et al. Strategies to enhance rational use of antibiotics in hospital: a guideline by the German Society for Infectious Diseases. Infection. 2016;44:395–439.
35. Federal Statistical Office: https://www.destatis.de/DE/ZahlenFakten/GesellschaftStaat/Gesundheit/Krankenhaeuser/Tabellen/KrankenhaeuserJahreVeraenderung.html. 2013.

Hospital acquired vancomycin resistant enterococci in surgical intensive care patients

Stefanie Kampmeier[1*†], Annelene Kossow[1†], Larissa Monika Clausen[1], Dennis Knaack[2], Christian Ertmer[3], Antje Gottschalk[3], Hendrik Freise[3] and Alexander Mellmann[1]

Abstract

Background: Vancomycin resistant enterococci (VRE) occur with enhanced frequency in hospitalised patients. This study elucidates the prevalence of VRE on admission among surgical intensive care unit (SICU) patients, whether these patients are at special risk for VRE acquisition and which risk factors support this process.

Methods: Patients admitted to SICUs of the University Hospital Münster were examined during August–October 2017. VRE screening was performed within 48 h after admission and directly prior to discharge of patients. In parallel risk factors were recorded to estimate their effect on VRE acquisition during SICU stay.

Results: In total, 374 patients (68% male) with a median age of 66 years were admitted to one of the SICUs during the investigation period. Of all, 336 patients (89.8%) were screened on admission and 268 (71.7%) on discharge. Nine patients were admitted with previously known VRE colonisation. Twelve (3.6%) further patients were VRE positive on admission. During ICU stay, eight (3.0%) additional patients turned out to be VRE colonised. Risk factors found to be significantly associated with VRE acquisition were median length of stay on the ICU (14 vs. 3 days; $p = 0.01$), long-term dialysis (12.5% vs. 2.0% of patients; $p = 0.05$), and antibiotic treatment with flucloxacillin (28.6% vs. 7.2% of patients; $p = 0.01$) or piperacillin/tazobactam (57.1% vs. 26.6% of patients; $p = 0.01$).

Conclusions: SICU patients are not at special risk for VRE acquisition. Previous stay on a SICU should therefore not be considered as specific risk factor for VRE colonisation.

Keywords: Vancomycin resistant enterococci, Hospital-acquisition, Risk factors, Surgical intensive care patients

Background

Enterococci are an emerging pathogen in hospitalised patients [1]. These pathogens ubiquitously occur in the hospital environment and show a high tenacity on inanimate surfaces [2–4]. As a result, enterococcal infections emerge with a rising frequency. Additionally, enterococci have the ability of acquiring resistances to multiple antimicrobial agents and the capacity to transfer resistances to other pathogens via mobile genetic elements [5–7]. For this reason the prevalence of vancomycin resistant enterococci (VRE) has increased intensively [1]. Vancomycin resistance is associated with enhanced mortality, e.g. among patients with enterococcal blood stream infections [8]. Within hospital settings prevention of VRE transmission is therefore a major objective.

Infection control strategies to control VRE vary, depending on local guidelines. Usually bundle strategies are applied to prevent transmission of VRE between two patients [9]. These include contact precautions, intensified disinfection strategies, the usage of personal protective equipment and active surveillance [10, 11]. In this context, screening strategies are controversially discussed [12]. Both, generalised screening and a risk-adaptive screening, are possible approaches. Regarding the latter, the question arises, which patient groups should be included. Acquisition of VRE in critical ill patients has been associated with prolonged duration of hospital stay, previous hospitalisations, antibiotic

* Correspondence: Stefanie.Kampmeier@ukmuenster.de
[†]Stefanie Kampmeier and Annelene Kossow contributed equally to this work.
[1]Institute of Hygiene, University Hospital Münster, Robert-Koch-Strasse 41, 48149 Münster, Germany
Full list of author information is available at the end of the article

treatment, long-term dialysis and immunosuppression [13–15]. Surgical intensive care patients host a variety of these risk factors, although not explicitly mentioned as risk clientele. Whether surgical intensive care patients per se are at a special risk to acquire VRE and should therefore be included in a risk adapted screening upon subsequent admission to a hospital has not yet been investigated. The present work addresses these questions and investigates risk factors making a VRE acquisition more probable.

Methods

Clinical setting and infection control measures

The 1500-bed University Hospital Münster comprises four interdisciplinary SICUs, hosting abdominal-, trauma-, neuro-, vascular- and thoracic-surgery patients. In total, capacity of all ICUs is 43 beds at its maximum distributed over 26 patient rooms.

Routinely, screening for multidrug-resistant organisms includes an admission-screening for methicillin-resistant *Staphylococcus aureus* (MRSA) and multidrug-resistant Gram-negative bacteria according to the national German guidelines is established [16, 17]. After coincidental detection of VRE in screening swabs and clinical samples of SICU patients, a prospective investigation was initiated, concentrating on VRE acquisition during a stay on a SICU.

Extended hygiene measures in case of VRE detection include contact isolation in a separate room; cohorting of multiple VRE patients is possible. Sanitary facilities are strictly separated and staff is instructed to wear personal protective equipment in case of entering a patient room, consisting of gloves, and gowns. Surface cleaning disinfection was performed once a day.

Detection of risk factors for VRE acquisition

During the 2-month study period (August – October 2017), risk factors for VRE acquisition were prospectively recorded during the entire in-patient stay. These risk factors included demographic data (age, gender), the duration of stay on the respective SICU, underlying diseases (haemato-oncological, immunosuppressive diseases [e.g. autoimmune-disease, malignancies, HIV-infection, immunomodulatory drug treatment], hepatic insufficiency, liver transplantation, renal insufficiency, long-term dialysis) and medication (systemic glucocorticoid and antibiotic treatment) attributed to VRE acquisition and previous contacts to the healthcare system (admission from a foreign or domestic hospital, admission from an (in-house) ICU) [13–15, 18]. Patients with a pre-existing VRE status were not included in the analysis, in order to detect risk factors of VRE acquisition on the SICU ward.

VRE screening, culture, antibiotic resistances, PCR testing methods

VRE screening was performed upon patients' admission on the SICU as well as upon discharge of patients from the SICU in order to detect VRE acquisition during SICU stay. Hospital-acquired VRE was defined as acquisition > 48 h after hospitalisation on the SICU. All VRE not acquired during SICU stay were defined as pre-existing VRE. Swabs were obtained rectally (5 cm *ab ano*) (Transwab® m40 compliant, mwe, Corsham, Wiltshire, UK) and subsequently streaked onto chromogenic selective agar (VRESelect™, Biorad, Hercules, California, USA). Suspected colonies were confirmed via MALDI-TOF-MS (Bruker Corporation, Bremen, Germany). Susceptibility testing was performed in accordance with the current European Committee on Antimicrobial Susceptibility Testing (EUCAST) standards for clinical breakpoints (version 7.0) using the VITEK® 2 system (BioMérieux, Nürtingen, Germany). Vancomycin resistance was confirmed by the detection of *vanA*, *vanB*, *vanC1* and *vanC2/3* using the GenoType Enterococcus system (Hain Lifescience, Nehren, Germany). Additionally, subsequent whole genome sequence-based typing confirmed presence of *van*--genes in these isolates.

Whole genome sequence-based typing

In order to elucidate the clonal relationship of VRE -strains, isolates were compared genetically via whole genome sequencing (WGS) using the Illumina MiSeq platform (Illumina Inc., San Diego, USA) and laboratory procedures as described previously [19]. Coding regions were compared in a gene-by-gene approach (core genome multilocus sequence typing, cgMLST) using the SeqSphere+ software version 4.1 (Ridom GmbH, Münster, Germany) [20]. To visualize the clonal relationship a minimum-spanning tree was generated using the same software. Genotypes that differed in ≤3 cgMLST targets were rated as closely related and highly suspected for a hospital-acquired transmission. For backwards compatibility with classical molecular typing, i. e. MLST, the MLST sequence types (ST) were extracted from the WGS data in silico.

Statistical analysis

All data are expressed as absolute numbers or percentage, if not stated otherwise. Independent risk factors were determined in a two-step analysis. First, a univariate analysis was performed, selecting potential risk factors. Chi-Square test was used for categorical and the two-sided student's t-test for comparison of numerical data. Second, a logistic regression was performed to ascertain the independency of risk factors. Statistical significance was declared at $p \leq 0.05$.

Results

Screening adherence, acquired VRE, genotypes

Table 1 shows the detailed results of screening data. Of 374 admitted patients, 336 were screened on admission and 268 on discharge respectively, not considering patients with a confirmed VRE status prior to admission or discharge. In total eight hospital-acquired VRE could be detected. Of all pre-existing VRE (on admission), six presented a *vanA*, 14 a *vanB* and one both genotypes. Of all hospital-acquired VRE, one hosted a *vanA* and seven a *vanB* genotype.

Antimicrobial resistance expressions

In total, 29 VRE isolates of 26 patients (one patient was readmitted twice and one patient once) were tested for antimicrobial resistance expressions. Table 2 gives a detailed overview of tested substances.

Whole genome sequence-based typing and VRE transmission

Of all 29 isolates 25 were subjected to whole genome sequencing. In patients with repetitive VRE detections and the same antimicrobial resistance expression, only the first isolate was undertaken the sequencing procedure. One isolate was not sequenced. Analysing the MLST ST of all sequenced isolates, ST117 was most prevalent (64.0%) followed by ST80 (24.0%) and ST721 (11.0%) (see also Table 2). A genetical comparison with the help of the cgMLST scheme, based on 1423 genes present in all isolates, revealed six clusters, comprising two, three, five and six isolates respectively (Fig. 1). Two of these clusters contain genotypes of pre-existing isolates and isolates detected in both screenings. Six out of eight VRE isolates (204, 283, 291, 314, 361, 372) detected in patients on discharge, who were previously tested negative for VRE on admission, are genetically closely related to isolates detected in other patients, suggesting a transmission of one VRE clone on ward in these cases (see also Fig. 2). The other two isolates (300, 302) detected on discharge are genetically unrelated to other isolates, which can be attributed to selection of VRE e.g. via antibiotic application in these patients or a false-negative screening result on admission.

Analysis of risk factors in SICU patients

Risk factors were compared between the group of hospital-acquired VRE-patients and all patients being not VRE-colonised or infected hospital-acquired. Patients with a pre-existing VRE status were not included in the analysis, in order to detect risk factors of VRE acquisition on the SICU ward. Risk factors to have a significant influence on VRE acquisition in this patient clientele were found to be long-term dialysis ($p = 0.05$), the median duration of stay ($p = 0.01$), and an antibiotic treatment with flucloxacillin (duration of treatment for 5.3 days [$p = 0.01$]) or piperacillin/tazobactam (duration of treatment for 4.6 days [$p = 0.01$]), while an antibiotic treatment per se did not show a significant risk profile. Further results of the risk factor analyses can be found in Table 3. The multivariate analysis found the duration of stay and flucloxacillin treatment to be statistically significant as shown in Table 4.

Discussion

Control of VRE is an emerging topic, patients and healthcare workers have to cope with. An important aspect for prevention of transmission is the early recognition of VRE via screening strategies. Here, the question was addressed, whether SICU patients acquire VRE during their stay and which factors put them at special risk for acquisition. VRE acquisition rate (3.0%) on the SICU was lower than the initial prevalence (3.6%) on admission of all patients. Additionally, no hospital-acquired infection but only colonisations occurred. Distribution of detected *van*-genotypes and MLST ST (*vanB*-genotype and ST117 were most prevalent) are thereby in accordance with national results and trends published for German healthcare institutions recently [21]. In contrast to another retrospective study investigating hospital-acquired VRE, where the acquisition rate was 28.6%, on different wards including surgical and internal ICUs and lacking a generalised VRE screening, acquisition of VRE in our investigation was comparably low [22]. Further investigations on haemato-oncological patients revealed one third of these patients to develop hospital-acquired VRE [18]. SICU patients should per se not be considered as a specific risk clientele for VRE acquisition in comparison with these patients.

Table 1 Screening data of SICU-admitted patients ($n = 374$) during August to October 2017

	Screening result				
	Positive			Negative	Total
	vanA genotype	*vanB* genotype	*vanA* and *vanB* genotype		
Pre-existing VRE	6 (66.7%)	3 (33.3%)	0 (0%)	/	9
Screening on admission	0 (0%)	11 (3.3%)	1 (0.3%)	324 (96.4%)	336
Screening on discharge	1 (0.4%)	7 (2.6%)	0 (0%)	260 (97.0%)	268

Table 2 Collection dates, *van*-genotypes, MLST sequence types and antimicrobial resistance expression of VRE strains detected in SICU patients. Each row represents a single patient

Isolate no.	Collection date	Positive result	MLST ST	*Van* - genotype	AMP	SAM	AX	AMC	PRL	TPZ	IPM	CIP	LEV	VAN	TEC	QD	TGC	LNZ	CN-HLR	S-HLR
001	15/08/2017	On admission	ST80	*vanB*	r	r	r	r	r	r	r	r	r	r	s	s	s	r	–	–
123	01/09/2017	Pre-existing	ST80	*vanB*																
021	07/07/2017	Pre-existing	ST721	*vanA*	r	r	r	r	r	r	r	r	r	r	r	s	s	s	+	–
119	31/08/2017	Pre-existing	ST721	*vanA*																
143	04/09/2017	Pre-existing	ST721	*vanA*																
025	02/07/2017	Pre-existing	ST117	*vanB*	r	r	r	r	r	r	r	r	r	r	s	s	s	s	–	–
076	25/08/2017	On admission	ST117	*vanB*	r	r	r	r	r	r	r	r	r	r	s	s	s	s	–	+
085	02/08/2017	Pre-existing	ST721	*vanA*	r	r	r	r	r	r	r	r	r	r	r	s	s	s	+	+
126	05/09/2017	On admission	ST117	*vanB*	r	r	r	r	r	r	r	r	r	r	s	s	s	s	–	–
189	12/09/2017	On admission	ST80	*vanB*	r	r	r	r	r	r	r	r	r	r	s	s	s	s	–	+
204	26/09/2017	On discharge	ST80	*vanB*	r	r	r	r	r	r	r	r	r	r	s	s	s	s	–	+
235	20/09/2017	On admission	ST117	*vanB*	r	r	r	r	r	r	r	r	r	r	s	s	s	s	–	–
248	27/03/2017	Pre-existing	ST721	*vanA*	r	r	r	r	r	r	r	r	r	r	r	s	s	s	+	–
251	22/09/2017	On admission	NS	*vanA + B*	r	r	r	r	r	r	r	r	r	r	r	r	s	s	+	+
256	22/09/2017	On admission	ST117	*vanB*	r	r	r	r	r	r	r	r	r	r	s	s	s	s	–	–
283	02/10/2017	On discharge	ST117	*vanB*	r	r	r	r	r	r	r	r	r	r	s	s	s	s	–	–
291	05/10/2017	On discharge	ST80	*vanB*	r	r	r	r	r	r	r	r	r	r	s	s	s	s	–	–
300	04/10/2017	On discharge	ST80	*vanA*	r	r	r	r	r	r	r	r	r	r	r	r	s	s	–	+
302	25/10/2017	On discharge	ST117	*vanB*	r	r	r	r	r	r	r	r	r	r	s	s	s	s	–	–
314	13/10/2017	On discharge	ST117	*vanB*	r	r	r	r	r	r	r	r	r	r	s	s	s	s	–	–
330	06/10/2017	On admission	ST117	*vanB*	r	r	r	r	r	r	r	r	r	r	s	s	s	s	–	+
335	04/10/2017	Pre-existing	ST80	*vanB*	r	r	r	r	r	r	r	r	r	r	s	s	s	s	–	–
338	09/10/2017	On admission	ST117	*vanB*	r	r	r	r	r	r	r	r	r	r	s	s	s	s	–	–
348	11/10/2017	On admission	ST117	*vanB*	r	r	r	r	r	r	r	r	r	r	s	r	s	s	–	+
351	11/10/2017	On admission	ST117	*vanB*	r	r	r	r	r	r	r	r	r	r	s	s	s	s	–	–
352	02/04/2013	Pre-existing	ST117	*vanA*	r	r	r	r	r	r	r	r	r	r	r	r	s	s	+	+
361	22/10/2017	On discharge	ST117	*vanB*	r	r	r	r	r	r	r	r	r	r	s	s	s	s	–	–
366	13/10/2017	On admission	ST117	*vanB*	r	r	r	r	r	r	r	r	r	r	s	s	s	s	–	–
372	30/10/2017	On discharge	ST117	*vanB*	r	r	r	r	r	r	r	r	r	r	s	s	s	s	–	–

MLST Multilocus sequence typing; *AMP* Ampicillin, *SAM* Ampicillin/sulbactam, *AX* Amoxicillin, *AMC* Amoxicillin/clavulanic acid, *PRL* Piperacillin, *TPZ* Piperacillin/tazobactam, *IPM* Imipenem, *CIP* Ciprofloxacin, *LEV* Levofloxacin, *VAN* Vancomycin, *TEC* Teicoplanin, *QD* Quinopristin/dalfopristin, *TGC* Tigecyclin, *LNZ* Linezolid, *CN-HLR* Gentamicin-high level resistance, *S-HLR* Streptomycin-high level resistance; *r* Resistant, *s* Susceptible, + – positive, – - negative, *NS* not sequenced

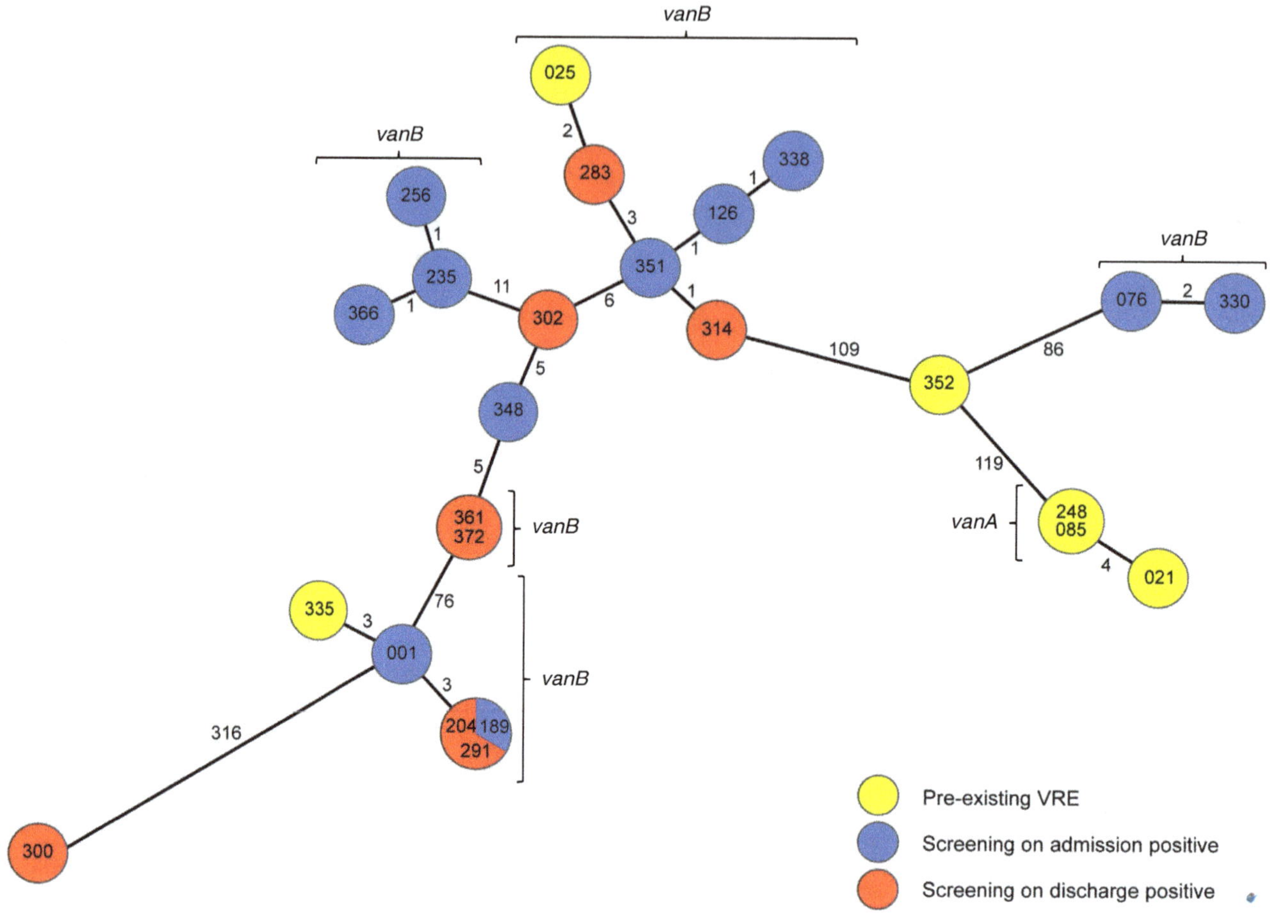

Fig. 1 Minimum spanning tree of VRE isolates illustrating their genotypic relationship. Minimum spanning tree of 25 VRE strains isolated from intensive care unit patients with VRE anamnesis (*yellow*) and detected during screening on admission (*blue*) and on discharge (*red*) during August and October 2017 based on 1423 cgMLST target genes [20], pairwise ignoring missing values. Genotypes are numbered chronologically in order of patients' admission on ICU. Each dot represents one genotype. Size of dots correlates with the number of identical genotypes. Numbers near to the connecting lines show the number of alleles differing between two genotypes. Whole Genome Sequencing revealed six clusters of VRE, one *vanA*-cluster and five *vanB*-clusters

Nevertheless, since hospital-acquired VRE colonisations occurred in our patients, risk factors supporting a VRE acquisition in this group of patients were assessed. Here, the median duration of stay, long-term dialysis and the antibiotic treatment with flucloxacillin or piperacillin/tazobactam were found to be the predominant risk factors. These data correspond with previously investigated risk factors and certainly cannot be considered independently but presuppose each other [23, 24], as also verified by the multivariate analysis. Other risk factors that were found to play an important role in VRE acquisition in other patient clientele could not be verified for our SICU patients. Here, the attributed risk of VRE acquisition after cephalosporin treatment needs to be mentioned. Due to perioperative antibiotic prophylaxis standards, especially referring to cardiac surgery patients, approximately 60% of all admitted patients received cefuroxime; however, this did not lead to an increased VRE acquisition rate. This is noteworthy, since cephalosporine use promotes selection of enterococci and thereby VRE due to intrinsic resistance mechanisms. Nevertheless, previous studies could confirm, that cephalosporine use per se during hospitalization does not result in an enhanced VRE carriage [14]. Interestingly, since the duration of application of flucloxacillin and piperacillin/tazobactam did not vary significantly among the hospital-acquired VRE and the non VRE group, the present results suggest that few antibiotic applications can be sufficient to potentially select VRE. The impact of relatively low numbers of antibiotic administrations on selection of certain pathogens corroborates similar findings for the selection of *Clostridium difficile* [25].

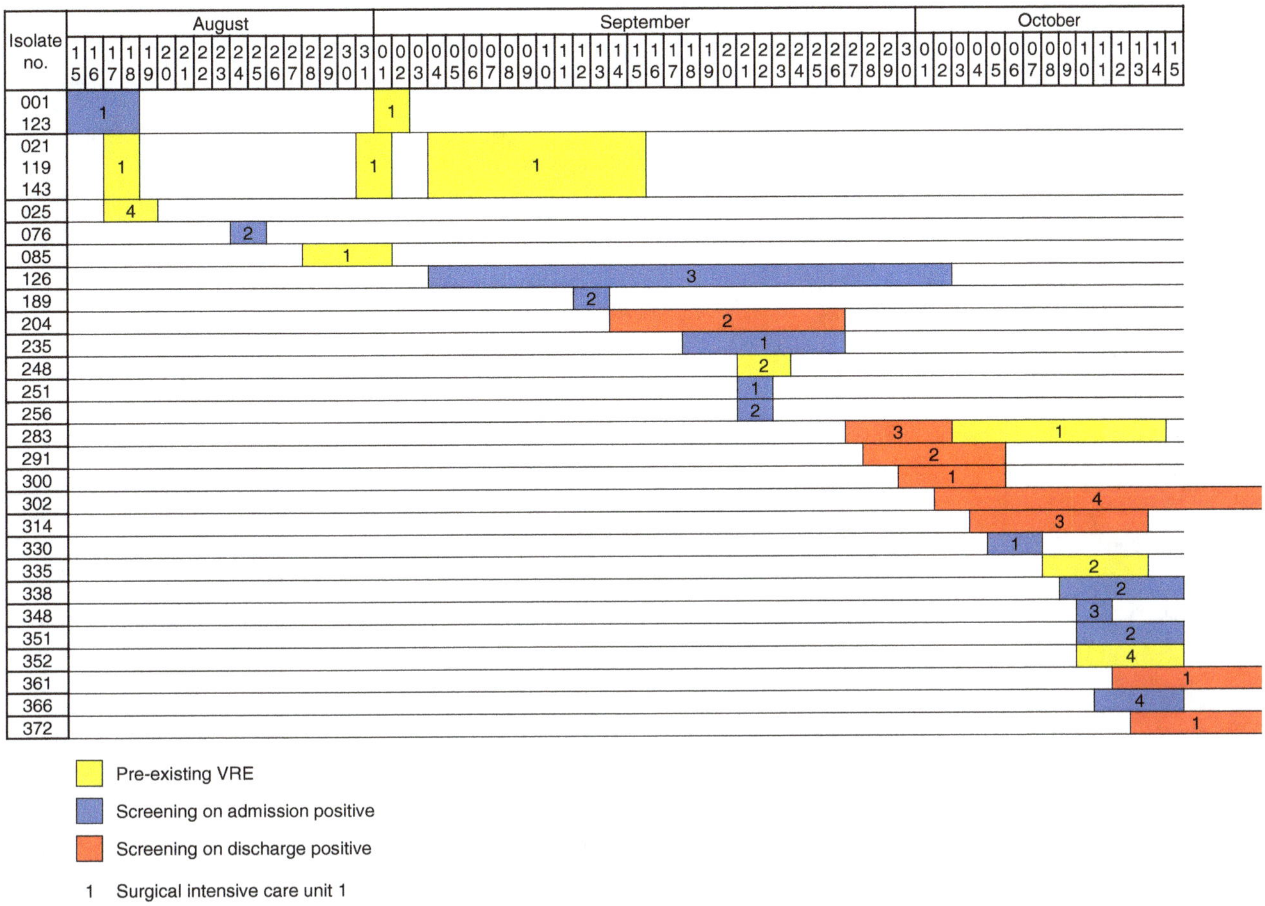

Fig. 2 Timeline of detected VRE isolates illustrating time overlap. Timeline of 29 VRE strains isolated from intensive care unit patients with VRE anamnesis (*yellow*) and detected during screening on admission (*blue*) and on discharge (*red*) during August and October 2017. Each row represents one patient. Numbers within coloured boxes indicate the surgical intensive care unit the patient was admitted to. Isolates 302, 361 and 372, detected in screening on discharge, were identified after end the of study period, but included, as the patients, strains were isolated from, were admitted during the observation period

Previous contacts to VRE confirmed patients are often mentioned as a major risk factor in VRE acquisition [26]. Considering the present core genome analysis of isolates, transmission of VRE on ward could not explicitly be excluded in some cases. This may be due to the transmission of this pathogen on inanimate surfaces in advance to the final diagnosis of the VRE status. Hence in case of a confirmed VRE status, adequate basic and, if necessary, intensified hygienic measures consisting of bundle strategies including contact precautions, usage of personal protective equipment, appropriate disinfection strategies, screening of contact patients and antibiotic stewardship should be implemented to avoid transmissions as good as possible.

Our study has limitations. First, the study period was relatively short. Additional risk factors might have been revealed in case of a longer study period. Moreover, distribution of detected MLST ST in found VRE could have been different. Second, we evaluated risk factors promoting VRE carriage, e.g. flucloxacillin and piperacillin/tazobactam application, but did not investigate the pathophysiological background. Future (prospective) studies are needed to reveal underlying mechanisms. Nevertheless, our findings are in accordance with results published previously [27]. Environmental sampling was not performed during the present study, which could have uncovered the role of inanimate surfaces in VRE transmission, especially in cases of clonality of isolates. Another limitation is the problem of screening sensitivity. Here, only one rectal swab was applied on admission and on discharge respectively, which can lead underestimation of VRE prevalence. However, since screening was performed the same way on admission and on discharge, acquisition rate of VRE during SICU stay can still be assessed precisely.

Table 3 Characteristics and risk factors of admitted surgical intensive care patients with and without hospital-acquired VRE

Characteristic	All admitted patients (n = 374)	Patients with acquired VRE (*n* = 8)	Patients without acquired/ pre-existing VRE (*n* = 345)	*p*-value
Demographic data				
Median age (years)	66 (range: 14–91)	71.5 (range: 50–78)	65 (range: 14–91)	0.43
Male gender	254 (67.9%)	4 (50.0%)	241 (69.9%)	0.23
Median duration of stay (days)	3 (range: 1–45)	14 (range: 7–30)	3 (range: 1–45)	*0.01*
Underlying disease/treatment				
Haemato-oncological disease	62 (16.6%)	1 (12.5%)	58 (16.8%)	0.74
Immunosuppressive disease	71 (19.0%)	1 (12.5%)	66 (19.1%)	0.63
Hepatic insufficiency	17 (4.5%)	0 (0%)	15 (4.3%)	0.55
Liver transplantation	8 (2.1%)	0 (0%)	8 (2.3%)	0.66
Renal insufficiency	51 (13.6%)	2 (25.0%)	41 (11.9%)	0.26
Long-term dialysis	10 (2.7%)	1 (12.5%)	7 (2.0%)	*0.05*
Systemic glucocorticoid treatment	36 (9.6%)	1 (12.5%)	32 (9.2%)	0.76
Antibiotic treatment	218 (58.3%)	7 (87.5%)	207 (60.0%)	0.11
Ampicillin	7 (3.2%)	0 (0%)	4 (1.9%)	0.76
Amoxicillin	14 (6.4%)	0 (0%)	13 (6.3%)	0.58
Flucloxacillin	20 (9.2%)	2 (28.6%)	15 (7.2%)	*0.01*
Piperacillin/tazobactam	62 (28.4%)	4 (57.1%)	55 (26.6%)	*0.01*
Cefuroxime	130 (59.6%)	1 (14.2%)	127 (61.4%)	0.16
Ceftriaxone	7 (3.2%)	0 (0%)	3 (1.4%)	0.79
Meropenem	41 (18.8%)	2 (28.6%)	36 (17.4%)	0.19
Clindamycin	7 (3.2%)	0 (0%)	7 (3.4%)	0.68
Daptomycin	8 (3.7%)	0 (0%)	5 (2.4%)	0.73
Linezolid	3 (1.4%)	0 (0%)	3 (1.4%)	0.79
Rifampicin	13 (6.0%)	0 (0%)	10 (4.8%)	0.63
Erythromycin	7 (3.2%)	0 (0%)	6 (2.9%)	0.71
Vancomycin	19 (8.7%)	0 (0%)	16 (7.7%)	0.53
Fosfomycin	7 (3.2%)	0 (0%)	6 (2.9%)	0.71
Trimethoprim/Sulfamethoxazole	6 (2.8%)	0 (0%)	6 (2.9%)	0.71
Metronidazole	8 (3.7%)	0 (0%)	7 (3.4%)	0.68
Previous contact to healthcare system				
Admission from a foreign hospital	1 (0.3%)	0 (0%)	1 (0.3%)	0.88
Admission from a domestic hospital	188 (50.2%)	5 (62.5%)	173 (50.0%)	0.49
Admission from an intensive care unit	90 (24.1%)	4 (50.0%)	76 (22.0%)	0.06

Statistical significance was declared at $p \leq 0.05$ (see italicized entries)

Table 4 Multivariate analysis: risk factors associated with VRE acquisition

Risk factors ($p \leq 0.05$)	Odds Ratio	95% CI
Duration of stay	0.90	0.84–0.96
Long-term-dialysis	0.08	0.01–1.10
Flucloxacillin treatment	0.09	0.01–0.60
Piperacillin/tazobactam treatment	0.24	0.05–1.13

Conclusion

Compared to patient clienteles previously investigated [23, 28–30], SICU patients per se are not at higher risk of VRE acquisition if hygiene measures are applied as recommended. If a risk adapted screening policy is applied as practised in other national institutions [22], stay on a SICU should not be considered as a risk factor for screening upon admission to a healthcare facility.

Abbreviations

SICU: Surgical intensive care unit; VRE: Vancomycin resistant enterococci

Authors' contributions
SK and AK: Conception and design of the study, acquisition, analysis and interpretation of data, drafting article. LMC and DK: Acquisition, analysis and interpretation of data, revising article critically. CE, AG and HF: Interpretation of data, revising article critically. AM: Conception and design of the study, interpretation of data, revising article critically. All authors have seen and approved the final version of the manuscript.

Consent for publication
Not applicable.

Competing interests
The authors declare that they have no competing interests.

Author details
[1]Institute of Hygiene, University Hospital Münster, Robert-Koch-Strasse 41, 48149 Münster, Germany. [2]Institute of Medical Microbiology, University Hospital Münster, Münster, Germany. [3]Department of Anaesthesiology, Intensive Care and Pain Medicine, University Hospital Münster, Münster, Germany.

References
1. European Center for Disease Prevention and Control. Data from the ECDC Surveillance Atlas - Antimicrobial resistance. https://ecdc.europa.eu/en/antimicrobial-resistance/surveillance-and-disease-data/data-ecdc. Accessed 05 Nov 2017.
2. Kramer A, Schwebke I, Kampf G. How long do nosocomial pathogens persist on inanimate surfaces? A systematic review. BMC Infect Dis. 2006;6:130.
3. Sample ML, Gravel D, Oxley C, Toye B, Garber G, Ramotar K. An outbreak of vancomycin-resistant enterococci in a hematology-oncology unit: control by patient cohorting and terminal cleaning of the environment. Infect Control Hosp Epidemiol. 2002;23:468–70.
4. McDermott H, Skally M, O'Rourke J, Humphreys H, Fitzgerald-Hughes D. Vancomycin-resistant enterococci (VRE) in the intensive care unit in a nonoutbreak setting: identification of potential reservoirs and epidemiological associations between patient and environmental VRE. Infect Control Hosp Epidemiol. 2018;39:40–5.
5. Pinholt M, Gumpert H, Bayliss S, Nielsen JB, Vorobieva V, Pedersen M, et al. Genomic analysis of 495 vancomycin-resistant enterococcus faecium reveals broad dissemination of a vanA plasmid in more than 19 clones from Copenhagen, Denmark. J Antimicrob Chemother. 2017;72:40–7.
6. Bender JK, Kalmbach A, Fleige C, Klare I, Fuchs S, Werner G. Population structure and acquisition of the *vanB* resistance determinant in German clinical isolates of *Enterococcus faecium* ST192. Sci Rep. 2016;6:21847.
7. Gawryszewska I, Zabicka D, Hryniewicz W, Sadowy E. Linezolid-resistant enterococci in polish hospitals: species, clonality and determinants of linezolid resistance. Eur J Clin Microbiol Infect Dis. 2017;36:1279–86.
8. DiazGranados CA, Zimmer SM, Klein M, Jernigan JA. Comparison of mortality associated with vancomycin-resistant and vancomycin-susceptible enterococcal bloodstream infections: a meta-analysis. Clin Infect Dis. 2005;41:327–33.
9. Reyes K, Bardossy AC, Zervos M. Vancomycin-Resistant Enterococci. Epidemiology, Infection Prevention, and Control Infect Dis Clin North Am. 2016;30:953–65.
10. Derde LP, Cooper BS, Goossens H, Malhotra-Kumar S, Willems RJ, Gniadkowski M, et al. Interventions to reduce colonisation and transmission of antimicrobial-resistant bacteria in intensive care units: an interrupted time series study and cluster randomised trial. Lancet Infect Dis. 2014;14:31–9.
11. Price CS, Paule S, Noskin GA, Peterson LR. Active surveillance reduces the incidence of vancomycin-resistant enterococcal bacteremia. Clin Infect Dis. 2003;37:921–8.
12. Faron ML, Ledeboer NA, Buchan BW. Resistance mechanisms, epidemiology, and approaches to screening for vancomycin-resistant enterococcus in the health care setting. J Clin Microbiol. 2016;54:2436–47.
13. Zacharioudakis IM, Zervou FN, Ziakas PD, Rice LB, Mylonakis E. Vancomycin-resistant enterococci colonization among dialysis patients: a meta-analysis of prevalence, risk factors, and significance. Am J Kidney Dis. 2015;65:88–97.
14. Papadimitriou-Olivgeris M, Drougka E, Fligou F, Kolonitsiou F, Liakopoulos A, Dodou V, et al. Risk factors for enterococcal infection and colonization by vancomycin-resistant enterococci in critically ill patients. Infection. 2014;42:1013–22.
15. Ford CD, Lopansri BK, Haydoura S, Snow G, Dascomb KK, Asch J, et al. Frequency, risk factors, and outcomes of vancomycin-resistant enterococcus colonization and infection in patients with newly diagnosed acute leukemia: different patterns in patients with acute myelogenous and acute lymphoblastic leukemia. Infect Control Hosp Epidemiol. 2015;36:47–53.
16. Robert Koch Institut. Empfehlungen zur Prävention und Kontrolle von Methicillin-resistenten *Staphylococcus aureus*-Stämmen (MRSA) in medizinischen und pflegerischen Einrichtungen. Epi Bull. 2014;57:696–732.
17. Robert Koch Institut. Hygienemaßnahmen bei Infektionen oder Besiedlung mit multiresistenten gramnegativen Stäbchen. Epi Bull. 2012;55:1311–54.
18. Ford CD, Lopansri BK, Gazdik MA, Webb B, Snow GL, Hoda D, et al. Room contamination, patient colonization pressure, and the risk of vancomycin-resistant enterococcus colonization on a unit dedicated to the treatment of hematologic malignancies and hematopoietic stem cell transplantation. Am J Infect Control. 2016;44:1110–5.
19. Mellmann A, Bletz S, Boking T, Kipp F, Becker K, Schultes A, et al. Real-time genome sequencing of resistant Bacteria provides precision infection control in an institutional setting. J Clin Microbiol. 2016;54:2874–81.
20. de Been M, Pinholt M, Top J, Bletz S, Mellmann A, van Schaik W, et al. Core genome multilocus sequence typing scheme for high- resolution typing of *Enterococcus faecium*. J Clin Microbiol. 2015;53:3788–97.
21. Robert Koch Institut. Eigenschaften, Häufigkeit und Verbreitung von Vancomycin-resistenten Enterokokken (VRE) in Deutschland - Update 2015/2016. Epi Bull. 2017;46:519–27.
22. Remschmidt C, Behnke M, Kola A, Pena Diaz LA, Rohde AM, Gastmeier P, et al. The effect of antibiotic use on prevalence of nosocomial vancomycin-resistant enterococci- an ecologic study. Antimicrob Resist Infect Control. 2017;6:95.
23. D'Agata EM, Green WK, Schulman G, Li H, Tang YW, Schaffner W. Vancomycin-resistant enterococci among chronic hemodialysis patients: a prospective study of acquisition. Clin Infect Dis. 2001;32:23–9.
24. Pan SC, Wang JT, Chen YC, Chang YY, Chen ML, Chang SC. Incidence of and risk factors for infection or colonization of vancomycin-resistant enterococci in patients in the intensive care unit. PLoS One. 2012;7:e47297.
25. Hensgens MP, Goorhuis A, Dekkers OM, Kuijper EJ. Time interval of increased risk for Clostridium difficile infection after exposure to antibiotics. J Antimicrob Chemother. 2012;67:742–8.
26. Tacconelli E, Cataldo MA. Vancomycin-resistant enterococci (VRE): transmission and control. Int J Antimicrob Agents. 2008;31:99–106.
27. Karki S, Land G, Aitchison S, Kennon J, Johnson PD, Ballard SA, et al. Long-term carriage of vancomycin-resistant enterococci in patients discharged from hospitals: a 12-year retrospective cohort study. J Clin Microbiol. 2013;51:3374–9.
28. Vydra J, Shanley RM, George I, Ustun C, Smith AR, Weisdorf DJ, et al. Enterococcal bacteremia is associated with increased risk of mortality in recipients of allogeneic hematopoietic stem cell transplantation. Clin Infect Dis. 2012;55:764–70.
29. Flokas ME, Karageorgos SA, Detsis M, Alevizakos M, Mylonakis E. Vancomycin-resistant enterococci colonisation, risk factors and risk for infection among hospitalised paediatric patients: a systematic review and meta-analysis. Int J Antimicrob Agents. 2017;49:565–72.
30. Ziakas PD, Pliakos EE, Zervou FN, Knoll BM, Rice LB, Mylonakis E. MRSA and VRE colonization in solid organ transplantation: a meta-analysis of published studies. Am J Transplant. 2014;14:1887–94.

A systematic review of the epidemiology of carbapenem-resistant Enterobacteriaceae in the United States

Daniel J. Livorsi[1,2*†], Margaret L. Chorazy[3†], Marin L. Schweizer[1,2], Erin C. Balkenende[1], Amy E. Blevins[4,5], Rajeshwari Nair[1,2], Matthew H. Samore[6,7], Richard E. Nelson[6,7], Karim Khader[6,7] and Eli N. Perencevich[1,2]

Abstract

Background: Carbapenem-resistant Enterobacteriaceae (CRE) pose an urgent public health threat in the United States. An important step in planning and monitoring a national response to CRE is understanding its epidemiology and associated outcomes. We conducted a systematic literature review of studies that investigated incidence and outcomes of CRE infection in the US.

Methods: We performed searches in MEDLINE via Ovid, CDSR, DARE, CENTRAL, NHS EED, Scopus, and Web of Science for articles published from 1/1/2000 to 2/1/2016 about the incidence and outcomes of CRE at US sites.

Results: Five studies evaluated incidence, but many used differing definitions for cases. Across the entire US population, the reported incidence of CRE was 0.3–2.93 infections per 100,000 person-years. Infection rates were highest in long-term acute-care (LTAC) hospitals. There was insufficient data to assess trends in infection rates over time. Four studies evaluated outcomes. Mortality was higher in CRE patients in some but not all studies.

Conclusion: While the incidence of CRE infections in the United States remains low on a national level, the incidence is highest in LTACs. Studies assessing outcomes in CRE-infected patients are limited in number, small in size, and have reached conflicting results. Future research should measure a variety of clinical outcomes and adequately adjust for confounders to better assess the full burden of CRE.

Keywords: Carbapenem-resistant Enterobacteriaceae, United States, Epidemiology

Background

The Centers for Disease Control and Prevention (CDC) in the United States has deemed carbapenem-resistant Enterobacteriaceae (CRE) an urgent public health threat that requires immediate and aggressive action [1]. The reason for this urgency is clear: CRE infections are resistant to nearly all antibiotics and are associated with poor clinical outcomes [2].

Carbapenem-resistance in Enterobacteriaceae can result from a variety of mechanisms [3]. In the US, CRE isolates commonly produce carbapenemases; these enzymes are carried on plasmids and can be easily shared with other gram-negative bacteria. The *Klebsiella pneumoniae* carbapenemase (KPC) was first recognized in North Carolina in 1996 and has since spread around the world [4]. Other examples of carbapenemases include the New Delhi Metallo-β-lactamase (NDM), Verona Integron-encoded Metallo-β-lactamase (VIM), Oxacillinase-48-type carbapenemases (OXA-48), and imipenemase (IMP).

CRE infections are typically seen in patients with prior healthcare exposure, and medical devices are a common risk factor for CRE acquisition [5]. According to 2009–2010 data from the National Healthcare Safety Network (NHSN), 20% of hospitals reporting central line-associated bloodstream infections (CLABSIs) or catheter-associated urinary tract infections (CAUTIs) due to *Klebsiella* spp. reported at least 1 carbapenem-resistant strain [6]. In 2013,

* Correspondence: daniel-livorsi@uiowa.edu
†Equal contributors
[1]Center for Comprehensive Access Delivery & Research, Iowa City VA Health Care System, Iowa City, USA
[2]Department of Internal Medicine, Carver College of Medicine, University of Iowa, Iowa City, USA
Full list of author information is available at the end of the article

an outbreak of NDM-producing *Escherichia coli* was associated with duodenoscopes at an Illinois hospital [7].

Despite ongoing control efforts, CRE has become prevalent in several US regions, including Orange County, California and the Chicago metropolitan area [8, 9]. CRE has been endemic in the New York/New Jersey area since the early 2000s [10]. According to the 2013 CDC Antibiotic Resistance Threat Report, there are 9000 healthcare-associated CRE infections every year in the US, resulting in 600 deaths (mortality rate 6.6%) [1]. However, such a low proportion of deaths may be an underestimation due to how infections were defined.

The CDC has published toolkits on preventing the spread of CRE within and between healthcare facilities [3, 11]. While these toolkits have aided efforts at CRE prevention, a better understanding of the epidemiology and burden of CRE is critical to encourage increased investments in the study and prevention of these pathogens. To this end, we conducted a systematic review and evaluation of studies which investigated incidence and outcomes of CRE infection at US sites.

Methods

Search strategy

This systematic literature review was performed according to the MOOSE and PRISMA guidelines [12, 13]. An experienced health sciences librarian conducted systematic searches in MEDLINE via Ovid, Cochrane Database of Systematic Reviews via Wiley (CDSR), Database of Abstracts of Reviews of Effects via Wiley (DARE), Cochrane Central Register of Controlled Trials via Wiley (CENTRAL), NHS Economic Evaluation Database (NHS EED) via Wiley, Scopus, and Web of Science. We searched for articles published between the dates January 1, 2000 and February 1, 2016. Search terms included Medical Subject Headings (MeSH) and keywords for carbapenem resistance, Enterobacteriaceae, adverse events, incidence, prevalence, and economics. Additional file 1 includes a description of the complete search strategy. We reviewed the reference lists from each article to identify additional studies.

Inclusion and exclusion criteria

Studies were included if they (1) were conducted in the United States; (2) evaluated incidence of CRE or outcomes attributed to CRE infections including mortality, length of stay (LOS), discharge to a long-term acute-care (LTAC) hospitals, readmission, recurrence, and costs; (3) included at least 7 study sites (incidence studies only); and (4) used either the CDC's original or revised definition for CRE [3, 11]. In the original definition, an Enterobacteriaceae isolate qualified as CRE if it was non-susceptible to imipenem, meropenem or doripenem AND resistant to all of the following third-generation cephalosporins: ceftriaxone, cefotaxime and ceftazidime [11]. In the revised 2015 definition, an Enterobacteriaceae isolate qualified as CRE if it was resistant to imipenem, meropenem, or doripenem, (minimum inhibitory concentration [MIC] ≥ 4 mcg/mL) OR resistant to ertapenem (MIC ≥2 mcg/mL) OR had documented production of a carbapenemase [3]. In 2010, the Clinical and Laboratory Standards Institute (CLSI) lowered the breakpoints for carbapenems by a factor of 4, so in reviewing each study, we made note of which version of the CLSI breakpoints was used.

We excluded studies that (1) were less than 6 months in duration; (2) used International Classification of Diseases Clinical Modification diagnosis codes to define CRE infections; (3) used surveillance cultures from non-sterile body sites to detect CRE; (4) did not have a denominator or control group; (5) took place during an outbreak; (6) were mathematical models; (7) did not contain original data; and (8) were published in a language other than English. We excluded studies evaluating LOS or costs if they did not measure post-infection LOS or costs, or if they did not match infected cases and uninfected controls on time at risk (time from admission to infection for cases, time from admission to discharge for uninfected controls) or did not match on propensity scores.

Data extraction and quality assessment

One investigator (MLC) reviewed the titles and abstracts of all articles for inclusion and exclusion criteria. Two of four reviewers (MLC, RN, ENP, MLS) independently abstracted data for each included study. Disagreements between reviewers were resolved by consensus.

The reviewers abstracted data on the following items: study design, population and setting, location, definition of CRE infection, incidence data, prevalence data, mortality, LOS, discharge to LTAC, readmission, recurrence, and cost. Additional data were collected regarding tests used to identify CRE infection, identification of different species that were identified as CRE, and definitions of resistance.

Risk of bias was assessed using the Newcastle-Ottawa scale for included studies [14].

Results

We screened 18,178 unique studies for eligibility (Fig. 1). Nine studies were eligible for inclusion, including 5 multicenter studies reporting the incidence of CRE infections [15–19] and 4 studies (2 multicenter and 2 single center) evaluating relevant outcomes [20–23]. Included studies were of moderate-to-high risk of bias according to the Newcastle-Ottawa tool (Table 1). Included studies had low risk of bias when it came to representativeness and ascertainment of CRE infected patients and controls. However, most of the included studies had high risk of

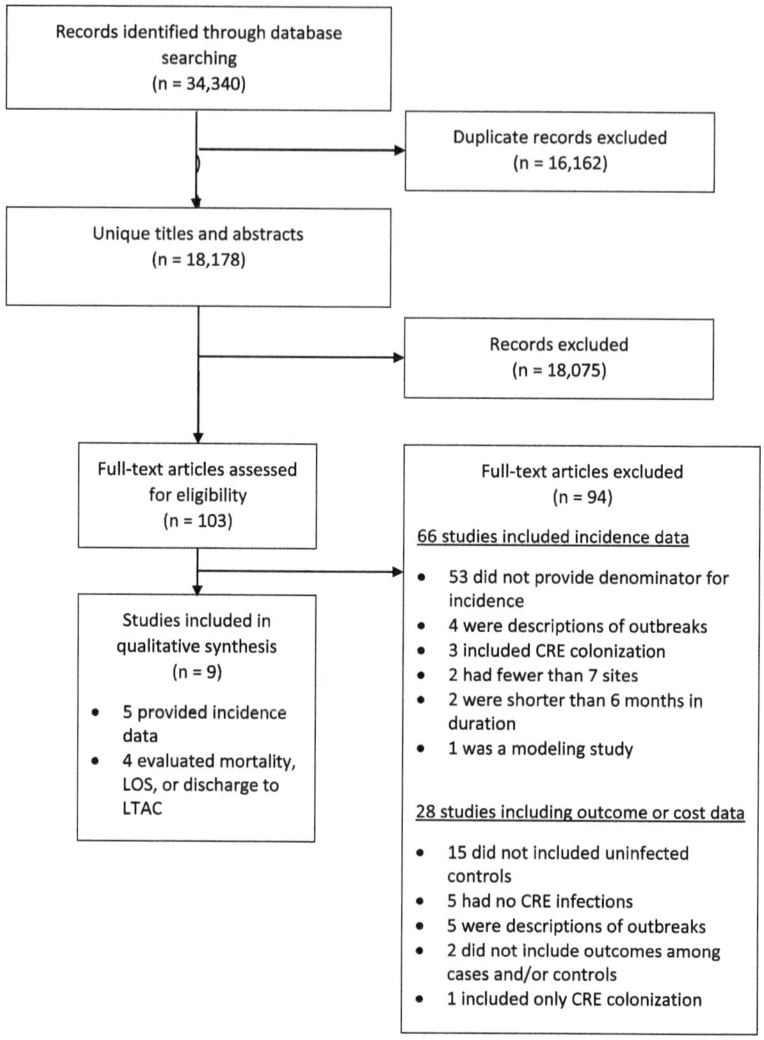

Fig. 1 Flow diagram of search strategy. Legend: CRE, Carbapenem-resistant *Enterobacteriaceae*; LOS, length of stay; LTAC, long-term acute-care hospital

bias in terms of adequacy of follow-up, cohort design and analysis, and assessment of outcomes.

Incidence of CRE infections

There were 5 studies (Table 2) that measured the incidence of CRE: 4 studies used the lower CLSI breakpoints (i.e. 2010 and later) [15–18] while one study largely used the pre-2010 breakpoints [19]. All studies included clinical cultures from sterile and non-sterile body sites, but one study limited non-sterile cultures to only urine samples [18].

Three studies used the denominator of patient-days [15, 17, 19], but these 3 studies could not be pooled because definitions varied: 1 study included all species of Enterobacteriaceae while 2 studies used less inclusive definitions. Among these 3 studies, the incidence of CRE ranged from 0.46 CRE infections per 10,000 patient-days to 4.17 CRE infections per 10,000 patient-days. Two studies stratified by long-term acute care (LTAC) hospitals and acute care hospitals [15, 17]. One of these studies–which took place in Los Angeles County, California—found that the incidence of CRE infections in acute care hospitals was 0.31 per 10,000 patients-days and the incidence of CRE infections in LTAC hospitals was 2.54 per 10,000 patient-days [17]. The other study, which took place in Michigan, found a similar incidence of CRE infections in LTAC hospitals (2.93 per 10,000 patient-days) but the incidence of CRE infections among the acute care hospitals (1.01 per 10,000 patient-days) was higher than that of the Los Angeles County study [15].

Two studies included both inpatients and outpatients, reflected in a denominator of person-years [16, 18]. In a study of the civilian component of the US military health care system, the incidence of CRE remained steady at 0. 49 infections per 100,000 person-years between 2005

Table 1 Risk of bias assessment of CRE studies using Newcastle Ottawa tool (Stang 2010). Receiving a star (*) represents that the study has low risk of bias and high quality in that category

	Selection				Comparability	Outcome		
Author (Year)	Representative-ness of the exposed cohort	Selection of the non-exposed cohort	Ascertainment of exposure	Demonstration that outcome of interest was not present at start of study	Comparability of cohorts on the basis of design or analysis	Assessment of outcome	Was follow-up long enough for outcomes to occur	Adequacy of follow-up of cohorts
Bogan (2014) [20]	*	*	*	*	*	*	*	–
Brennan (2014) [15]	*	*	*	*	–	–	–	–
Gasink (2009) [21]	*	*	*	*	*	*	*	–
Guh (2015) [18]	*	*	*	*	–	–	–	–
Lesho (2015) [16]	*	*	*	*	–	–	–	–
Marquez (2013) [17]	*	*	*	–	–	–	–	–
Patel (2008) [22]	*	*	*	*	*	*	*	–
Thaden (2014) [19]	*	*	*	*	–	–	–	–
Kalpoe (2012) [23]	*	*	*	*	*	*	*	*

and 2012; the peak incidence was 0.67 per 100,000 person years in the year 2010 [16]. A study across 7 metropolitan areas estimated an incidence of 2.94 cases per 100,000 persons in 2012 and 2.93 per 100,000 persons in 2013. Site-specific incidence rates ranged from 0.82 cases per 100,000 persons in Oregon to 4.80 cases per 100,000 persons in Maryland [18].

Carbapenemase production was assessed in 2 studies [15, 18]. One study only included isolates with a positive or unknown result on the Modified-Hodge Test (MHT), but a breakdown of MHT results was not provided [15]. In another study, 90 of 188 (47.9%) isolates across 6 sites produced a carbapenemase, all of which were KPCs [18].

Outcomes attributable to CRE infections

Each of the 5 outcomes studies included data from 2009 or earlier (Table 3). Two studies evaluated outcomes in CRE patients compared to uninfected controls [20, 23]. In the earliest study, all patients who underwent liver transplantation at a single center were followed for 1 year after transplantation [23]. That study found that 71% of the patients infected with carbapenem-resistant *K. pneumoniae* (CRKP) died compared to 14% of the uninfected patients (log rank $p < 0.001$). Based on a multivariate Cox proportional hazards analysis, mortality at 1-year was significantly higher in patients who developed CRKP infections compared to uninfected patients (hazard ratio = 4.9, 95% CI 1.5–15.6). In the second study, patients with and without infections were matched by hospital or facility, unit or clinic, calendar year, and time at risk (i.e., from admission to culture). This study found higher odds of dying among CRE patients compared with uninfected controls, but the difference was not statistically significant (OR = 1.6; 95% CI: 0.7–3.3) [20]. The study also found that CRE infected patients had significantly higher odds of being discharged to a LTAC after being admitted from home (OR = 13.7; 95% CI: 4.3–44.4). There was no difference in LOS between CRE and uninfected patients.

Three studies evaluated outcomes in patients with CRE compared to carbapenem-susceptible Enterobacteriaceae (CSE) [20–22]. Two studies only included isolates of *K. pneumoniae* while the third study included all types of CSE not producing extended-

Table 2 Studies that Evaluated CRE Incidence

First Author (Year)	Study Population	CLSI protocol	Study Period	Culture type	# of Infections	IncidenceRate
Brennan (2014) [15]	CRE Surveillance and Prevention Initiative in Michigan	M100-S22 2012	09/2012–02/2013	All cultures positive for carbapenem non-susceptible *K. pneumoniae* or *E.coli*. All cases had a positive or unknown modified Hodge-Test result. Only 1 case per patient per 30-day period.	102	Per 10,000 patient-days Overall: 1.07 Acute care: 1.01 LTAC: 2.93 East: 1.24 West: 0.52 Mid-North: 0.36
Lesho (2015) [16]	Tricare, i.e.civilian component of the US military health care system	M100-S20–2010	01/2005–12/2012	All CRE-positive cultures (*E.coli*, *Klebsiella* spp., *Enterobacter* spp.). For each year of surveillance, the first CRE-positive culture per patient was included.	368	Per 100,000 person-years All Years: 0.487 2012: 0.394 2011: 0.528 2010: 0.672 2009: 0.607 2008: 0.439 2007: 0.424 2006: 0.490 2005: 0.335
Marquez (2013) [17]	Los Angeles County	M100-S20 2010	06/2010–05/2011	All cultures positive for carbapenem-resistant *K. pneumoniae*. Only 1 isolate allowed per patient per calendar month.	675	Per 1000 patient-days Acute and LTAC: 0.46 LTAC only: 2.54 Acute only: 0.31
Thaden (2014) [19]	Duke Infection Control Outreach Network (DICON)	M100-S20 2010 (20%) sites; earlier CLSI definitions (80% sites)	01/2008–12/2012	All CRE-positive cultures. Only 1 culture was allowed per patient for the entire surveillance period.	180	Per 100,000 patient-days 2008: 0.26 2012: 1.4
Guh (2015) [18]	Multi-site Gram-negative Surveillance Initiative	M100-S22 2012	1/2012–12/2013	All CRE non-susceptible cultures (*E.coli*, *Klebsiella* spp., *Enterobacter* spp.) from a normally sterile site or urine. An incident case was defined as the first isolate from a patient per 30-day period.	599	Per 100,000 persons 2012: 2.94 2013: 2.93

CLSI Clinical and Laboratory Standards Institute, *CRE* carbapenem-resistant Enterobacteriaceae, *LTAC* long-term acute-care hospital

spectrum beta-lactamases (ESBLs). Two studies used multivariable analysis to adjust for important predictors of mortality; only one of these studies adjusted for severity of illness [21] while the other matched cases-and-controls on baseline factors [20]. The third study matched patients with CRE to those with CSE based on body-site of infection [22].

In both studies that exclusively evaluated *K. pneumoniae*, cases with carbapenem-resistance had significantly higher odds of all-cause in-hospital mortality (OR = 2.28 and OR = 3.71; Table 3) [21, 22]. One of these studies also found that the odds of attributable in-hospital mortality were more than 4-fold higher among CRKP-infected patients compared with carbapenem-susceptible *K. pneumoniae* infected controls [22]. In the study that included all types of Enterobacteriaceae, carbapenem-resistance was not significantly associated with either an increase in hospital mortality (adjusted OR 2.7, 95% CI 0.8–9.4) or a longer LOS. However, carbapenem-resistance was associated with being discharged to a LTAC after being admitted from home (OR = 14.5, 95% CI 2.7–79.8).

Discussion

Estimating the incidence of CRE is an important step in designing a national public health response to this emerging pathogen [24]. Our review found that the reported incidence of CRE in the US was 0.3–2.93 infections per 100,000 person-years. The incidence of CRE is relatively higher in LTACs compared to acute-care hospitals and community settings. In 1 population-based study, nearly half of CRE isolates produced a carbapenemase. Carbapenemase-producing CRE are of the greatest epidemiologic concern, because these enzymes are typically carried on mobile genetic elements that can be shared with other bacteria [25].

Based on our findings, CRE is still relatively uncommon in the US compared to other antibiotic-resistant pathogens. For example, the estimated incidence of invasive methicillin-resistant *Staphylococcus aureus* (MRSA)

Table 3 Studies of the Association between CRE Infection and Outcome

First Author (Year)	Study Population	CLSI protocol	Study Period	No. of Patients	Types of infections	Mortality: CRE versus control (%) HR or OR (95% CI)	Length of stay (LOS), median (IQR), days	Discharge to a LTAC after being admitted from home (%), OR (95% CI)
CRE infected patients versus uninfected controls								
Bogan (2014) [20]	Detroit Medical Center, 8 hospitals	M100-S19 2009	09/2008–08/2009	91 cases, 91 controls (matched)	All classified by NHSN definitions.[1]	All-cause in-hospital 38.3% versus 16.7% ($p = 0.006$), adjusted OR = 1.6 (0.2–14.8)[2]	CRE Infected Pts Median = 10 days (IQR: 4–23) Uninfected Pts Median = 13 days (IQR: 3–25)	OR = 15.1 (3.1–73.5)
Kalpoe (2012) [23]	Mount Sinai Hospital, New York City	Not stated	10/2005–10/2006	14 cases, 161 controls	Cultures positive for carbapenem-resistant *K.pneumoniae* from normally sterile body-sites	All-cause mortality at 1-year: 71% versus 14% (log rank $p < 0.001$) HR = 4.9 (1.5–15.6)		
Carbapenem-resistant *Enterobacteriaceae (CRE)* versus carbapenem-susceptible *Enterobacteriaceae (CSE)*								
Gasink (2009) [21]	University of Pennsylvania (2 hospitals)	KPC-production[3]	10/2006–4/2008	56 cases, 863 controls	Clinical cultures with *K.pneumoniae*[4]	All-cause in-hospital: 32.1% versus 9.9% ($p < 0.001$), adjusted OR 2.28 (1.18–4.40)		
Patel (2008) [22]	Mount Sinai Hospital, New York City	M100-S16 2006	7/2004–6/2006	99 cases, 99 controls (matched)	Cultures positive for *K. pneumoniae* from normally sterile body-sites	All-cause in-hospital: 48% versus 20%, OR 3.71 (1.97–7.01) Attributable in-hospital: OR 4.50 (2.16–9.35)		
Bogan (2014) [20]	Detroit Medical Center, 8 hospitals	M100-S19 2009	09/2008–08/2009	91 cases, 91 controls (matched)	CRE or non-ESBL CSE. All infections classified by NHSN definitions.[1]	All-cause in-hospital: 38.3% versus 16.7% ($p = 0.004$), adjusted OR 2.7 (0.8–9.4)	Among CRE Pts Median = 10 days (IQR: 4–23) Among CSE Pts Median = 7 days (IQR: 5–16)	OR = 14.5 (2.7–79.8)

CI confidence interval, *CRE* carbapenem-resistant Enterobacteriaceae, *CSE* carbapenem-susceptible Enterobacteriaceae, *HR* hazard ratio, *IQR* interquartile range, *KPC Klebsiella pneumoniae* carbapenemase, *LTAC* long-term acute-care facility, *NHSN* National Healthcare Safety Network, *OR* odds ratio

[1]Infectious clinical syndrome for CRE cases: 28.2% colonization, 19.7% UTI, 19.7% pneumonia, remaining syndromes not stated

[2]Excludes uninfected colonized-only CRE patients and their matched controls

[3]All cases had confirmed production of a *Klebsiella pneumoniae* carbapenemase (KPC) by either PCR for bla_{KPC} or the Modified Hodge Test

[4]Body site of positive-culture: urine 59.9%, blood 17.3%, respiratory tract 12.1%, abdomen 8.1%, other 6.6%

infections in 2011 across the US was 25 per 100,000 persons, or at least 8 times more common than CRE [26]. In the Veterans Health Administration during 2009–2013, the overall incidence of *C. difficile* was approximately 200 infections per 100,000 patient-years, which was at least 65 times more common than CRE [27]. It is important to note that, even though the current incidence of CRE is low, CRE has been rapidly spreading across the US. Prior to 1996, carbapenemase-producing CRE was not reported in the US, but as of August 2017, this pathogen has been reported in every US state but Idaho [28].

Despite its low incidence, CRE remains a public health threat due to its limited treatment options and worse clinical outcomes [1]. Based on the studies that compared outcomes between CRE and uninfected patients, infection with CRE was associated with a higher risk of being discharged to a LTAC and a higher risk of death within the year after liver transplantation [20, 23]. Studies consistently reported an unadjusted CRE-related mortality rate that was higher than the 6.6% estimate from the CDC [1].

Surprisingly, however, patients with CRE were not always found to have an increased risk for death compared with controls. Studies that compared CRE to uninfected patients reached different conclusions on mortality, albeit using different definitions of mortality [20, 23]. Conflicting results on mortality were also seen in studies that compared CRE to CSE. Two studies found that patients with carbapenem-resistant *K. pneumoniae* had 2–3 times the odds of in-hospital death as patients with carbapenem-susceptible *K. pneumoniae*, but a similar difference in mortality was not seen in a study that included all types of Enterobacteriaceae (i.e., CRE compared with CSE). In contrast, evidence from outside the United States shows increased mortality with CRE. A case-control study from Israel found that, after adjusting for severity of illness, patients with infections from carbapenem-resistant *K. pneumoniae* had 4 times the risk of death as patients infected with carbapenem-susceptible *K. pneumoniae* [29].

While it seems intuitive that CRE would be associated with worse outcomes, the lack of consistency across the literature raises several important questions about how CRE cases are defined and how CRE outcomes are measured. First, only 2 studies in this systematic literature review restricted cases to patients with CRE-positive cultures from normally sterile body sites. As a result, there is potential that patients colonized with CRE (i.e., a positive culture from a non-sterile site in the absence of signs or symptoms of infection) were included as "infected" cases. Such a misclassification bias could obscure differences in outcomes. As with any bacteria, the body site of infection is a key determinant of outcomes. A CRE bacteremia, for example, would be expected to have a higher mortality rate than a CRE urinary tract infection. In fact, a case-control study from Israel found that carbapenem-resistant *K. pneumoniae* bacteremia has an attributable mortality of 50%, or 3 times the risk of death compared with non-bacteremic controls [30]. Second, patients with CRE may have a higher risk of death for reasons beyond the infection itself. For example, CRE-positive patients may have a higher burden of comorbidities and, due to these comorbidities, be more acutely ill when they do become infected. These factors were not adequately accounted for in all studies. Third, it is possible that outcomes other than mortality are worse in patients with CRE, but these alternate outcomes have gone unmeasured. For example, none of the studies measured hospital re-admissions and costs.

Another potential explanation for the conflicting mortality results is that the current studies were underpowered to find statistically significant results. Each of the 4 studies that evaluated mortality included fewer than 100 CRE-infected patients. In the future, larger well-designed studies should be performed to assess the association between CRE infection and mortality.

All the studies included in this systematic literature review evaluated outcomes before the Food and Drug Administration's (FDA) approval of ceftazidime-avibactam and meropenem-vaborbactam. Now that these new and potentially more efficacious agents are available, a re-evaluation of CRE-related outcomes is warranted.

There are several limitations to our meta-analysis. First, definitions of CRE varied across studies. This discrepancy reflects differences in how each study chose to define a CRE case; it also reflects changes in the CDC's definition for CRE and the CLSI's breakpoints for carbapenem-resistance. The original CDC definition for CRE did not include ertapenem, which limited its sensitivity for detecting OXA-48-producing CRE. Furthermore, studies that used the pre-2010 CLSI guidelines to define carbapenem-resistance or evaluated just certain species of Enterobacteriaceae may have underestimated the true incidence of CRE [19, 31]. Thus, we were unable to pool data using meta-analytic techniques. Second, while we excluded studies that used surveillance cultures, clinical cultures reflecting colonization of a non-sterile site were not consistently distinguished from true infections. This may have resulted in an overestimation of the incidence of infection and an underestimation of the risk of mortality. Third, our incidence rates were derived from a limited number of geographic regions and not the entire US. However, 2 studies included multiple states, which should increase the generalizability of our findings. Fourth, outcome studies were limited in both number and quality. For example, 3 of the 4 studies involved ≤2 hospitals, and only 1 adjusted for severity of illness, a key determinant of mortality.

Conclusions

In conclusion, while the incidence of CRE infections in the United States remains low on a national level, the incidence is highest in LTACs. Several studies have measured the incidence of CRE, but the percentage of CRE that results from carbapenemase-production needs to be better defined. Studies assessing outcomes in CRE-infected patients have been small and have reached conflicting results. Future research should measure a variety of clinical outcomes, should be adequately powered and should adequately adjust for confounders to better assess the full burden of CRE. Specifically, outcomes of CRE infections treated with recently FDA-approved antibiotics warrant further evaluation.

Without adequate studies measuring the burden of CRE infections, proper distribution of resources for research and prevention efforts will be impossible, thereby leaving patients vulnerable to this important emerging pathogen.

Abbreviations

CDC: Centers for Disease Control and Prevention; CLSI: Clinical and laboratory standards institute; CRE: carbapenem-resistant Enterobacteriaceae; CRKP: carbapenem-resistant *K. pneumoniae*; CSE: carbapenem-susceptible Enterobacteriaceae; KPC: *Klebsiella pneumoniae* carbapenemase; LOS: length of stay; LTCF: long-term care facility; MesH: Medical Subject Headings; MHT: Modified-Hodge Test; MIC: minimum inhibitory concentration; NHSN: National healthcare safety network

Funding

This study was funded by the Centers for Disease Control and Prevention, Safe Healthcare, Epidemiology, and Prevention Research Development (SHEPheRD) Program (contract 200-2011-42039 to M.S. and E.N.P.), by the VA Health Services Research and Development (HSR&D) Career Development Awards (award 16-204 to D.J.L., award 11-215 to M.L.S., award 11-210 to R.N), and by the VA HSR&D Centers of Innovation: Center for Comprehensive Access & Delivery Research Evaluation (CIN 13-412, PI: E.N.P.).

Authors' contributions

Study design: all authors. Data collection and analysis: MLC, MLS, ECB, AEB, RN, ENP Study supervision: MLS, ENP. Manuscript writing: DJL, MLC. Manuscript review: all authors. All authors read and approved the manuscript.

Competing interests

The authors declare that they have no competing interests.

Author details

[1]Center for Comprehensive Access Delivery & Research, Iowa City VA Health Care System, Iowa City, USA. [2]Department of Internal Medicine, Carver College of Medicine, University of Iowa, Iowa City, USA. [3]University of Iowa College of Public Health, Iowa City, USA. [4]Hardin Library for the Health Sciences, University of Iowa, Iowa City, USA. [5]Ruth Lilly Medical Library, Indiana University School of Medicine, Indianapolis, Indiana, USA. [6]Veterans Affairs Salt Lake City Health Care System, Salt Lake City, Utah, USA. [7]Department of Internal Medicine, University of Utah School of Medicine, Salt Lake City, Utah, USA.

References

1. Centers for Disease Control and Prevention. Antibiotic resistance threats in the United States. 2013; http://www.cdc.gov/drugresistance/threat-report-2013/. Accessed 17 Jan 2018.
2. Gupta N, Limbago BM, Patel JB, Kallen AJ. Carbapenem-resistant Enterobacteriaceae: epidemiology and prevention. Clin Infect Dis. 2011; 53(1):60–7.
3. Centers for Disease Control and Prevention. Facility Guidance for Control of Carbapenem-resistant Enterobacteriaceae (CRE): November 2015 Update - CRE Toolkit. https://www.cdc.gov/hai/pdfs/cre/CRE-guidance-508.pdf. Accessed 17 Jan 2018.
4. Molton JS, Tambyah PA, Ang BS, Ling ML, Fisher DA. The global spread of healthcare-associated multidrug-resistant bacteria: a perspective from Asia. Clin Infect Dis. 2013;56(9):1310–8.
5. van Loon K, Voor In't Holt AF, Vos MC. A systematic review and meta-analyses of the clinical epidemiology of carbapenem-resistant Enterobacteriaceae. Antimicrob Agents Chemother. 2018;62(1)
6. Sievert DM, Ricks P, Edwards JR, et al. Antimicrobial-resistant pathogens associated with healthcare-associated infections: summary of data reported to the national healthcare safety network at the centers for disease control and prevention, 2009-2010. Infect Control Hospital Epidemiology. 2013;34(1):1–14.
7. Epstein L, Hunter JC, Arwady MA, et al. New Delhi metallo-beta-lactamase-producing carbapenem-resistant Escherichia coli associated with exposure to duodenoscopes. JAMA. 2014;312(14):1447–55.
8. Gohil SK, Singh R, Chang J, et al. Emergence of carbapenem-resistant Enterobacteriaceae in Orange County, California, and support for early regional strategies to limit spread. Am J Infect Control. 2017;45(11):1177–82.
9. Ray MJ, Lin MY, Weinstein RA, Trick WE. Spread of carbapenem-resistant Enterobacteriaceae among Illinois healthcare facilities: the role of patient sharing. Clin Infect Dis. 2016;63(7):889–93.
10. Satlin MJ, Chen L, Patel G, et al. Multicenter clinical and molecular epidemiological analysis of bacteremia due to carbapenem-resistant Enterobacteriaceae (CRE) in the CRE epicenter of the United States. Antimicrob Agents Chemother. 2017;61(4)
11. Centers or Disease Control and Prevention. Guidance for Control of Carbapenem-resistant Enterobacteriaceae (CRE). https://stacks.cdc.gov/view/cdc/13205. Accessed 17 Jan 2018.
12. Stroup DF, Berlin JA, Morton SC, et al. Meta-analysis of observational studies in epidemiology: a proposal for reporting. Meta-analysis of observational studies in epidemiology (MOOSE) group. JAMA. 2000;283(15):2008–12.
13. Moher D, Liberati A, Tetzlaff J, Altman DG, Group P. Preferred reporting items for systematic reviews and meta-analyses: the PRISMA statement. Ann Intern Med. 2009;151(4):264–9. W264
14. Stang A. Critical evaluation of the Newcastle-Ottawa scale for the assessment of the quality of nonrandomized studies in meta-analyses. Eur J Epidemiol. 2010;25(9):603–5.
15. Brennan BM, Coyle JR, Marchaim D, et al. Statewide surveillance of carbapenem-resistant enterobacteriaceae in Michigan. Infect Control Hosp Epidemiol. 2014;35(4):342–9.
16. Lesho EP, Clifford RJ, Chukwuma U, et al. Carbapenem-resistant Enterobacteriaceae and the correlation between carbapenem and fluoroquinolone usage and resistance in the US military health system. Diagn Microbiol Infect Dis. 2015;81(2):119–25.
17. Marquez P, Terashita D, Dassey D, Mascola L. Population-based incidence of carbapenem-resistant Klebsiella pneumoniae along the continuum of care, Los Angeles County. Infect Control Hosp Epidemiol. 2013;34(2):144–50.
18. Guh AY, Bulens SN, Mu Y, et al. Epidemiology of carbapenem-resistant Enterobacteriaceae in 7 US communities, 2012-2013. JAMA. 2015; 314(14):1479–87.
19. Thaden JT, Lewis SS, Hazen KC, et al. Rising rates of carbapenem-resistant enterobacteriaceae in community hospitals: a mixed-methods review of epidemiology and microbiology practices in a network of community hospitals in the southeastern United States. Infect Control Hosp Epidemiol. 2014;35(8):978–83.
20. Bogan C, Kaye KS, Chopra T, et al. Outcomes of carbapenem-resistant Enterobacteriaceae isolation: matched analysis. Am J Infect Control. 2014; 42(6):612–20.
21. Gasink LB, Edelstein PH, Lautenbach E, Synnestvedt M, Fishman NO. Risk factors and clinical impact of Klebsiella pneumoniae carbapenemase-producing K. Pneumoniae. Infect Control Hosp Epidemiol. 2009;30(12):1180–5.

22. Patel G, Huprikar S, Factor SH, Jenkins SG, Calfee DP. Outcomes of carbapenem-resistant Klebsiella pneumoniae infection and the impact of antimicrobial and adjunctive therapies. Infect Control Hosp Epidemiol. 2008; 29(12):1099–106.
23. Kalpoe JS, Sonnenberg E, Factor SH, et al. Mortality associated with carbapenem-resistant Klebsiella pneumoniae infections in liver transplant recipients. Liver Transpl. 2012;18(4):468–74.
24. Schwaber MJ, Lev B, Israeli A, et al. Containment of a country-wide outbreak of carbapenem-resistant Klebsiella pneumoniae in Israeli hospitals via a nationally implemented intervention. Clin Infect Dis. 2011;52(7):848–55.
25. Mathers AJ, Stoesser N, Sheppard AE, et al. Klebsiella pneumoniae carbapenemase (KPC)-producing K. Pneumoniae at a single institution: insights into endemicity from whole-genome sequencing. Antimicrob Agents Chemother. 2015;59(3):1656–63.
26. Dantes R, Mu Y, Belflower R, et al. National burden of invasive methicillin-resistant Staphylococcus aureus infections, United States, 2011. JAMA Intern Med. 2013;173(21):1970–8.
27. Young-Xu Y, Kuntz JL, Gerding DN, et al. Clostridium difficile infection among veterans health administration patients. Infect Control Hosp Epidemiol. 2015;36(9):1038–45.
28. Centers for Disease Control and Prevention. Tracking CRE. 2017; https://www.cdc.gov/hai/organisms/cre/trackingcre.html. Accessed 8 Dec 2017.
29. Schwaber MJ, Klarfeld-Lidji S, Navon-Venezia S, Schwartz D, Leavitt A, Carmeli Y. Predictors of carbapenem-resistant Klebsiella pneumoniae acquisition among hospitalized adults and effect of acquisition on mortality. Antimicrob Agents Chemother. 2008;52(3):1028–33.
30. Borer A, Saidel-Odes L, Riesenberg K, et al. Attributable mortality rate for carbapenem-resistant Klebsiella pneumoniae bacteremia. Infect Control Hosp Epidemiol. 2009;30(10):972–6.
31. Hombach M, Bloemberg GV, Bottger EC. Effects of clinical breakpoint changes in CLSI guidelines 2010/2011 and EUCAST guidelines 2011 on antibiotic susceptibility test reporting of gram-negative bacilli. J Antimicrob Chemother. 2012;67(3):622–32.

22

Incidence of infections due to third generation cephalosporin-resistant *Enterobacteriaceae* - a prospective multicentre cohort study in six German university hospitals

Anna M. Rohde[1,2*], Janine Zweigner[1,2,3], Miriam Wiese-Posselt[1,2], Frank Schwab[1,2], Michael Behnke[1,2], Axel Kola[1,2], Birgit Obermann[1,4], Johannes K.-M. Knobloch[1,4,11], Susanne Feihl[1,5], Christiane Querbach[1,5], Friedemann Gebhardt[1,5], Alexander Mischnik[1,6], Vera Ihle[1,6], Wiebke Schröder[1,7], Sabina Armean[1,7], Silke Peter[1,8], Evelina Tacconelli[1,7], Axel Hamprecht[1,9], Harald Seifert[1,9], Maria J. G. T. Vehreschild[1,10], Winfried V. Kern[1,6], Petra Gastmeier[1,2] and on behalf of the DZIF-ATHOS study group[1]

Abstract

Background: Infections caused by third generation cephalosporin-resistant *Enterobacteriaceae* (3GCREB) are an increasing healthcare problem. We aim to describe the 3GCREB infection incidence and compare it to prevalence upon admission. In addition, we aim to describe infections caused by 3GCREB, which are also carbapenem resistant (CRE).

Methods: In 2014–2015, we performed prospective 3GCREB surveillance in clinically relevant patient specimens (screening specimens excluded). Infections counted as hospital-acquired (HAI) when the 3GCREB was detected after the third day following admission, otherwise as community-acquired infection (CAI).

Results: Of 578,420 hospitalized patients under surveillance, 3367 had a 3GCREB infection (0.58%). We observed a similar 3GCREB CAI and HAI incidence (0.28 and 0.31 per 100 patients, respectively). The most frequent pathogen was 3GCR *E. coli*, in CAI and HAI (0.15 and 0.12 per 100 patients). We observed a CRE CAI incidence of 0.006 and a HAI incidence of 0.008 per 100 patients (0.014 per 1000 patient days).

Conclusions: Comparing the known 3GCREB admission prevalence of the participating hospitals (9.5%) with the percentage of patients with a 3GCREB infection (0.58%), we conclude the prevalence of 3GCREB in university hospitals to be about 16 times higher than suggested when only patients with 3GCREB infections are considered. Moreover, we find the HAI and CAI incidence caused by CRE in Germany to be relatively low.

Keywords: Fluoroquinolone, Carbapenem, Gram-negative, ESBL, *Enterobacter* spp., *Klebsiella* spp., *E. coli*, CRE, Hospital-acquired infections, Community-acquired infections

* Correspondence: Anna.rohde@charite.de
[1]German Center for Infection Research (DZIF), Inhoffenstraße 7, 38124 Braunschweig, Germany
[2]Charité – Universitätsmedizin Berlin, Institute of Hygiene and Environmental Medicine, Hindenburgstraße 27, 12203 Berlin, Germany
Full list of author information is available at the end of the article

Background

Emerging multidrug-resistant Gram-negative bacteria are a global health concern, especially those harbouring extended-spectrum beta-lactamases (ESBL), which render *Enterobacteriaceae* resistant to third generation cephalosporins (3GC) and extended-spectrum penicillins [1]. Third generation cephalosporin resistant *Enterobacteriaceae* (3GCREB) infections are a special threat to patient safety, as resistance may cause a delay in effective antimicrobial therapy and thereby lead to worsening patient outcomes [2]. EU surveillance data shows that the 3GC resistance rate of *E. coli* in blood and cerebrospinal fluid samples has increased in many EU countries (EU mean 2012: 11.9%, 2015: 13.1%) [3]. The incidence density of 3GCREB in clinical specimens in German intensive care units (ICUs) rose from 2001 to 2015 (*E. coli*: 0.16 to 3.83/1000 patient days, *K. pneumoniae*: 0.25 to 1.41/1000 patient days) [4]. The percentage of hospital-acquired infections (HAI) caused by ESBL-producing *Enterobacteriaceae* in German ICUs and surgical departments increased as well (2007: 10.9% to 2012: 15.5%) [5].

The ATHOS (Antibiotic Therapy Optimization Study) project aimed at assessing the 3GCREB admission prevalence and 3GCREB incidence of community-acquired and hospital-acquired infections (CAI, HAI) in six German university hospitals in 2014 and 2015. The prevalence data was published previously [6]. Here, we describe the incidence of 3GCREB infections in the same hospitals and relate the data to the 3GCREB admission prevalence. Furthermore, we analyse the distribution of additional resistance phenotype patterns in those 3GCREB that caused infections.

Methods

Study design and data sources

The ATHOS project was a prospective observational cohort study that monitored hospitalized patients in general wards and ICUs for their first 3GCREB detection in clinical specimens (active surveillance). Each microbiology finding was followed by checking the health record or by contacting the wards and clinicians directly. The study was performed in six German university hospitals from January 1, 2014 to December 31, 2015. Patients hospitalized in the departments of dermatology, gynaecology/obstetrics, ophthalmology, otorhinolaryngology, paediatrics and psychiatry were excluded from surveillance.

Microbiological analysis

Gram-negative bacteria were identified down to species level using either MALDI-TOF MS or VITEK®2 (bioMérieux, Nürtingen, Germany). Antimicrobial susceptibility testing was performed using VITEK®2. *Enterobacteriaceae* were classified as susceptible or resistant based on minimal inhibitory concentrations according to EUCAST breakpoints [7]. Non-susceptibility was regarded as resistance. Indicator antimicrobials for third generation cephalosporin resistance were cefotaxime and ceftazidime, indicators for carbapenem resistance were imipenem and meropenem.

Definitions

A 3GCREB case was defined as the first 3GCREB isolate detected in clinical specimens (e.g. urine, wound swab, blood culture, tracheobronchial secretion or other clinical specimens) in a patient during a single hospital stay. Readmission followed by another 3GCREB detection created a new case.. Cases were distinguished in colonisations and cases with infections. Infections were defined as the detection of 3GCREB in a clinical specimen with additional signs and symptoms of infection as determined by a clinician followed by adequate antimicrobial therapy. A single case could present several 3GCREB species, each with several infections (though counting only by infection type). Acquisition was defined as follows: detection on day 1–3 (admission day = day 1) counted as community-acquired (CA), later detections counted as hospital-acquired (HA) [8]. We stratified for the following infection types: urinary tract infection (UTI), lower respiratory tract infection (LRTI), surgical site infection (SSI) and bloodstream infection (BSI). Other infection types were pooled in the category "other infections". We analysed HAI caused by HA-3GCREB and CAI caused by CA-3GCREB. Cases with an ambiguous acquisition (CA-3GCREB with HAI and HA-3GCREB on top of existing CAI) were discarded.

Statistical analysis

Infection incidence was calculated as infections per 100 patients, incidence density as infections per 1000 patient days. Both were stratified by species, resistance phenotype and infection type. Then 95% confidence intervals were calculated. The species distribution over infection types was tested with X^2 test (R x C table). The comparison of resistance phenotypes among 3GCREB responsible for different infection types was tested with Fisher's exact test (2 × 2 table, carbapenem-resistant versus -susceptible). *P*-values < 0.05 were considered significant. Statistical analysis was performed with SAS 9.4 (SAS Institute, Cary, NC, USA) and OpenEpi (Open Source Epidemiologic Statistics for Public Health, V3.01 http://www.openepi.com).

Ethics and data protection

3GCREB surveillance was performed in accordance with the German Infection Protection Act [9]. The ethics committee at Charité, University Medicine Berlin, Germany, approved this study (EA/018/14). Data from the six hospitals was entered into an online accessible database approved by the data protection commissioner.

Results

The ATHOS project was conducted at six German university hospitals comprising a total of 283 wards and 4957 beds in the surveillance area. The majority were general wards with surgical specialty (n = 104) followed by medical specialty (n = 83), intensive care units (ICU, n = 49), haematology/oncology (n = 35) and intermediate care wards (n = 12).

In the period 2014–2015, 578,420 patient admissions with 3,385,112 patient days were under surveillance. After excluding invalid data and cases of colonization (n = 2262), 3367 clinical cases with one or more 3GCREB infections (0.58% of the patients) were analysed (Fig. 1a). The median age was 69 (IQR 58–77 years) and 55% of the cases were male. Of the cases, 92% had one infection, 7% had two infections and 1% had three or four infections.

To compare different infection types, cases were broken down into single infections and those with ambiguous acquisition were discarded, yielding 3370 single infections. The majority of infections were hospital-acquired (3GCREB HAI, Fig. 1b). We observed a difference in infection incidence among the university hospitals, e.g. the 3GCREB HAI incidence ranged from 0.17–0.42 per 100 patients. Therefore, the data of the individual hospitals was pooled for further analysis. The absolute numbers of infections stratified by species, resistance phenotype, and infection type are shown in Table 1, the infection incidences and incidence densities in Table 2. The 3GCREB CAI incidence was 0.28 per 100 patients, and that of HAI 0.31 per 100 patients. The majority of CAI were caused by 3GCREB which were also fluoroquinolone resistant (FQR, 0.17 per 100 patients), in HAI that incidence was lower (0.14 per 100

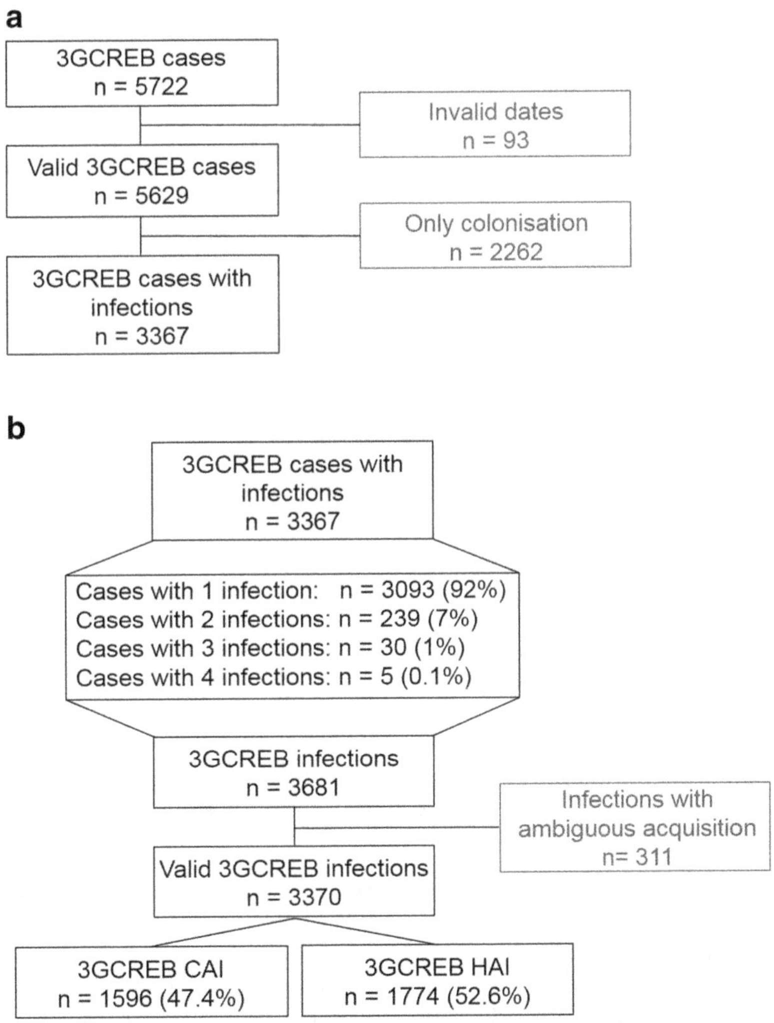

Fig. 1 Flow chart of third generation cephalosporin resistant *Enterobacteriaceae* (3GCREB) cases (**a**) and infections (**b**). **a**) Readmission followed by 3GCREB detection created a second case. **b**) Each case could represent several infections but only one per infection type

Table 1 Distribution of third generation cephalosporin resistant *Enterobacteriaceae* (3GCREB) infections in the ATHOS project, 2014–2015, Germany

Parameter	Category	3GCREB infections *n* (%)	3GCREB CAI *n* (%)	3GCREB HAI *n* (%)
3GCREB	total	3370 (100%)	1596 (100%)	1774 (100%)
Species	*E. coli*	1624 (48%)	910 (57%)	714 (40%)
	Enterobacter spp.	702 (21%)	221 (14%)	481 (27%)
	Klebsiella spp.	562 (17%)	264 (17%)	298 (17%)
	Citrobacter spp.	209 (6%)	76 (5%)	133 (7%)
	Other species [a]	273 (8%)	125 (8%)	148 (8%)
Resistance	all 3GCREB			
	only 3GCR	1488 (44%)	580 (36%)	908 (51%)
	+ FQR	1796 (53%)	979 (61%)	817 (46%)
	+ CR	86 (3%)	37 (2%)	49 (3%)
	E. coli	1624 (100%)	910 (100%)	714 (100%)
	only 3GCR	409 (25%)	209 (23%)	200 (28%)
	+ FQR	1203 (74%)	698 (77%)	505 (71%)
	+ CR	12 (1%)	3 (0%)	9 (1%)
	Enterobacter spp.	702 (100%)	221 (100%)	481 (100%)
	only 3GCR	553 (79%)	168 (76%)	385 (80%)
	+ FQR	122 (17%)	45 (20%)	77 (16%)
	+ CR	27 (4%)	8 (4%)	19 (4%)
	Klebsiella spp.	562 (100%)	264 (100%)	298 (100%)
	only 3GCR	157 (28%)	59 (22%)	98 (33%)
	+ FQR	362 (64%)	181 (69%)	181 (61%)
	+ CR	43 (8%)	24 (9%)	19 (6%)
Infections	SSI	401 (12%)	99 (6%)	302 (17%)
	UTI	1528 (45%)	872 (55%)	656 (37%)
	LRTI	571 (17%)	158 (10%)	413 (23%)
	BSI	459 (14%)	220 (14%)	239 (13%)
	Other infections [b]	411 (12%)	247 (15%)	164 (9%)
Year	2014	1784 (53%)	847 (53%)	937 (53%)
	2015	1586 (47%)	749 (47%)	837 (47%)
Ward type	General ward	2174 (65%)	1102 (69%)	1072 (60%)
	ICU/interm. Care	1196 (35%)	494 (31%)	702 (40%)
Specialty	Surgical	1407 (42%)	522 (33%)	885 (50%)
	Non-surgical	1963 (58%)	1074 (67%)	889 (50%)

3GCREB infections among 578,420 patient admissions and 3,385,112 patient days in six German university hospitals. [a] "Other *Enterobacteriaceae* species" include *Cedecea, Hafnia, Morganella, Pantoea, Proteus, Providencia, Raoultella,* and *Serratia* species. [b] "Other infections" includes all other infection types. 3GCREB = third generation cephalosporin-resistant *Enterobacteriaceae*, *3GCR* third generation cephalosporin resistance, *FQR* fluoroquinolone resistance, *CR* carbapenem resistance, *CA* community-acquired, *HA* hospital-acquired, *SSI* surgical site infection, *UTI* urinary tract infection, *LRTI* lower respiratory tract infection, *BSI* bloodstream infection, *ICU* intensive care unit, *interm. Care* intermediate care. Column percentages were calculated for each parameter with respect to "3GCREB total"

patients). 3GCREB that were also carbapenem resistant caused 0.006 CAI and 0.008 HAI per 100 patients.

Among 3GCREB species, *E. coli* caused the highest incidence of CAI (0.15 per 100 patients) and HAI (0.12 per 100 patients). The most frequent infections were UTIs irrespective of the acquisition; the incidence of 3GCREB CA-UTI exceeded that of 3GCREB HA-UTI (0.15 vs. 0.11 per 100 patients). For SSI and LRTI, the incidence of 3GCREB HAI exceeded that of CAI (Table 2).

Figure 2 shows the distribution of 3GCREB infections stratified by CAI/HAI and by species. Species distribution differed significantly in UTI, LRTI and BSI: HA-UTI, -LRTI and -BSI were caused more frequently

Table 2 Incidence (densities) of infections with third generation cephalosporin-resistant *Enterobacteriaceae* (3GCREB), ATHOS project, 2014–2015, Germany

Parameter	Category	3GCREB CAI incidence per 100,000 admissions (95% CI)	3GCREB CAI incidence per 100 admissions (95% CI)	3GCREB HAI incidence per 100 admissions (95% CI)	3GCREB HAI incidence density per 1000 patient days (95% CI)
3GCREB	total	276 (263–290)	0.28 (0.26–0.29)	0.31 (0.29–0.32)	0.52 (0.50–0.55)
Species	*E. coli*	157 (147–168)	0.16 (0.15–0.17)	0.12 (0.12–0.13)	0.21 (0.20–0.23)
	Enterobacter spp.	38 (33–44)	0.04 (0.03–0.04)	0.08 (0.08–0.09)	0.14 (0.13–0.16)
	Klebsiella spp.	45 (40–52)	0.05 (0.04–0.05)	0.05 (0.05–0.06)	0.09 (0.08–0.10)
	Citrobacter spp.	13 (10–16)	0.01 (0.01–0.02)	0.02 (0.02–0.03)	0.04 (0.03–0.05)
	Other species [a]	22 (18–26)	0.02 (0.02–0.03)	0.03 (0.02–0.03)	0.04 (0.04–0.05)
Resistance	all 3GCREB				
	only 3GCR	100 (92–109)	0.10 (0.09–0.11)	0.16 (0.15–0.17)	0.27 (0.25–0.29)
	+ FQR	169 (159–180)	0.17 (0.16–0.18)	0.14 (0.13–0.15)	0.24 (0.23–0.26)
	+ CR	6 (5–9)	0.006 (0.005–0.009)	0.008 (0.006–0.011)	0.014 (0.011–0.019)
	E. coli				
	only 3GCR	36 (31–41)	0.04 (0.03–0.04)	0.04 (0.03–0.04)	0.06 (0.05–0.07)
	+ FQR	121 (112–130)	0.12 (0.11–0.13)	0.09 (0.08–0.10)	0.15 (0.14–0.16)
	+ CR	1 (0–2)	0.001 (0.000–0.002)	0.002 (0.001–0.003)	0.003 (0.001–0.005)
	Enterobacter spp.				
	only 3GCR	29 (25–34)	0.03 (0.03–0.03)	0.07 (0.06–0.07)	0.11 (0.10–0.13)
	+ FQR	8 (6–10)	0.01 (0.01–0.01)	0.01 (0.01–0.02)	0.02 (0.02–0.03)
	+ CR	1 (1–3)	0.001 (0.001–0.003)	0.003 (0.002–0.005)	0.006 (0.003–0.009)
	Klebsiella spp.				
	only 3GCR	10 (8–13)	0.01 (0.01–0.01)	0.02 (0.01–0.02)	0.03 (0.02–0.04)
	+ FQR	31 (27–36)	0.03 (0.03–0.04)	0.03 (0.03–0.04)	0.05 (0.05–0.06)
	+ CR	4 (3–6)	0.004 (0.003–0.006)	0.003 (0.002–0.005)	0.006 (0.003–0.009)
Infections	SSI	17 (14–21)	0.02 (0.01–0.02)	0.05 (0.05–0.06)	0.09 (0.08–0.10)
	UTI	151 (141–161)	0.15 (0.14–0.16)	0.11 (0.11–0.12)	0.19 (0.18–0.21)
	LRTI	27 (23–32)	0.03 (0.02–0.03)	0.07 (0.07–0.08)	0.12 (0.11–0.13)
	BSI	38 (33–43)	0.04 (0.03–0.04)	0.04 (0.04–0.05)	0.07 (0.06–0.08)
	Other infections [b]	43 (38–48)	0.04 (0.04–0.05)	0.03 (0.02–0.03)	0.05 (0.04–0.06)

[a] "Other *Enterobacteriaceae* species" include *Cedecea, Hafnia, Morganella, Pantoea, Proteus, Providencia, Raoultella,* and *Serratia* species. [b] "Other infections" includes all other infection types. 3GCREB = third generation cephalosporin-resistant *Enterobacteriaceae*, *3GCR* third generation cephalosporin resistance, *FQR* fluoroquinolone resistance, *CR* carbapenem resistance, *3GCR + CR* carbapenem resistant *Enterobacteriaceae* (CRE), *CAI* community-acquired infection, *HAI* hospital-acquired infection, *SSI* surgical site infection, *UTI* urinary tract infection, *LRTI* lower respiratory tract infection, *BSI* bloodstream infection, *95% CI* 95% confidence interval

by *Enterobacter* spp.. HA-BSI were also caused to a higher percentage by *Klebsiella* spp. than CA-BSI. Figure 3 shows the distribution of resistance phenotypes by infection type. The resistance phenotypes of 3GCR *E. coli* isolates did not differ between CAI and HAI (Fig. 3a). In contrast, 3GCR *Klebsiella* spp. showed a higher proportion of carbapenem resistance in all CAI except UTI. Twenty percent of the 3GCR *Klebsiella* spp. that caused CA-BSI and 28% of those that caused CA-LRTI were carbapenem resistant. A high percentage of 3GCR *Klebsiella* spp. that caused surgical site infections were also carbapenem resistant, irrespective of the acquisition (15% in CA-SSI and 13% in HA-SSI) (Fig. 3b).

Discussion

The incidence of 3GCREB infections among patients admitted to German university hospitals in 2014/15 was < 1%. Additional fluoroquinolone resistance was frequent in particular in CAI, while additional carbapenem resistance was rare, both in CAI and HAI (0.006 and 0.008 per 100 patients; HAI incidence density 0.014 per 1000 patient days). An interesting finding was that among CA-LRTI caused by 3GCR *Klebsiella* spp., the percentage of additional carbapenem resistance (28%) was substantial and significantly higher than in 3GCR *Klebsiella* spp. causing HA-LRTI (6%, $p = 0.015$).

In an admission prevalence study performed in parallel, we screened a minimum of 500 patients per hospital for

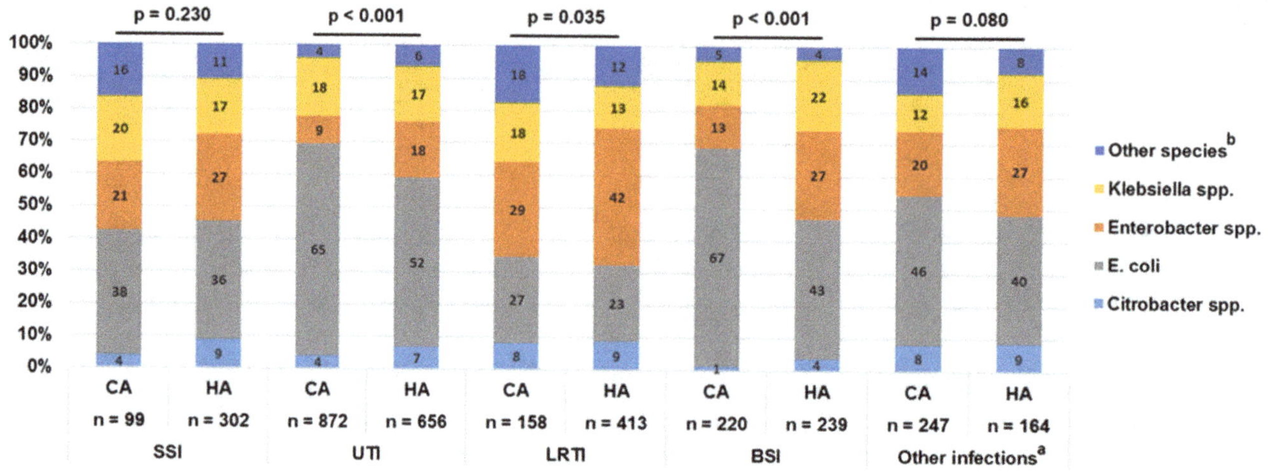

Fig. 2 Relative species distribution in third generation cephalosporin-resistant *Enterobacteriaceae* (3GCREB) infections, stratified for infection type and acquisition, ATHOS project, 2014–2015, Germany. [a] *"Other infections" includes all infection types other than: SSI = surgical site infection, UTI = urinary tract infection, LRTI = lower respiratory tract infection, BSI = bloodstream infection. CA = community-acquired, HA = hospital-acquired.* [b] *"Other Enterobacteriaceae species" include Cedecea, Hafnia, Morganella, Pantoea, Proteus, Providencia, Raoultella, and Serratia species. X2-tests (5 × 2 table) were performed for each infection type to test for differences between CAI and HAI*

rectal 3GCREB carriage on admission (day 1–3, admission day = day 1). This study showed a 3GCREB colonization prevalence of 9.5% [6]. Therefore, we conclude that the colonization rate of patients in university hospitals is about 16 times higher (=9.5%/0.58% patients with 3GCREB infection) than suggested when only patients with 3GCREB infections are considered. The reason for this high colonization prevalence and for a CAI incidence comparable to HAI is most likely the case mix in tertiary care university hospitals due to their position at the end of the treatment chain. On admission, many patients most likely have received previous antimicrobial treatment and have higher co-morbidity scores than patients in other hospital types.

The incidence of CAI causing 3GCREB that were also resistant to fluoroquinolones exceeded that of HAI (Table 2). One reason for this may be the high antibiotic use reported by patients admitted to the participating hospitals (34% of the 3GCREB-negative and 53% of the 3GCREB-positive patients) [6]. Another reason may be an enhanced use of fluoroquinolones in outpatient care [10]. This excess of fluoroquinolone use might be caused (among other reasons) by over prescription and non-adherence to antibiotic prescription guidelines in outpatient care [11–13]. A reduction of fluoroquinolone prescriptions would be desirable.

In 2013/14, the EU mean of carbapenemase-producing (CP) *E. coli* and *K. pneumoniae* was found to be 0.025 per 1000 patient days and 0.006 per 1000 patient days were reported for Germany (EuSCAPE study) [14]. We observed a CRE HAI incidence density for *Klebsiella* spp. of 0.006 (95% CI 0.000–0.008) and for *E. coli* of 0.003 per 1000 patient days (95% CI 0.001–0.005). The EuSCAPE study showed that among CRE, 70% of the *K. pneumoniae* and 30% of the *E. coli* produced carbapenemases [14]. Combining these percentages of CPE among CRE with our CRE data yields an estimated CPE incidence density for *Klebsiella* spp. and *E. coli* of 0.005 per 1000 patient days (*Klebsiella* spp. 0.004 and *E. coli* 0.001 per 1000 patient days). Thus, our data is comparable to the EuSCAPE data for Germany [14].

In contrast to other *Enterobacteriaceae* species, 3GCR *Klebsiella* spp. showed a high percentage of carbapenem resistance among CA infections, especially in LRTI and BSI. In a UK study, the prevalence of carbapenem resistance in clinically relevant *K. pneumoniae* specimens was also due primarily to community-acquired isolates (70%) [15]. The EU mean of carbapenem resistance in invasive *K. pneumoniae* isolates increased from 2012 to 2015 to 8%. In two European countries, carbapenem resistance was observed in over 25% of *K. pneumoniae* (Italy 34% and Greece 62%). In isolates from Germany, carbapenem resistance was rare (0.1%) [3]. Surveillance in German ICUs showed that the carbapenem resistance rate of *K. pneumoniae* in clinically relevant specimens increased from 2001 to 2015 to 1.5% [4]. A large admission prevalence study found a low CRE admission prevalence in Germany (comparable to UK, both 0.1%) [6, 16]. In light of this data, we conclude that even with increasing trends Germany currently still is a low CRE prevalence region.

The ATHOS project was a prospective observational study. One major limitation is the lack of patient-based information on previous healthcare contacts. Therefore, a classification into the important "healthcare-associated"

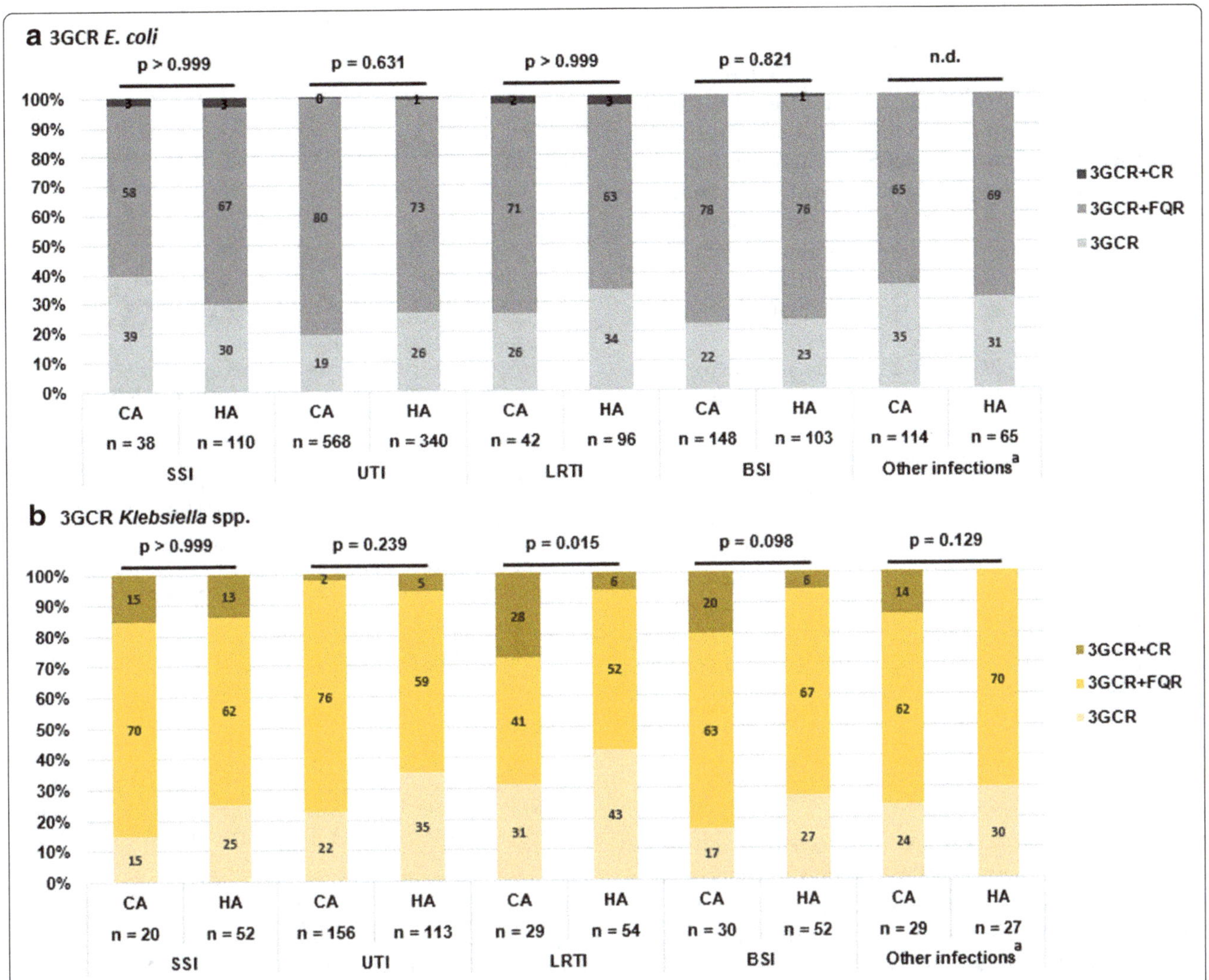

Fig. 3 Relative distribution of resistance phenotypes of third generation cephalosporin-resistant (3GCR) *E. coli* (**a**) and *Klebsiella* spp. (**b**) depending on infection type and acquisition, ATHOS project, 2014–2015, Germany. [a] *"Other infections" includes all infection types other than: SSI = surgical site infection, UTI = urinary tract infection, LRTI = lower respiratory tract infection, BSI = bloodstream infection. 3GCR = third generation cephalosporin resistance, FQR = fluoroquinolone resistance, CR = carbapenem resistance, 3GCR + CR = carbapenem-resistant Enterobacteriaceae (CRE), CA = community-acquired, HA = hospital-acquired. Fishers exact-tests (2 × 2 table, carbapenem-resistant versus -susceptible) were performed for each infection type to test for differences between CAI and HAI, p < 0.05 was considered significant. "n.d." = not defined, p-value cannot be calculated due to missing events in both groups*

category was not possible. Instead, the somewhat arbitrary day 3 limit for classification into CA and HA was applied, as it is commonly used for surveillance of HAI [8]. Nonetheless, we have some insight into the healthcare contacts of our patient mix from our patients in the admission prevalence study sample, 9% of whom had stayed in a rehabilitation centre, 5% in a long-term care facility and 26% in another hospital in the 6 months prior to admission [6]. Some CAI may, in fact, be healthcare-associated and thus the incidence of CAI may be overestimated in our analysis. This CA/HA classificiation was also used for SSI. We cannot exclude that some CA-SSI cases may be readmitted cases. An advantage of the study is the inclusion of general wards. We can describe the incidence of 3GCREB infections in German university hospitals comprehensively and are not limited to ICU data. However, due to the hospital-wide surveillance, we lack ward-specific denominator data and are not able to calculate department-specific incidences.

One strength of the study is the inclusion of most *Enterobacteriaceae* species, since other studies are often restricted to *E. coli* or *K. pneumoniae*. Such studies are likely to underestimate the real incidence of CRE. We found a major part of CRE-HAI caused by *Enterobacter* spp. (0.006 per 1000 patient days, 95% CI 0.000–0.008). Imipenem resistance of *E. cloacae* complex has increased over the last years in German ICUs [4]. In addition, long-term surveillance by the US Veterans Health

Administration of CRE in patients also showed a steady increase of carbapenem resistance in *E. cloacae* [17]. However, we have noticed that Vitek®2 frequently over-reported imipenem resistance. For future CRE studies, we suggest including *Enterobacter* spp. and using additional, more reliable diagnostic methods (e.g. disk diffusion test or agar gradient diffusion) to determine if the high frequency of Vitek®2 imipenem resistance represents the true epidemiology. Another drawback of using routine diagnostic methods is that we were unable to compare sequence types of 3GCREB causing CAI and HAI.

As a result of the 3GCREB admission prevalence study performed in parallel [6] and the surveillance data for infections, we can for the first time estimate the 3GCREB prevalence to be about 16-times higher than indicated by the 3GCREB infection incidence (0.58%). This will enable other university hospitals with a similar patient mix to estimate roughly the dimension of colonization prevalence present in their patients. Furthermore, we conclude that very few 3GCREB carriers are identified using clinically indicated diagnostic procedures. Therefore, we believe the majority of hospitals underestimate the extent of 3GCREB prevalence. This study gives a comprehensive description of the incidence of CRE found in German university hospitals.

Conclusion

Overall, our analysis showed that German university hospitals have a low 3GCREB infection incidence when compared to the admission prevalence. As we observed a comparable incidence of 3GCREB CAI and HAI, it is important that clinicians consider cephalosporin resistance in their empirical treatment decisions, irrespective of the acquisition type (CA vs. HA) of the infection.

Abbreviations

3GC (3GCR): 3rd generation cephalosporin (–resistant); 3GCREB: 3rd generation cephalosporin-resistant *Enterobacteriaceae*; ATHOS: Antibiotic therapy optimisation study; BSI: Bloodstream infection; CA (CAI): Community-acquired (infection); CP (CPE): Carbapenemase-producing (*Enterobacteriaceae*); CR (CRE): Carbapenemase-resistant (*Enterobacteriaceae*); *E. cloacae*: *Enterobacter cloacae*; *E. coli*: *Escherichia coli*; ESBL: extended spectrum β-lactamase; EU: European Union; EUCAST: European committee on antimicrobial susceptibility testing; HA (HAI): Hospital-acquired (infection); ICU: Intensive care unit; IQR: Interquartile range; *K. pneumonia*: *Klebsiella pneumonia*; LRTI: Lower respiratory tract infection; MALDI-TOF MS: Matrix-assisted laser desorption/ionization-time of flight mass spectrometry; spp.: species; SSI: Surgical site infection; UK: United Kingdom; US: United States; UTI: Urinary tract infection

Acknowledgements

We would like to acknowledge all other members of the ATHOS study group:
Michael Buhl, Tübingen; Dirk Busch, Munich; Simone Eisenbeis, Tübingen; Gesche Först, Freiburg; Federico Foschi, Tübingen; Meyke Gillis, Cologne; Dorothea Hansen, Cologne; Georg Häcker, Freiburg; Markus Heim, Munich; Martin Hug, Freiburg; Klaus Kaier, Freiburg; Fabian Küpper, Freiburg; Georg Langebartels, Cologne; Andrea Liekweg, Cologne; Hans-Peter Lipp, Tübingen; Nayana Märtin, Berlin; Mathias Nordmann, Berlin; Andrea Pelzer, Cologne; Luis-Alberto Peña-Diaz, Berlin; Jan Rupp, Lübeck; Christin Schröder, Berlin; Katrin Spohn, Tübingen; Michaela Steib-Bauert, Freiburg; Jörg J. Vehreschild, Cologne; Ulrich vor dem Esche, Freiburg and Solvy Wolke, Berlin.

Funding

The German Centre for Infection Research (DZIF) funded the ATHOS project (TTU 08.801).

Authors' contributions

AMR local site coordinator, local data collection, supervision of data collection in partner sites, data analysis, drafting and revising manuscript. JZ study design, surveillance protocol, local site coordinator. MWP study design, surveillance protocol, local site coordinator. FS study design, data analysis. MB database setup, supervision of data collection in partner sites. AK microbiological analysis. BO local data collection. JKMK local principal investigator, microbiological analysis. SF microgiological analysis, local data collection. CQ local data collection. FG local site coordinator. AM microbiological analysis. VI local data collection. WS local site coordinator, local data collection. SA local data collection. SP microbiological analysis. ET local principal investigator. AH microbiological analysis. HS principal investigator of the study, study design, surveillance protocol. MJGTV local site coordination, local data collection. WVK principal investigator of the project, study design, surveillance protocol. PG principal investigator of the study, study design, surveillance protocol. All authors contributed to writing the manuscript through commenting and approved the final document.

Consent for publication

Not applicable.

Competing interests

No competing interests unless stated.
MJGTV is a consultant to: Alb Fils Kliniken, Astellas Pharma, MaaT Pharma, MSD/Merck; has served with the speakers' bureau of: Astellas Pharma, Basilea, Gilead Sciences, Merck/MSD, Organobalance and Pfizer; received research funding from: 3 M, Astellas Pharma, DaVolterra, Gilead Sciences, Merck/MSD, Morphochem, Organobalance, and Seres Therapeutics.
HS reports grants from Bundesministerium für Bildung und Forschung (BMBF), the German Center for Infection Research (DZIF), Cubist, and Novartis, and personal fees from Astellas-Basilea, Cubist, Durata, Genentech, Gilead, MSD, Roche Pharma, and Tetraphase.
JKMK received research and travel grants from Novartis, bioMérieux, Bayer Vital, and Alere and served as consultant or speaker for bioMérieux, Novartis,and Pfizer.
JZ received a speaker's honorarium from Pfizer.

Author details

[1]German Center for Infection Research (DZIF), Inhoffenstraße 7, 38124 Braunschweig, Germany. [2]Charité – Universitätsmedizin Berlin, Institute of Hygiene and Environmental Medicine, Hindenburgstraße 27, 12203 Berlin, Germany. [3]Department of Infection Control and Hygiene, University Hospital Cologne, Kerpener Straße 62, 50937 Köln, Germany. [4]Department of Infectious Diseases and Microbiology, Institute for Medical Microbiology, University Hospital Schleswig-Holstein, Ratzeburger Allee 160, 23562 Lübeck, Germany. [5]Institute for Medical Microbiology, Immunology and Hygiene, Klinikum Rechts der Isar, Technische Universität München, Munich, Germany. [6]Division of Infectious Diseases, Department of Medicine II, Medical Center and Faculty of Medicine, University of Freiburg, Hugstetter Strasse 55, 79106 Freiburg, Germany. [7]Division of Infectious Diseases, Department of Internal Medicine 1, University Hospital Tübingen, Otfried-Müller-Straße 12, 72076 Tübingen, Germany. [8]Institute for Medical Microbiology and Hygiene, University Hospital Tübingen, Elfriede-Aulhorn-Straße 6, 72076 Tübingen, Germany. [9]Institute for Medical Microbiology, Immunology and Hygiene, University Hospital Cologne, Goldenfelsstrasse 19-21, 50935 Köln, Germany. [10]Department I of Internal Medicine, University Hospital of Cologne, Herderstraße 52-54, 50931 Köln, Germany. [11]Institute for Medical Microbiology, Virology and Hygiene, University Medical Center Hamburg-Eppendorf, Martinistraße 52, 20246 Hamburg, Germany.

References

1. World Health Organization: Antimicrobial resistance: global report on surveillance. In. WHO Library Cataloguing-in-Publication Data: World Health Organisation 2014.
2. Rottier WC, Ammerlaan HS, Bonten MJ. Effects of confounders and intermediates on the association of bacteraemia caused by extended-spectrum beta-lactamase-producing Enterobacteriaceae and patient outcome: a meta-analysis. J Antimicrob Chemother. 2012;67(6):1311–20.
3. European Centre for Disease Prevention and Control: Antimicrobial resistance surveillance in Europe 2015. Annual Report of the European Antimicrobial Resistance Surveillance Network (EARS-Net). In. Stockholm: ECDC; 2017.
4. Remschmidt C, Schneider S, Meyer E, Schroeren-Boersch B, Gastmeier P, Schwab F. Surveillance of antibiotic use and resistance in intensive care units (SARI). Dtsch Arztebl Int. 2017;114(50):858–65.
5. Leistner R, Schroder C, Geffers C, Breier AC, Gastmeier P, Behnke M. Regional distribution of nosocomial infections due to ESBL-positive Enterobacteriaceae in Germany: data from the German National Reference Center for the surveillance of nosocomial infections (KISS). Clin Microbiol Infect. 2015;21(3):255 e251–5.
6. Hamprecht A, Rohde AM, Behnke M, Feihl S, Gastmeier P, Gebhardt F, Kern WV, Knobloch JK, Mischnik A, Obermann B, et al. Colonization with third-generation cephalosporin-resistant Enterobacteriaceae on hospital admission: prevalence and risk factors. J Antimicrob Chemother. 2016;71(10): 2957–63. https://doi.org/10.1093/jac/dkw216.
7. Breakpoint tables for interpretation of MICs and zone diameters. Version 4.0. http://www.eucast.org.
8. Multidrug-Resistant Organism & Clostridium difficile Infection (MDRO/CDI) Module. https://www.cdc.gov/nhsn/pdfs/pscmanual/12pscmdro_cdadcurrent.pdf.
9. Federal Ministry of Justice and Consumer Protection: German Infection Protection Act, §23. In.; 2001.
10. Dingle KE, Didelot X, Quan TP, Eyre DW, Stoesser N, Golubchik T, Harding RM, Wilson DJ, Griffiths D, Vaughan A, et al. Effects of control interventions on Clostridium difficile infection in England: an observational study. Lancet Infect Dis. 2017;17(4):411–21.
11. Pouwels KB, Dolk FCK, Smith DRM, Robotham JV, Smieszek T. Actual versus 'ideal' antibiotic prescribing for common conditions in English primary care. J Antimicrob Chemother. 2018;73(suppl_2):19–26.
12. Smieszek T, Pouwels KB, Dolk FCK, Smith DRM, Hopkins S, Sharland M, Hay AD, Moore MV, Robotham JV. Potential for reducing inappropriate antibiotic prescribing in English primary care. J Antimicrob Chemother. 2018; 73(suppl_2):ii36–43.
13. Zweigner J, Meyer E, Gastmeier P, Schwab F. Rate of antibiotic prescriptions in German outpatient care - are the guidelines followed or are they still exceeded? GMS Hyg Infect Control. 2018;13 Doc04.
14. Grundmann H, Glasner C, Albiger B, Aanensen DM, Tomlinson CT, Andrasevic AT, Canton R, Carmeli Y, Friedrich AW, Giske CG, et al. Occurrence of carbapenemase-producing Klebsiella pneumoniae and Escherichia coli in the European survey of carbapenemase-producing Enterobacteriaceae (EuSCAPE): a prospective, multinational study. Lancet Infect Dis. 2017;17(2):153–63.
15. Trepanier P, Mallard K, Meunier D, Pike R, Brown D, Ashby JP, Donaldson H. Awad-El-Kariem FM, Balakrishnan I, Cubbon M *et al*: Carbapenemase-producing Enterobacteriaceae in the UK: a national study (EuSCAPE-UK) on prevalence, incidence, laboratory detection methods and infection control measures. J Antimicrob Chemother. 2017;72(2):596–603.
16. Otter JA, Dyakova E, Bisnauthsing KN, Querol-Rubiera A, Patel A, Ahanonu C, Tosas Auguet O, Edgeworth JD, Goldenberg SD. Universal hospital admission screening for carbapenemase-producing organisms in a low-prevalence setting. J Antimicrob Chemother. 2016;71(12):3556–61.
17. Kaase M, Schimanski S, Schiller R, Beyreiss B, Thurmer A, Steinmann J, Kempf VA, Hess C, Sobottka I, Fenner I, et al. Multicentre investigation of carbapenemase-producing Escherichia coli and Klebsiella pneumoniae in German hospitals. Int J Med Microbiol. 2016.

23

Prevalence of antibiotic resistant *Escherichia coli* isolates from fecal samples of food handlers in Qatar

Nahla O. Eltai[1], Hadi M. Yassine[1,2], Asmaa A. Al Thani[1,2], Marwan A. Abu Madi[2], Ahmed Ismail[3], Emad Ibrahim[4] and Walid Q. Alali[5,6*]

Abstract

Background: It is well documented that food handlers harbor and shed enteric foodborne pathogens causing foodborne disease outbreaks. However, little known on enteric antibiotic resistant (AR) bacteria carriage in food handlers. The objective of this study was to establish a baseline prevalence of fecal AR *E. coli* among food handlers in Qatar.

Methods: Fecal samples were collected from 456 migrant food handlers of different nationalities arriving in Qatar on a work permit between January 2015 and December 2016. These samples (25 g each) were collected based on the availability and examination schedule at the Medical Commission facility from those consented to participate. Isolated *E. coli* bacteria were tested for antibiotic susceptibility against nine antibiotics using the E-test method and Double Disc Synergy Test (DDST) for extended-spectrum beta-lactamase (ESBL) production.

Results: From the 78 *E. coli* positive samples (17.1%, $n = 456$), 60% of the isolates were resistant to at least one antibiotic, whereas, 27% were multi-drug resistant (MDR). Seven isolates (9%, $n = 78$) were ESBL producers of which five were MDR. Individual AR *E. coli* frequencies to the nine antibiotics were not significantly ($P > 0.05$) different by nationality.

Conclusions: Based on our findings, we revealed that individual resistant *E. coli* and MDR resistant *E. coli* were common in fecal samples of food handlers in Qatar. This may indicate that food handlers can potentially contaminate foods with AR *E. coli*, a possible public health concern.

Keywords: Food handlers, *E. coli*, Antibiotic resistance, Multi-drug resistant, ESBL

Background

Antibiotic resistance (AR) continues to pose a great threat to public health in both developed and developing countries [1, 2]. Infections caused by AR bacteria, especially multi-drug resistant organisms, can lead to serious health problems such as prolonged hospitalization, treatment failure and deaths [1, 2]. A worrying increase in multi-drug resistant phenotypes in enterobacteriaceae including *E. coli* and particularly to third-generation cephalosporins as well as to colistin (last resort antibiotic used to treat carbapenem-resistant enterobacteriaceae) has been reported [3–8]. The emergence, development, and spread of AR bacteria is a complex issue that involves multiple factors such as the use and misuse of antibiotics, poor infection control practices, inadequate sanitary conditions, and inappropriate food-handling practices [9–12]. Accordingly, food handlers with poor personal hygiene and inadequate food safety knowledge working in food service establishments can be a potential source for food contamination that can lead to foodborne disease and outbreaks [13, 14]. Likewise, food handlers who harbor AR bacteria in their gastrointestinal tract may contaminate foods which is considered as a potential route AR bacteria transmission to consumers [15].

* Correspondence: walidalali@gmail.com
[5]College of Public Health, Hamad Bin Khalifa University, Doha, Qatar
[6]Present Address: Department of Veterinary Medicine, College of Food and Agriculture, United Arab Emirates University, Alain, United Arab Emirates
Full list of author information is available at the end of the article

Food handlers have been linked to a large number of foodborne outbreaks worldwide. A total of 816 foodborne outbreaks with 80,682 foodborne illnesses occurred between 1927 and 2006 were linked to food handlers (Greig et al., 2007). Likewise, The Centre for Disease Control and Prevention (CDC) revealed that 52% of 9040 foodborne disease outbreaks reported between 1998 and 2004 were associated with food services (i.e., restaurants, cafeterias, and hotels) [16]. Approximately, bacterial agents caused 13% of these outbreaks. The majority of foodborne outbreaks associated with food services were associated with unsanitary conditions of the food handlers [17, 18].

Escherichia coli bacteria are very abundant in the human gastrointestinal tract and can serve as carriers/reservoirs of AR genes. These bacteria are also able to share AR genetic material with their fellow bacteria of the same and/or different species [19, 20]. The incidence of AR bacteria are rapidly increasing in humans in Qatar (Personal communication with the Microbiological diagnostic Laboratory of Hamad Medical Corporation, Doha, Qatar). A hospital-based AR bacteria surveillance system exists in Qatar to monitor the incidence of a number of AR bacteria from outpatient and in-patient clinics (Hamad Medical Corporation, Doha, Qatar). However, there is no available information on the AR enteric bacteria such as *E. coli* from non-clinical samples [21–23].

There is a large and continuous influx of migrant labor workers in Qatar; largely from south-east Asian countries [24]. A group of those migrant workers comes to Qatar on a work permit designated for jobs within the food industry such as food handling and service. Many of the food handlers have limited knowledge of risks associated with food contamination. Nonetheless, they may harbor and shed AR commensal *E. coli* during handling of food leading to food contamination. Hence, resistant bacteria can spread to the public through consumption of contaminated food. Research studies have shown that multi-drug resistant *E. coli* can be present in 'healthy' individual in community settings [25–29] even with the absence of antibiotic use [30]. Furthermore, several studies have revealed that AR *E. coli* from food source can spread to humans, colonize human gut, and potentially cause infections such as urinary tract infections [31–35].

There is currently limited information on AR phenotypes in commensal enteric organisms, from non-clinical human populations in Qatar. A first step to assess the AR risk associated with food handlers is to obtain a baseline prevalence of AR *E. coli* (an indicator organism) in fecal samples collected from this cohort. Therefore, the objective of this study was to determine the prevalence of the AR *E. coli* isolates from fecal samples of migrant food handlers in Qatar.

Methods

Study population and sampling scheme

All migrant workers including food handlers arriving to Qatar on work permit have to go through a mandatory medical screening at the Medical Commission, Department of Ministry of Public Health, Doha, Qatar [36]. Individual fecal samples were collected randomly from apparently healthy food handlers within one week of arrival to Qatar. The collection of the fecal samples was conducted between January 2015 and December 2016 as part of another research study that focused on presence of enteric parasites (Abu Madi et al., College of Health Sciences, Qatar University). All participants were provided with informed consent form explaining the purpose of the study and clearly reassured no obligation to participate; moreover, they have been comforted that all collected data will be treated with high confidentiality. The fecal samples (25 g each) were collected based on the availability and examination schedule at the Medical Commission Department from those consented to participate. Nationality information was obtained for each food handler. Portions of the fecal samples were used for the parasite analysis, while the leftover samples (~ 10 g) were stored in the freezer at – 20 °C. For this study, all available frozen fecal samples ($n = 456$) representing 456 food handlers collected over two year period (January 2015 to December 2016) were used i. These samples were utilized for *E. coli* isolation and antibiotic susceptibility testing. The food handlers included in this study were all males between the ages of 20 and 35 year old. There were 139, 118, 110, 40, 25, 16, 5, and 3 fecal samples from food handlers that originated from India, Bangladesh, Nepal, Philippine, Sir Lanka, Indonesia, Kenya, and Thailand, respectively. There were no reports of acute or chronic infections in the food handlers. No additional identifiable information were available for this study. Moreover, historical antibiotic use data associated with the study subjects were not available. The Institutional Review Board (IRB) of Ministry of Public Health (Doha, Qatar) approved this study in June 2017.

E. coli isolation and identification

To isolate *E. coli*, fecal samples were thawed at room temperature (25 °C), streaked directly onto a selective medium CHROMagar™ *E. coli* plates (Difco, Becton Dickenson, Sparks, MD) using sterile cotton-tipped swabs, and then incubated at 37 °C for 18–24 h. A typical *E. coli* colony (green color with smooth surface) was randomly selected and subsequently streaked onto 5% sheep blood agar (Difco, BD) plates, then incubated at 37 °C for 18–24 h to obtain pure single colonies. For confirmation, suspected *E. coli* colonies were transferred onto MacConkey agar (Difco, BD) plates and incubated (37 °C, 18–24 h). Thereafter, colonies were streaked onto fresh blood agar plates and incubated (37 °C, 18–24 h) for isolation. Up to three colonies from the blood agar were tested for lactose fermentation using the Indole spot test (Remel, Thermoscientific, Lenexa, KS, USA). *Escherichia coli* isolates were transferred to Cryovial tubes (TechnicalService, Lancashire, U.K.) and stored at – 80 °C until further analysis.

Antibiotic susceptibility testing of *E. coli* isolates

Frozen *E. coli* isolates were revived from the Cryovials on blood agar plates. A single *E. coli* isolate was randomly selected from the blood agar plate and suspended in 0.85% saline (Difco, BD) to achieve an inoculum equivalent to 0.5 McFarland standard as measured by DensiCHEK™ Plus spectrophotometer (Biomérieux, Marcy, France). The suspension was swabbed on a Mueller-Hinton agar plate (MH; Difco, BD) using a sterile cotton-tip and allowed to dry completely at room temperature. An antibiotic susceptibility test strip (E-test strip, BioMerieux) was then applied to the MH agar surface with sterile forceps and the plate was incubated at 37 °C for 18–24 h. Thereafter, the minimum inhibitory concentration (MIC) was read directly from the test strip where the elliptical zone of inhibition intersected with the MIC scale on the strip, according to the manufacturer's instructions. The MIC values were interpreted according to the Clinical & Laboratory Standards Institute (CLSI) guidelines [37]. *Escherichia coli* strains ATCC® 25,922 and 35,218 were used as controls. The nine antibiotics utilized for antibiotic susceptibility testing of *E. coli* isolates and their breakpoints are shown in Table 1.

Double disc synergy test (DDST)

All *E. coli* isolates that showed resistant to 3rd generation cephalosporins (i.e., ceftriaxone in this study) with MIC ≥4 based on the E-test strip results were further screened for extended-spectrum beta-lactamase (ESBL) production via the Double Disc Synergy Test (DDST) as described elsewhere [37]. Briefly, *E. coli* isolates from blood agar plate were suspended in 0.85% saline to achieve an inoculum equivalent to 0.5 McFarland standard as described earlier. The suspension was then plated on an MH agar plate and a disc containing amoxicillin-clavulanate (20/10 μg, BD- Sensi Disc™) was placed in the center of the plate. Next, one disc of ceftriaxone (30 μg, BD- Sensi Disc™) and another disk of ceftazidime (30 μg, BD- Sensi Disc™) were placed 15 mm apart from the edge of amoxicillin-clavulanate disc as shown in Fig. 1. The cefoxitin (30 μg, BD- Sensi Disc™) disc was placed in any available space remaining on the plate [37, 38]. The MH plates with the four antibiotic discs were incubated at 37 °C for 18–24 h. Any *E. coli* isolate that showed an increase in the zone of inhibition around either ceftazidime or ceftriaxone (i.e., > 5 mm towards the disc of amoxicillin-clavulanate) together with susceptibility to cefoxitin was interpreted as positive for the ESBL production. *Escherichia coli* ATCC® 51,446 and 25,922 were used as control strains for positive and negative ESBL production, respectively.

Data analysis

The antibiotic resistance outcomes (resistance or susceptible [i.e., binary]) and multidrug-resistant (MDR)

Table 1 Minimum inhibitory concentration (MIC) range and interpretation for antibiotics used to test susceptibility of *E. coli* isolates ($n = 78$) from food handlers' fecal samples

Antibiotic	Abbreviation	MIC range tested (μg/mL)	MIC Interpretive Standard (μg/mL)[a]		
			S	I	R
Penicillin & Penicillin β-lactamase inhibitor combinations					
Ampicillin	AM	0.016–256	≤8	16	≥32
Amoxicillin/Clavulanic acid	XL	0.016–256	≤8/4	16/8	≥32/16
Aminoglycosides					
Gentamicin	GM	0.016–256	≤4	8	≥16
Quinolone					
Ciprofloxacin	CI	0.002–32	≤0.006	0.12–0.5	≥1
Chloramphenicol					
Chloramphenicol	CL	0.016–256	≤8	16	≥32
Tetracycline					
Tetracycline	TC	0.016–256	≤4	8	≥16
Folate pathway inhibitors					
Trimethoprim	TR	0.002–32	≤8	–	≥16
Sulphamethoxazole	SX	0.064–1024	≤258		≥512
Cephalosporin					
Ceftriaxone	TX	0.016–256	≤1	2	≥4

[a] The MIC values interpretation into sensitive (S), intermediate (I), and resistant (R) was according to the Clinical & Laboratory Standards Institute (CLSI) guidelines

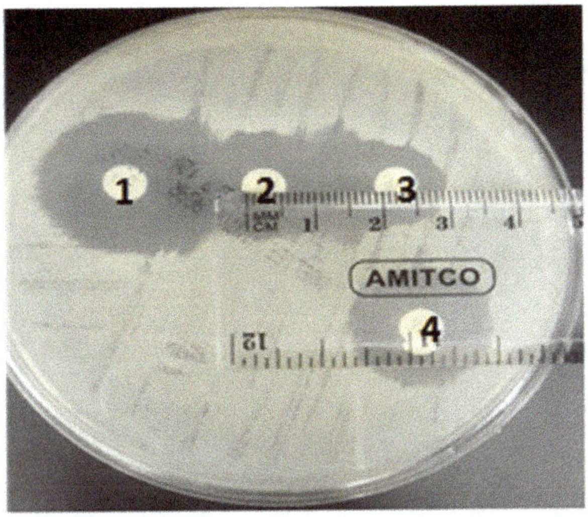

Fig. 1 Double Disc Synergy Test (DDST) confirming ESBL-Producing *E. coli* isolates from fecal samples of food handlers (Antibiotic discs and concentrations used were as follows: 1. Ceftazidime (30 µg); 2. Amoxicillin/Clavulanic acid (20/10 µg); 3. Ceftriaxone (30 µg); and 4. cefoxitin (30 µg))

isolates (those resistant to three or more antimicrobial classes) were cross tabulated with nationality using a Fisher's exact test or 2-by-n likelihood ratio chi-square test, as appropriate, in STATA 14.1 software (Stata Corp., College Station, TX).

Results

From the 456 food handler fecal samples tested, 78 (17.1%) were positive for *E. coli*. In general, isolates were frequently resistant to sulfamethoxazole (33.3%), followed by ampicillin (32.1%), trimethoprim (30.8%), and tetracycline (25.6%). The *E. coli* isolates were less resistant to ciprofloxacin (14.2%), ceftriaxone (9%), and chloramphenicol (3.9%).

Table 2 Distribution of fecal *E. coli* isolates ($n = 78$) by food handler's nationality

Nationality	Frequency	Percentage [a]
Indian	30	38.5
Bangladesh	19	24.4
Nepalese	13	16.7
Philippine	8	10.3
Indonesian	3	3.8
Kenyan	2	2.6
Siri Lankan	2	2.6
Thai	1	1.3

[a] Percentages of antibiotic resistant *E. coli* isolates by nationality were not significantly different ($P > 0.05$) based on chi-square test in STATA 14.1 software

The distribution of *E. coli* isolates by nationality is shown in Table 2. The individual antibiotic resistant *E. coli* frequencies were not significantly ($P > 0.05$) different by nationality. The antibiotic resistance profiles among the 78 *E. coli* isolates are summarized in Table 3. The distribution of phenotypic antibiotic resistance to the 9 antibiotics is shown in Fig.2. Approximately, 59% of the isolates were resistant to at least one antibiotic, whereas 11.5, 15.4%, 11.5, 11.5, 6.4 and 2.6% isolates showed resistance to one, two, three, four, five and six antibiotics, respectively (Fig. 2). Twenty-seven percent ($n = 78$) of all

Table 3 Phenotypic resistant profiles of *E. coli* isolates from food handlers' fecal samples ($n = 78$)

Resistant phenotype	Frequency	Percentage [c]
No resistance	32	41
Resistant to only one antibiotic	9	11.5
Trimethoprim; Sulfamethoxazole	5	6.4
Ampicillin; Trimethoprim; Sulfamethoxazole	4	5.12
[a] [b] Ciprofloxacin; Ampicillin; Ceftriaxone; Trimethoprim; Sulfamethoxazole; Tetracycline	2	2.6
[a] Trimethoprim; Sulfamethoxazole; Tetracycline; Ampicillin	3	3.8
[a] Tetracycline; Ciprofloxacin; Trimethoprim; Sulfamethoxazole	3	3.8
[a] Ampicillin; Trimethoprim; Sulfamethoxazole; Tetracycline; Ciprofloxacin	2	2.6
[a] [b] Ampicillin; Trimethoprim; Ceftriaxone; Tetracycline; Ciprofloxacin	1	1.3
[a] Chloramphenicol; Sulphamethoxazole; Tetracycline	2	2.6
[a] Ampicillin; Trimethoprim; Tetracycline	2	2.6
[b] Ampicillin; Ceftriaxone	2	2.6
Ampicillin; Tetracycline	2	2.6
Ampicillin; Trimethoprim	1	1.3
Trimethoprim; Tetracycline	1	1.3
Trimethoprim; Sulfamexazole; Ciprofloxacin	1	1.3
Ampicillin; trimethoprim; Sulfamethxazole; Amoxcicillin-Clavulanic acid	1	1.3
Ampicillin; Sulfamethoxazole	1	1.3
[a] [b] Ampicillin; Sulfamethoxazole; Ceftriaxone; Ciprofloxacin	1	1.3
[a] Ampicillin; Trimethoprim, Sulfamethoxazole; Ciprofloxacin	1	1.3
[a] [b] Ampicillin; Tetracycline; Trimethoprim; Sulfamethoxazole; Ceftriaxone	1	1.3
Ampicillin; Chloramphenicol; Tetracycline; Trimethoprim; Sulfamethoxazole	1	1.3

MDR multi drug resistant, *ESBL* extended spectrum beta lactamase producer
[a]MDR ($n = 19$)
[b]ESBL isolates; ESBL + MDR (21)
[c]Percentages of phenotypic resistant profiles of *E. coli* were significantly different ($P < 0.05$) based on chi-square test in STATA 14.1 software

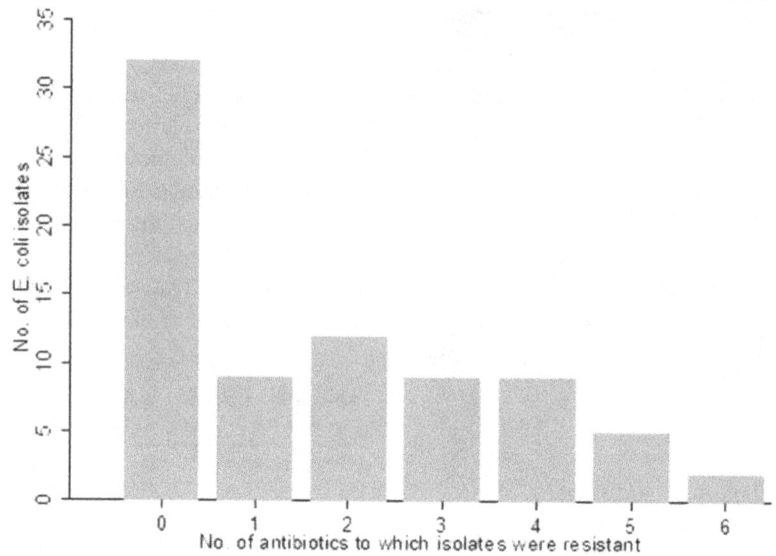

Fig. 2 Frequency bar chart illustrating the distribution of phenotypic antibiotic resistance to up to six antibiotics among *E. coli* isolates ($n = 79$) from food handlers' fecal samples in Qatar

E. coli isolates were multi drug resistant (MDR). Moreover, 9% (seven) of the *E. coli* isolates ($n = 78$) were ESBL producers; of which five were MDR isolates.

Discussion

The incidence of AR bacteria in public hospital and clinics is monitored by the Hamad Medical Corporation (HMC), which is Qatar's main health care provider. According to recent reports by HMC, a notable increase in the incidence of AR bacteria in individuals attending out- and in-patient facilities has been observed [39, 40]. However, there are limited AR bacteria data on individuals in non-hospital (i.e., community) settings such as food handlers. To the best of our knowledge, this is the first study to investigate the prevalence of AR enteric *E. coli* in apparently healthy food handlers. In this pilot study, we reported remarkable percentages of *E. coli* isolates resistant to at least one antibiotic (i.e., 59%) with 27% being MDR and 9% being ESBL producing isolates. The majority of the food handlers in this study had limited knowledge of risk associated with food contamination (personal communication with the Medical Commission staff). This group may harbor and shed AR enteric *E. coli* bacteria that can contaminate food prepared for and consumed by people in Qatar. Thus, these findings suggest that resistant *E. coli* isolates are present in the community; hence, aggravating the public health concerns regarding the spread of AR bacteria. A one-health approach ought to be considered to address this food safety and public health problem.

There are over 1300 food service establishments (restaurant and hotels) in Qatar that employ more than 50,000 workers with the majority being food handlers [41]. Food handlers have been linked to large number of foodborne outbreaks worldwide. The majority of foodborne outbreaks associated with food services are due to unsanitary conditions of the food handlers [17, 18] . Therefore, they can easily contaminate the food they handle with pathogens and non-pathogens. In agreement with our findings, several studies have shown that multi-drug resistant *E. coli* including commensal isolates harboring ESBLs can be present in healthy individuals [42–44]. Garedew-Kifelew L, Wondafrash N and Feleke A [45] examined stool specimens of food handlers from Ethiopia and revealed that 3.1% of the subjects were infected with AR *Salmonella*. Similarly, Greig JD, Todd EC, Bartleson CA and Michaels BS [46] concluded that most of the foodborne outbreaks were associated with food handlers who were asymptomatic carrier and excrete the pathogen unknowingly while working, or they were sick but continue to prepare food.

One of the limitations of this study was the low recovery percentage of *E. coli* from fecal sample (~ 17%) which could be due to the long storage of fecal samples in − 20 °C over 2 year period and the direct plating method of the samples on the selective medium. Another limitation was that the sample collection was from the participants conducted as part of another research study that focused on presence of enteric parasites; hence, we had no control over the sampling scheme. Moreover, the results regarding the AR *E. coli* by nationality need to be interpreted with caution as the number of isolates from some nationalities was low.

Conclusions

In conclusion, food handlers that are apparently healthy individuals could harbor and shed AR enteric *E. coli,* posing a significant public health risk to the general population in Qatar. This may occur via dissemination of AR *E. coli* through contaminated food. Despite the potential effect encountered by the transmission of the opportunistic bacteria through food handlers, this is the first pilot study to screen the AR *E. coli* among apparently healthy food handlers. More research studies are needed to longitudinally follow AR commensal and pathogenic bacteria in food handlers and the relationship with unique and common strains found in hospital settings. A better infection control and improved food safety plans could reduce the risk of AR bacteria contamination of food in Qatar. This could be through delivering proper training to food handlers in order to prevent the contamination of foods. In addition, one-health approach with collaboration between food safety, public health, and veterinary service entities can further address this concern.

Abbreviations

AR: Antibiotic resistant; DDST: Double Disc Synergy Test; ESBL: Extended-spectrum beta-lactamase; MDR: Multi-drug resistant

Funding

This work was supported by internal funds from Hamad Bin Khalifa University to Dr. Walid Alali.

Authors' contributions

NOE, WQA, HMY, AAA, AI, EI and MAA designed the study and drafted the manuscript. NOE performed the experimental work. NOE and WQA analyzed the data. All authors read and approved the final manuscript.

Consent for publication

Not applicable.

Competing interests

The authors declare that they have no competing interests.

Author details

[1]Biomedical Research Center, Qatar University, Doha, Qatar. [2]College of Health Sciences, Qatar University, Doha, Qatar. [3]Laboratory Services, Medical Commission, Ministry of Public Health, Doha, Qatar. [4]Department of Lab Medicine and Pathology, Hamad Medical Hospital, Doha, Qatar. [5]College of Public Health, Hamad Bin Khalifa University, Doha, Qatar. [6]Present Address: Department of Veterinary Medicine, College of Food and Agriculture, United Arab Emirates University, Alain, United Arab Emirates.

References

1. WHO. Antimicrobial resistance global report on surveillance. 2014. http://www.who.int/drugresistance/documents/surveillancereport/en/. Accessed 8 Sept 2017.
2. WHO. Global action plan on antimicrobial Resistance. 2015. http://www.wpro.who.int/entity/drug_resistance/resources/global_action_plan_eng.pdf. Accessed 14 Oct 2017.
3. Burow E, Simoneit C, Tenhagen BA, Käsbohrer A. Oral antimicrobials increase antimicrobial resistance in porcine *E. coli*–a systematic review. Prev Vet Med. 2014;113:364–75.
4. Cannatelli A, Giani T, Antonelli A, Principe L, Luzzaro F, Rossolini GM. First detection of the mcr-1 colistin resistance gene in *Escherichia coli* in Italy. Antimicrob Agents Chemother. 2016;60:3257–8.
5. Hasman H, Hammerum AM, Hansen F, Hendriksen RS, Olesen B, Agersø Y, Zankari E, Leekitcharoenphon P, Stegger M, Kaas RS. Detection of mcr-1 encoding plasmid-mediated colistin-resistant *Escherichia coli* isolates from human bloodstream infection and imported chicken meat, Denmark 2015. Euro Surveill. 2015;20:1–5.
6. Poirel L, Kieffer N, Liassine N, Thanh D, Nordmann P. Plasmid-mediated carbapenem and colistin resistance in a clinical isolate of *Escherichia coli.* Lancet Infect Dis. 2016;16:00006–2.
7. McGann P, Snesrud E, Maybank R, Corey B, Ong AC, Clifford R, Hinkle M, Whitman T, Lesho E, Schaecher KE. *Escherichia coli* harboring mcr-1 and blaCTX-M on a novel IncF plasmid: first report of mcr-1 in the United States. Antimicrob Agents Chemother. 2016;60:4420–1.
8. Borg MA, Scicluna E, De Kraker M, Van De Sande-Bruinsma N, Tiemersma E, Gür D, Ben RS, Rasslan O, Elnassar Z, Benbachir M. Antibiotic resistance in the southeastern Mediterranean–preliminary results from the ARMed project. Euro Surveill. 2006;11:164–7.
9. Gould IM, Bal AM. New antibiotic agents in the pipeline and how they can help overcome microbial resistance. Virulence. 2013;4:185–91.
10. Wright GD. Something old, something new: revisiting natural products in antibiotic drug discovery 1. Can J Infect Dis. 2014;60:147–54.
11. Institute of Medicine Forum on Emerging Infections. The National Academies Collection: Reports funded by National Institutes of Health. In: Knobler SL, Lemon SM, Najafi M, Burroughs T, editors. The resistance phenomenon in microbes and infectious disease vectors: Implications for Human Health and Strategies for Containment: Workshop Summary. Washington (DC): National Academies Press (US); 2003.
12. Tanwar J, Das S, Fatima Z, Hameed S. Multidrug resistance: an emerging crisis. Interdiscip Perspect Infect Dis. 2014;2014:1–7.
13. Andargie G, Kassu A, Moges F, Tiruneh M, Huruy K. Prevalence of bacteria and intestinal parasites among food-handlers in Gondar town, Northwest Ethiopia. J Health Popul Nutr. 2008;26:451–5.
14. WHO. Health surveillance and management procedures for food-handling personnel: report of a WHO consultation [held in Geneva from 18 to 22 April 1988]. 1989. http://apps.who.int/iris/handle/10665/39610. Accessed 4 Oct 2017.
15. Käferstein F, Abdussalam M. Food safety in the 21st century. Bull World Health Organ. 1999;77:347.
16. Angulo FJ, Jones TF, Angulo FJ. Eating in restaurants: a risk factor for foodborne disease? Clin Infect Dis. 2006;43:1324–8.
17. Egan MB, Raats MM, Grubb SM, Eves A, Lumbers ML, Dean MS, Adams MR. A review of food safety and food hygiene training studies in the commercial sector. Food Control. 2007;18:1180–90.
18. Shinbaum S, Crandall PG, O'Bryan CA. Evaluating your obligations for employee training according to the food safety modernization act. Food Control. 2016;60:12–7.
19. Bennett PM. Plasmid encoded antibiotic resistance: acquisition and transfer of antibiotic resistance genes in bacteria. Br J Pharmacol. 2008;153:S347–57.
20. Huddleston JR. Horizontal gene transfer in the human gastrointestinal tract: potential spread of antibiotic resistance genes. Infect Drug Resist. 2014;7:167–76.
21. Khan FY, Elshafie SS, Almaslamani M, Abu-Khattab M, El Hiday AH, Errayes M, Almaslamani E. Epidemiology of bacteraemia in Hamad general hospital, Qatar: a one year hospital-based study. Travel Med Infect Dis. 2010;8:377–87.
22. Rolain JM, Loucif L, Al-Maslamani M, Elmagboul E, Al-Ansari N, Taj-Aldeen S, Shaukat A, Ahmedullah H, Hamed M. Emergence of multidrug-resistant Acinetobacter baumannii producing OXA-23 Carbapenemase in Qatar. New Microbes New Infect. 2016;11:47–51.
23. Samawi A, Saad M, Khan FY, Eldeeb Y, Almaslamani M, Alkhal A, Alsoub H, Ghadban W, Howady F, Hashim S. Acinetobacter infections among adult patients in Qatar: a 2-year hospital-based study. Can J Infect Dis Med Microbiol. 2016;2016:1–5.
24. Snoj J. Population of Qatar by nationality. 2017. http://priyadsouza.com/population-of-qatar-by-nationality-in-2017/. Accessed 10 Aug 2017.
25. Pitout JDD, Nordmann P, Laupland KB, Poirel L. Emergence of Enterobacteriaceae producing extended-spectrum β-lactamases (ESBLs) in the community. J Antimicrob Chemother. 2005;56:52–9.
26. Garau J, Xercavins M, Rodríguez-Carballeira M, Gómez-Vera JR, Coll I, Vidal D, Llovet T, Ruíz-Bremón A. Emergence and dissemination of quinolone-resistant *Escherichia coli* in the community. Antimicrob Agents Chemother.

1999;43:2736–41.
27. Ahmed SF, Ali MMM, Mohamed ZK, Moussa TA, Klena JD. Fecal carriage of extended-spectrum β-lactamases and AmpC-producing *Escherichia coli* in a Libyan community. Ann Clin Microbiol Antimicrob. 2014;13:1–8.
28. Al-Agamy MH, El Mahdy TS, Shibl AM. Fecal colonization with extended-Spectrum Beta-lactamase and AmpC-producing *Escherichia coli*. Biomed Res Int. 2016;2016:7.
29. Azap OK, Arslan H, Serefhanoglu K, Colakoglu S, Erdogan H, Timurkaynak F, Senger SS. Risk factors for extended-spectrum beta-lactamase positivity in uropathogenic *Escherichia coli* isolated from community-acquired urinary tract infections. Clin Microbiol Infect. 2010;16:147–51.
30. Murray BE, Mathewson JJ, DuPont HL, Ericsson CD, Reves RR. Emergence of resistant fecal *Escherichia coli* in travelers not taking prophylactic antimicrobial agents. Antimicrob Agents Chemother. 1990;34:515–8.
31. Linton AH, Howe K, Bennett PM, Richmond MH, Whiteside EJ. The colonization of the human gut by antibiotic resistant *Escherichia coli* from chickens. J Appl Bacteriol. 1977;43:465–9.
32. Carlet J. The gut is the epicentre of antibiotic resistance. Antimicrob Resist Infect Control. 2012;1:1–7.
33. Szmolka A, Nagy B. Multidrug resistant commensal *Escherichia coli* in animals and its impact for public health. Front Microbiol. 2013;4:258.
34. Vincent C, Boerlin P, Daignault D, Dozois CM, Dutil L, Galanakis C, Reid-Smith RJ, Tellier P-P, Tellis PA, Ziebell K, et al. Food reservoir for *Escherichia coli* causing urinary tract infections. Emerg Infect Dis. 2010;16:88–95.
35. Hooton TM, Samadpour M. Is acute uncomplicated urinary tract infection a foodborne illness, and are animals the source? Clin Infect Dis. 2005;40:258–9.
36. Houkoomi Qatar. Medical comission procedure: keeping Qatar disease free. 2017. http://portal.www.gov.qa/wps/portal/topics/Health/medicalcommissionprocedures. Accessed 27 Aug 2017.
37. CLSI. Clinical and Laboratory Standards Institute. Performance standards for antimicrobial susceptibility testing. M100S. 2016;26:1–129.
38. Giriyapur RS, Nandihal NW, Krishna BVS, Patil AB, Chandrasekhar MR. Comparison of disc diffusion methods for the detection of extended-spectrum beta lactamase-producing Enterobacteriaceae. J Lab Physicians. 2011;3:33.
39. Al Soub H. HMC expert warns against improper use of antimicrobial drugs. Hamad Medical Corporation news 2015. https://www.hamad.qa/EN/news/2015/August/Pages/HMC-Expert-Warns-Against-Improper-Use-of-Antimicrobial-Drugs.aspx. Accessed 14 Nov 2017.
40. Aly M, Balkhy HH. The prevalence of antimicrobial resistance in clinical isolates from gulf corporation council countries. Antimicrob Resist Infect Control. 2012;1:26.
41. Ministry of Development Planning and Statistics. The Annual Bulletin of Hotels and Restaurants Statistics (accommodation and food services). 2017. http://www.mdps.gov.qa/en/statistics/Statistical%20Releases/Economic/HotelsandRestaurants/2014/Hotels_and_Resturants_MDPS_AnBu_AE_2014.pdf. Accessed 20 May 2017.
42. Luvsansharav U-O, Hirai I, Niki M, Sasaki T, Makimoto K, Komalamisra C, Maipanich W, Kusolsuk T, Sa-Nguankiat S, Pubampen S. Analysis of risk factors for a high prevalence of extended-spectrum β-lactamase-producing Enterobacteriaceae in asymptomatic individuals in rural Thailand. J Med Microbiol. 2011;60:619–24.
43. Rahman EMA, El-Sherif RH. High rates of intestinal colonization with extended-spectrum lactamase-producing Enterobacteriaceae among healthy individuals. J Investig Med. 2011;59:1284–6.
44. Sallem RB, Slama KB, Estepa V, Jouini A, Gharsa H, Klibi N, Sáenz Y, Ruiz-Larrea F, Boudabous A, Torres C. Prevalence and characterisation of extended-spectrum beta-lactamase (ESBL)-producing Escherichia coli isolates in healthy volunteers in Tunisia. Eur J Clin Microbiol Infect Dis. 2012;31:1511–6.
45. Garedew-Kifelew L, Wondafrash N, Feleke A. Identification of drug-resistant Salmonella from food handlers at the University of Gondar, Ethiopia. BMC Res Notes. 2014;7:545.
46. Greig JD, Todd EC, Bartleson CA, Michaels BS. Outbreaks where food workers have been implicated in the spread of foodborne disease. Part 1. Description of the problem, methods, and agents involved. J Food Prot. 2007;70:1752–61.

Permissions

All chapters in this book were first published in AR&IC, by BioMed Central; hereby published with permission under the Creative Commons Attribution License or equivalent. Every chapter published in this book has been scrutinized by our experts. Their significance has been extensively debated. The topics covered herein carry significant findings which will fuel the growth of the discipline. They may even be implemented as practical applications or may be referred to as a beginning point for another development.

The contributors of this book come from diverse backgrounds, making this book a truly international effort. This book will bring forth new frontiers with its revolutionizing research information and detailed analysis of the nascent developments around the world.

We would like to thank all the contributing authors for lending their expertise to make the book truly unique. They have played a crucial role in the development of this book. Without their invaluable contributions this book wouldn't have been possible. They have made vital efforts to compile up to date information on the varied aspects of this subject to make this book a valuable addition to the collection of many professionals and students.

This book was conceptualized with the vision of imparting up-to-date information and advanced data in this field. To ensure the same, a matchless editorial board was set up. Every individual on the board went through rigorous rounds of assessment to prove their worth. After which they invested a large part of their time researching and compiling the most relevant data for our readers.

The editorial board has been involved in producing this book since its inception. They have spent rigorous hours researching and exploring the diverse topics which have resulted in the successful publishing of this book. They have passed on their knowledge of decades through this book. To expedite this challenging task, the publisher supported the team at every step. A small team of assistant editors was also appointed to further simplify the editing procedure and attain best results for the readers.

Apart from the editorial board, the designing team has also invested a significant amount of their time in understanding the subject and creating the most relevant covers. They scrutinized every image to scout for the most suitable representation of the subject and create an appropriate cover for the book.

The publishing team has been an ardent support to the editorial, designing and production team. Their endless efforts to recruit the best for this project, has resulted in the accomplishment of this book. They are a veteran in the field of academics and their pool of knowledge is as vast as their experience in printing. Their expertise and guidance has proved useful at every step. Their uncompromising quality standards have made this book an exceptional effort. Their encouragement from time to time has been an inspiration for everyone.

The publisher and the editorial board hope that this book will prove to be a valuable piece of knowledge for researchers, students, practitioners and scholars across the globe.

List of Contributors

Marcelyn T. Magwenzi
College of Health Sciences, Department of Medical Microbiology, University of Zimbabwe, Harare, Zimbabwe

Valerie Robertson
College of Health Sciences, Department of Medical Microbiology, University of Zimbabwe, Harare, Zimbabwe
Biomedical Research and Training Institute, Harare, Zimbabwe

Muchaneta Gudza-Mugabe
National Microbiology Reference Laboratory, Harare Central Hospital, Harare, Zimbabwe

Hilda A. Mujuru
College of Health Sciences, Department of Paediatrics and Child Health, University of Zimbabwe, Harare, Zimbabwe
Harare Central Hospital, Harare, Zimbabwe

Mutsa Dangarembizi-Bwakura
College of Health Sciences, Department of Paediatrics and Child Health, University of Zimbabwe, Harare, Zimbabwe
Parirenyatwa Group of Hospitals, Harare, Zimbabwe

Alexander M. Aiken
Biomedical Research and Training Institute, Harare, Zimbabwe
London School of Hygiene and Tropical Medicine, London, UK

Allison Muller and Xavier Bertrand
University Hospital of Besançon, Infection Control Department, F-25030 Besançon, France
University Bourgogne-Franche-Comte, UMR 6249 Chrono-Environnement, F-25030 Besançon, France

Houssein Gbaguidi-Haore
University Hospital of Besançon, Infection Control Department, F-25030 Besançon, France
University Bourgogne-Franche-Comte, UMR 6249 Chrono-Environnement, F-25030 Besançon, France
Service d'Hygiène Hospitalière, Centre Hospitalier Régional Universitaire, Hôpital Jean Minjoz, 3 Bd Fleming, 25030, Besançon, Cedex, France

Anne-Marie Rogues and Catherine Dumartin
University Bordeaux, Inserm, Bordeaux Population Health Research Center, Team Pharmacoepidemiology, UMR 1219, F-33000 Bordeaux, France
CHU Bordeaux, Southwestern Centre for Infection Prevention and Control, F-33000 Bordeaux, France

Muriel Péfau
CHU Bordeaux, Southwestern Centre for Infection Prevention and Control, F-33000 Bordeaux, France

Serge Alfandari
Gustave Dron Hospital, Infectious Diseases Department, F-59208 Tourcoing, France

Rémy Gauzit
AP-HP, Cochin University Hospital, Infectious Diseases Department, F-75014 Paris, France

Courage Kosi Setsoafia Saba
Department of Biotechnology, Faculty of Agriculture, University for Development Studies, Tamale, Ghana

Jean Kwadwo Amenyona and Stephen Wilson Kpordze
Department of Ecotourism and Environmental Management, Faculty of Renewable Natural Resources, University for Development Studies, Tamale, Ghana

Serawit Deyno
Department of Pharmacology, School of Medicine, College of Medicine and Health Sciences, Hawassa University, Hawassa, Ethiopia

Sintayehu Fekadu
Department of Microbiology, Faculty of Medicine, Shimane University, Shimane, Japan

Ayalew Astatkie
School of Public and Environmental Health, College of Medicine and Health Sciences, Hawassa University, Hawassa, Ethiopia

Farhad Safarpoor Dehkordi, Hasan Gandomi, Afshin Akhondzadeh Basti and Ali Misaghi
Department of Food Hygiene and Quality Control, Faculty of Veterinary Medicine, University of Tehran, Tehran, Iran

Ebrahim Rahimi
Department of Food Hygiene and Public Health, Faculty of Veterinary Medicine, Shahrekord Branch, Islamic Azad University, Shahrekord, Iran

T. M. Rawson and E. Charani
National Institute for Health Research Health Protection Research Unit in Healthcare Associated Infections and Antimicrobial Resistance, Imperial College London, Hammersmith Campus, Du Cane Road, London W12 0NN, UK

L. S. P. Moore and A. H. Holmes
National Institute for Health Research Health Protection Research Unit in Healthcare Associated Infections and Antimicrobial Resistance, Imperial College London, Hammersmith Campus, Du Cane Road, London W12 0NN, UK
Imperial College Healthcare NHS Trust, Hammersmith Hospital, Du Cane Road, London W12 0HS, UK

A. M. Tivey and A. Tsao
Imperial College School of Medicine, Imperial College London, South Kensington Campus, London SW7 2AZ, UK

M. Gilchrist
Imperial College Healthcare NHS Trust, Hammersmith Hospital, Du Cane Road, London W12 0HS, UK

Seyda Ignak
Department of Medical Biology, Bahcesehir University School of Medicine, Sahrayıcedid Mah. Batman Sok. No:66-68, Yenisahra-Göztepe, Istanbul, Turkey

Yasar Nakipoglu and Bulent Gurler
Istanbul Faculty of Medicine, Department of Medical Microbiology, Istanbul University, Istanbul, Turkey

Jian-bo Chang, Hao Wu, Bai-tao Ma, Ren-zhi Wang and Jun-ji Wei
Department of Neurosurgery, Peking Union Medical College Hospital, Peking Union Medical College, Chinese Academy of Medical Sciences, No.1 Shuaifuyuan, Dongcheng District, Beijing 100730, China

He Wang
Department of Laboratory Medicine, Peking Union Medical College Hospital, Peking Union Medical College, Chinese Academy of Medical Sciences, No.1 Shuaifuyuan, Dongcheng District, Beijing 100730, China

Lamiaa Mohsen, Nermin Ramy, Dalia Saied, Dina Akmal and Niveen Salama
Department of Pediatrics, Faculty of Medicine, Cairo University, Cairo, Egypt
New Children Hospital, (Abu El Rish), Cairo University Hospitals, Ali Basha Ebrahim, Cairo, Egypt

Mona M. Abdel Haleim
Department of Clinical and Chemical Pathology, Cairo University, Cairo, Egypt
New Children Hospital, (Abu El Rish), Cairo University Hospitals, Ali Basha Ebrahim, Cairo, Egypt

Hany Aly
Division of Neonatology, the George Washington University and Children's National Health System, 900 23rd Street, N.W. Suite G2092, Washington, DC 20037, USA

Dilruba Ahmed, Md Ausrafuggaman Nahid, Abdullah Bashar Sami, Farhana Halim, Nasrin Akter, Tuhin Sadique, Md Sohel Rana, Md Shahriar Bin Elahi and Md Mahbubur Rahman
International Centre for Diarrhoeal Disease Research, Bangladesh (icddr,b), Dhaka 1212, Bangladesh

G. Ström and U. Magnusson
Department of Clinical Sciences, Swedish University of Agricultural Sciences, Uppsala, Sweden

S. Boqvist and L.-L. Fernström
Department of Biomedical Sciences and Veterinary Public Health, Swedish University of Agricultural Sciences, Uppsala, Sweden

A. Albihn
Department of Biomedical Sciences and Veterinary Public Health, Swedish University of Agricultural Sciences, Uppsala, Sweden
Department of Chemistry, Environment and Feed Hygiene, National Veterinary Institute, Uppsala, Sweden

A. Andersson Djurfeldt
Department of Human Geography, Lund University, Lund, Sweden

S. Sokerya
Centre for Livestock and Agriculture Development, Phnom Penh, Cambodia

T. Sothyra
National Animal Health and Production Research Institute, Phnom Penh, Cambodia

G. Ström, M. Halje, D. Karlsson and U. Magnusson
Department of Clinical Sciences, Swedish University of Agricultural Sciences, Uppsala, Sweden

J. Jiwakanon
Research Group for Preventive Technology in Livestock, Faculty of Veterinary Medicine, Khon Kaen University, Khon Kaen, Thailand

M. Pringle
National Veterinary Institute, Uppsala, Sweden

L.-L. Fernström
Department of Biomedical Sciences and Veterinary Public Health, Swedish University of Agricultural Sciences, Uppsala, Sweden

Tadesse Eguale
Aklilu Lemma Institute of Pathobiology, Addis Ababa University, Addis Ababa, Ethiopia

Josephine Birungi, Appolinaire Djikeng and Joyce Njuguna
Biosciences Eastern and Central Africa-International Livestock Research Institute (BecA-ILRI) Hub, Nairobi, Kenya

Daniel Asrat
Department of Microbiology, Immunology & Parasitology, School of Medicine, College of Health Sciences, Addis Ababa University, Churchill Avenue, Addis Ababa, Ethiopia

Moses N. Njahira
ICIPE-African Insect Science for Food and Health, Nairobi, Kenya

Wondwossen A. Gebreyes
Department of Veterinary Preventive Medicine, The Ohio State University, 1920 Coffey Rd., Columbus, OH 43210, USA

John S. Gunn
Department of Microbial Infection and Immunity, Center for Microbial Interface Biology, The Ohio State University, Biomedical Research Tower, 460 West 12th, Columbus, OH 432101214, USA

Ephrem Engidawork
Department of Pharmacology and Clinical Pharmacy, School of Pharmacy, College of Health Sciences, Addis Ababa University, Churchill Avenue, Addis Ababa, Ethiopia

Marko Oydanich, Claudia Ghisa and Penny Asbell
Department of Ophthalmology, Icahn School of Medicine at Mount Sinai, New York, NY, USA

Tanis C. Dingle and Camille L. Hamula
Department of Pathology, Icahn School of Medicine at Mount Sinai, New York, NY 10029, USA

Nichola R. Naylor, Nina Zhu, Anuja Chatterjee and Gwenan M. Knight
National Institute for Health Research Health Protection Research Unit in Healthcare Associated Infection and Antimicrobial Resistance at Imperial College, Hammersmith Campus, London W12 0NN, UK

Kavian Kulasabanathan
Imperial College London, Sir Alexander Fleming Building, South Kensington Campus, London, UK

Sachin Silva
Harvard University, 665 Huntington Avenue, Boston, MA 02115, USA

Rifat Atun
Harvard University, 665 Huntington Avenue, Boston, MA 02115, USA
National Institute for Health Research Health Protection Research Unit in Healthcare Associated Infection and Antimicrobial Resistance at Imperial College, Hammersmith Campus, London W12 0NN, UK

Julie V. Robotham
Modelling and Economics Unit, National Infection Service, Public Health England, 61 Colindale Avenue, London NW9 5EQ, UK
National Institute for Health Research Health Protection Research Unit in Healthcare Associated Infection and Antimicrobial Resistance at Imperial College, Hammersmith Campus, London W12 0NN, UK

Sabiha Yusuf Essack
Antimicrobial Research Unit, School of Health Sciences, College of Health Sciences, University of KwaZulu-Natal, Durban 4000, South Africa

Raspail Carrel Founou
Antimicrobial Research Unit, School of Health Sciences, College of Health Sciences, University of KwaZulu-Natal, Durban 4000, South Africa
Department of Clinical Microbiology, Centre of Expertise and Biological Diagnostic of Cameroon, (CEDBCAM), Yaoundé, Cameroon

Luria Leslie Founou
Antimicrobial Research Unit, School of Health Sciences, College of Health Sciences, University of KwaZulu-Natal, Durban 4000, South Africa
Department of Food Safety and Environmental Microbiology, Centre of Expertise and Biological Diagnostic of Cameroon, (CEDBCAM), Yaoundé, Cameroon

Cornelius Remschmidt, Christin Schröder, Michael Behnke, Petra Gastmeier, Christine Geffers and Tobias Siegfried Kramer
Institute of Hygiene and Environmental Medicine, Charité - University Medicine Berlin, Hindenburgdamm 27, 12203 Berlin, Germany
German National Reference Centre for Surveillance of Nosocomial Infections (NRZ), Hindenburgdamm 27, 12203 Berlin, Germany

Uwe Koppe, Ines Noll, Marcel Feig, Marc Schneider, Hermann Claus, Tim Eckmanns and Muna Abu Sin
Department of Infectious Disease Epidemiology, Robert Koch Institute, Seestr. 10, 13353 Berlin, Germany

Lars E. Kroll
Department of Epidemiology and Health Monitoring, Robert Koch Institute, General-Pape-Strasse 62-66, 12101 Berlin, Germany

Anja von Laer
Postgraduate Training for Applied Epidemiology, Department of Infectious Disease Epidemiology, Robert Koch Institute, Seestr. 10, 13353 Berlin, Germany

Stefanie Kampmeier, Annelene Kossow, Larissa Monika Clausen and Alexander Mellmann
Institute of Hygiene, University Hospital Münster, Robert-Koch-Strasse 41, 48149 Münster, Germany

Dennis Knaack
Institute of Medical Microbiology, University Hospital Münster, Münster, Germany

Christian Ertmer, Antje Gottschalk and Hendrik Freise
Department of Anaesthesiology, Intensive Care and Pain Medicine, University Hospital Münster, Münster, Germany

Erin C. Balkenende
Center for Comprehensive Access Delivery & Research, Iowa City VA Health Care System, Iowa City, USA

Daniel J. Livorsi, Marin L. Schweizer, Rajeshwari Nair and Eli N. Perencevich
Center for Comprehensive Access Delivery & Research, Iowa City VA Health Care System, Iowa City, USA
Department of Internal Medicine, Carver College of Medicine, University of Iowa, Iowa City, USA

Margaret L. Chorazy
University of Iowa College of Public Health, Iowa City, USA

Amy E. Blevins
Hardin Library for the Health Sciences, University of Iowa, Iowa City, USA
Ruth Lilly Medical Library, Indiana University School of Medicine, Indianapolis, Indiana, USA

Richard E. Nelson, Karim Khader and Matthew H. Samore
Veterans Affairs Salt Lake City Health Care System, Salt Lake City, Utah, USA
Department of Internal Medicine, University of Utah School of Medicine, Salt Lake City, Utah, USA

Janine Zweigner
German Center for Infection Research (DZIF), Inhoffenstraße 7, 38124 Braunschweig, Germany
Charité - Universitätsmedizin Berlin, Institute of Hygiene and Environmental Medicine, Hindenburgstraße 27, 12203 Berlin, Germany
Department of Infection Control and Hygiene, University Hospital Cologne, Kerpener Straße 62, 50937 Köln, Germany

Birgit Obermann
German Center for Infection Research (DZIF), Inhoffenstraße 7, 38124 Braunschweig, Germany
Department of Infectious Diseases and Microbiology, Institute for Medical Microbiology, University Hospital Schleswig-Holstein, Ratzeburger Allee 160, 23562 Lübeck, Germany

Evelina Tacconelli
German Center for Infection Research (DZIF), Inhoffenstraße 7, 38124 Braunschweig, Germany
Division of Infectious Diseases, Department of Internal Medicine 1, University Hospital Tübingen, Otfried-Müller-Straße 12, 72076 Tübingen, Germany

Nahla O. Eltai
Biomedical Research Center, Qatar University, Doha, Qatar

Hadi M. Yassine and Asmaa A. Al Thani
Biomedical Research Center, Qatar University, Doha, Qatar
College of Health Sciences, Qatar University, Doha, Qatar

Marwan A. Abu Madi
College of Health Sciences, Qatar University, Doha, Qatar

Ahmed Ismail
Laboratory Services, Medical Commission, Ministry of Public Health, Doha, Qatar

Emad Ibrahim
Department of Lab Medicine and Pathology, Hamad Medical Hospital, Doha, Qatar

Walid Q. Alali
College of Public Health, Hamad Bin Khalifa University, Doha, Qatar
Department of Veterinary Medicine, College of Food and Agriculture, United Arab Emirates University, Alain, United Arab Emirates

Index

www.ingramcontent.com/pod-product-compliance
Lightning Source LLC
LaVergne TN
LVHW080701210926
848485LV00003B/402